Perioperative Medicine for the Junior Clinician

Perioperative Medicine for the Junior Clinician

Edited by

Joel Symons
Anaesthetist and Head of Perioperative Medicine Education
Department of Anaesthesia and Perioperative Medicine
The Alfred Hospital and Monash University
Melbourne
Victoria, Australia

Paul Myles
Director, Department of Anaesthesia and Perioperative Medicine
The Alfred Hospital and Monash University
Melbourne
Victoria, Australia

Rishi Mehra
Anaesthetist and Senior Lecturer
Department of Anaesthesia and Perioperative Medicine
The Alfred Hospital and Monash University
Melbourne
Victoria, Australia

Christine Ball
Anaesthetist and Adjunct Senior Lecturer
Department of Anaesthesia and Perioperative Medicine
The Alfred Hospital and Monash University
Melbourne
Victoria, Australia

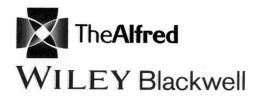

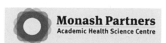

Contents

Part II Preoperative risk assessment 43

Part III Perioperative investigations 107

Part IV Specific medication management and prophylaxis 119

Part V Perioperative management of organ dysfunction and specific population groups 163

Part VIII Case studies (Online Only)

Part IX Investigation interpretation (Online Only)

Foreword

Perioperative medicine has matured over the past two decades to become a major specialty. Ageing populations in many parts of the world are presenting for ever more complex surgeries in greater numbers, with multiple co-morbidities and exposed to polypharmacy. The pace of change has demanded the development of perioperative physicians who are uniquely trained and skilled at supporting patients through the surgical pathway. *Perioperative Medicine for the Junior Clinician* is a testament to the maturation of the specialty, a comprehensive introduction to all aspects of perioperative care.

The fact that there are over 100 succinct chapters, packed with information and written by international experts, emphasises the breadth and depth of knowledge required to practise medicine in this rapidly developing field. Perioperative medicine also requires collaboration between many specialties, something which is epitomised by the multidisciplinary nature of the contributors to this book.

Despite the development of this specialty, the junior doctor is often the first point of consultation in the perioperative period. It is essential that junior doctors understand perioperative risk factors and can identify evolving emergencies; they need to know when to escalate care and who to call for assistance. This book has been carefully organised to allow it to be consulted in a variety of situations, and the addition of short, accessible videos provides another dimension to assist in education, assessment and planning. *Perioperative Medicine for the Junior Clinician* is intended as an introduction and a guide for the junior doctor but it also serves as a definitive quick reference for the more expert practitioner. I (will) relish my copy.

Michael (Monty) Mythen
Smiths Medical Professor of Anesthesia and Critical Care
Director, Centre for Anesthesia, University College London
Director, Research and Development, UCLH/UCL/RFH Research Support Centre
National Clinical Adviser, Department of Health, Enhanced Recovery Partnership
London, United Kingdom

Preface

The era of painless surgery began in the 1840s with the introduction of general anaesthesia, frequently described as the greatest medical discovery of all time. General anaesthesia provided greatly improved operating conditions for the surgeon and an ideal environment for the anaesthetist to appreciate the clinical applications of cardiorespiratory physiology and early drug pharmacology. These developments led to an urgent need for new equipment and improved antisepsis. All of these challenges were overcome by pioneers in anaesthesia, surgery, nursing and public health. Surgery offered cure or relief of symptoms for a rapidly growing number of conditions.

In the mid-20th century, recovery rooms and, later, intensive care units became established in most hospitals. But by the 1980s it was apparent that inadequate preoperative assessment and deficiencies in postoperative care were recurring features in reports from national anaesthetic and surgical mortality committees in many countries. The importance of optimising medical conditions before surgery, patient monitoring, pain management and the postoperative inflammatory process became better understood and appreciated. As outcomes continued to improve and more and more people were having surgery, more extensive surgery was being offered to older patients, often with concurrent medical diseases and drug treatments. The boundaries were constantly being tested, pushing the limits of who was or wasn't an operative candidate. An increasing need for higher acuity postoperative care developed which could not be met, despite innovations such as extended recovery and high-dependency units. As a result, postoperative patients at high risk of complications can now be found on the surgical wards of any hospital.

Excellence in perioperative care includes the seamless transition of an informed, medically optimised patient before surgery, through the operation, to a recovery period free of complications and with minimal discomfort, to optimal health. This cannot happen in a traditional model of medical specialty 'silos', with gaps in knowledge and care. It requires trained, multidisciplinary, team-based care, and should be embedded in a clinical care pathway focused on enhancing patient recovery.

We designed this book to provide up-to-date knowledge and advice from a broad range of medical specialists caring for surgical patients. It is intended to be succinct and practical, providing overviews to guide perioperative care. For e-book readers there is extra material with audio and video links. For junior doctors grappling with the complexity of perioperative care, the book can be read as a whole. For those needing information or advice on a specific problem, the book can be used as a ready reference.

This book is organised into nine sections. The first introductory section outlines some of the principles and practices of perioperative care. The following sections address preoperative risk assessment, laboratory investigations, medication management, specific medical conditions and complications concerning surgical patients, postoperative care and pain management. The book ends with some case scenarios, and finally a series of quizzes to test junior clinicians' knowledge of pertinent laboratory investigations.

To contribute to the care of patients undergoing anaesthesia and surgery is a great honour. We must never forget how much our patients depend on our knowledge, skills and vigilance.

Paul Myles, MBBS, MPH, MD, FCARCSI, FANZCA, FRCA, FAHMS
Melbourne, Australia
www.periopmedicine.org.au
www.masters.periopmedicine.org.au

Acknowledgements

Successful perioperative medicine requires collaboration between many disciplines. This book would not have happened without the co-operation and expertise of the many authors who are truly experts in their field. We would like to thank all involved, especially Arvinder Grover for his input into the ebook version. We would also like to acknowledge Dilan Kodltuwakku from the Monash University Department of Anaesthesia and Perioperative Medicine. Finally, we would like to thank our families for their support, patience and encouragement.

Joel Symons
Paul Myles
Rishi Mehra
Christine Ball

Melbourne, Australia

About the companion website

This book is accompanied by a companion website:

www.wiley.com/go/perioperativemed

The website includes:

- Videos
- Case studies
- Quizzes
- Appendix A: Unit conversions
- Appendix B: Basic airway management including bag-mask ventilation
- Appendix C: Opioid conversion table
- More information about the contributors
- Abbreviations used in the book
- Links to websites to further supplement information contained in this book

Part I
Introduction

The role of the perioperative medicine physician

Mike Grocott

University of Southampton, United Kingdom

The care of patients undergoing major surgery has evolved incrementally since anaesthesia revolutionised surgical care in the years following 1846. Whilst pharmacological and monitoring technologies have advanced, anaesthetists have remained predominantly focused on the operating room environment and have in general resisted moves outside this 'comfort zone'. Surgeons have been the principal care deliverers around the time of surgery. In the last two decades, this has begun to change, with a shift towards an expanded role in perioperative care for the anaesthetist. In parallel, physicians have become more interested in improving the perioperative care of some groups of patients. For example, the engagement of geriatricians in the care of patients undergoing hip fracture surgery has led to the concept of the 'ortho-geriatrician'. Meanwhile, manpower issues in surgical specialties have created pressure for many surgeons to concentrate on operating time, over and above other elements of the care of surgical patients. As a consequence, new labels have developed including perioperative medicine (1994), the perioperative physician (1996) and most recently the perioperative surgical home (2011).

So what has driven the increased focus on perioperative care? Primarily, there has been recognition of unmet need. With growth in the volume and scope of major surgery has come an epidemic of postoperative harm. This is an inevitable consequence of more adventurous, technically challenging surgery in an ageing population with multiple co-morbidities [1]. The global volume of major surgery is approaching 250 million cases per year. Short-term (hospital/30-day) mortality following major surgery, even in the developed world, may approach 4% and morbidity is more frequent by an order of magnitude [2,3]. Furthermore, the substantial impact of short-term postoperative morbidity on subsequent long-term survival is increasingly recognised as an important healthcare challenge [3]. Taken with the growing literature describing interventions that affect postoperative outcome [4], this suggests a significant burden of avoidable harm.

Perioperative Medicine for the Junior Clinician, First Edition. Edited by Joel Symons, Paul Myles, Rishi Mehra and Christine Ball.
© 2015 John Wiley & Sons, Ltd. Published 2015 by John Wiley & Sons, Ltd.
Companion website: www.wiley.com/go/perioperativemed

The scope of perioperative medicine

This spans the period from the moment that surgery is first contemplated through to complete recovery. The role of the perioperative physician includes preoperative risk evaluation, collaborative (shared) decision making [5], optimisation of all aspects of physiological function prior to surgery, individualised 'goal-directed' best intraoperative care, delivering the appropriate level of postoperative care and rehabilitation to normal function [4]. The preoperative period offers a unique opportunity to invest in improving physiological function in a short defined period of time, for example through physical prehabilitation, in patients who are likely to be highly motivated in the face of an imminent threat. Furthermore, the patient–perioperative physician interaction may be one of very few contacts that an individual patient has with medical professionals and offers an opportunity for general health messaging as well as implementation of primary and secondary prevention strategies.

In the post 'evidence-based medicine' era, the focus of medical practice will increasingly move towards personalised/stratified/precision medicine [6]. The technology available to quantify and classify perioperative risk is becoming increasingly sophisticated. In the future, this process is likely to involve a combination of clinical risk scores, objective evaluation of physiological reserve (e.g. cardiopulmonary exercise testing) and the use of specific plasma biomarkers, interpreted in the context of the patient's genotype (+/− epigenetic processes). Perioperative decision making will involve expertise in interpreting such data coupled with understanding of the planned operative procedure and a high degree of competence in collaborative decision making [5]. Improving the quality of decision making through the use of decision aids has been shown to reduce patient choices for discretionary surgery [7] and is likely to have a similar effect across all types of surgery. In the context of an extraordinarily high incidence of surgery during the final months of life [8], such an approach is likely to be beneficial for the quality of life of patients and their carers, as well as for an overburdened healthcare system.

The scope of decision making will include consideration of the extent of surgery, use of adjunctive therapies, and modification of pre-, intra- and postoperative care. Patients with limited physiological reserve may be prescribed general (prehabilitation) or specific (e.g. inspiratory muscle training) preoperative interventions. Intraoperative care may be focused on monitoring and interventions to address particular risks such as cardiac, pulmonary or cognitive dysfunction. The location and intensity of postoperative care will be based on the risk of harm assessed prior to surgery, modified by the response to the physiological challenge of surgery.

Postoperative intensive care has always been made available to patients requiring specific organ support. Increasingly, patients at elevated risk are being offered an enhanced level of postoperative care and monitoring to ensure early rapid and effective response to developing complications and avoid 'failure to rescue'.

Clinical data

The effective use of clinical data will be critical in the development of high-quality perioperative care and making best use of such data will be an important part of the perioperative physician's role [9]. National audit data have highlighted stark differences in quality of care and outcome for specific patient groups, most notably those undergoing emergency procedures such as hip fracture and emergency laparotomy surgery [10]. Systematic audit and quality improvement will serve to 'level the playing field' for patients undergoing diverse types of surgery. The data collected will also contribute to the development of increasingly sophisticated clinical risk tools that will, in turn, facilitate the delivery of precision medicine for this patient group.

The future

It is likely that in many contexts, anaesthetists will take the lead as perioperative physicians, due to their unique combination of competencies and experience. However, the role of the perioperative physician should be competency based and collaborative, and physicians and surgeons will also be involved in leading perioperative care. Irrespective of issues around professional identity, the primary aim of all perioperative physicians should be to improve the quantity and quality of life for patients undergoing major surgery. This will be best achieved by working closely with patients, surgeons and the extended perioperative care team to choose and deliver perioperative care of the highest quality through the interpretation of clinical evidence in the context of an individual patient's life and wishes [11].

References

1. Weiser TG, Regenbogen SE, Thompson KD, et al. An estimation of the global volume of surgery: a modelling strategy based on available data. *Lancet*, 2008;**372**:139–144. doi:10.1016/S0140-6736(08)60878-8

2. Pearse RM, Moreno RP, Bauer P, et al. Mortality after surgery in Europe: a 7 day cohort study. *Lancet*, 2012;**380**(9847):1059–1065. doi:10.1016/S0140-6736(12)61148-9

3. Khuri SF, Henderson WG, DePalma RG, et al. Determinants of long-term survival after major surgery and the adverse effect of postoperative complications. *Annals of Surgery*, 2005;**242**(3):326–341; discussion 41–43. doi:10.1097/01.sla.0000179621.33268.83

4. Pearse RM, Holt PJ, Grocott MP. Managing perioperative risk in patients undergoing elective non-cardiac surgery. *BMJ.* 2011;**343**:d5759. doi:10.1136/bmj.d5759

5. Glance LG, Osler TM, Neuman MD. Redesigning surgical decision making for high-risk patients. *New England Journal of Medicine*, 2014;**370**(15):1379–1381. doi:10.1056/NEJMp1315538

6. Mirnezami R, Nicholson J, Darzi A. Preparing for precision medicine. *New England Journal of Medicine*, 2012;**366**(6):489–491. doi:10.1056/NEJMp1114866

7. Stacey D, Bennett CL, Barry MJ, et al. Decision aids for people facing health treatment or screening decisions. *Cochrane Database of Systematic Reviews*, 2011;**10**:CD001431. doi:10.1002/14651858.CD001431.pub3

8. Kwok AC, Semel ME, Lipsitz SR, et al. The intensity and variation of surgical care at the end of life: a retrospective cohort study. *Lancet*, 2011;**378**(9800):1408–1413. doi:10.1016/S0140-6736(11)61268-3

9. White SM, Griffiths R, Holloway J, Shannon A. Anaesthesia for proximal femoral fracture in the UK: first report from the NHS Hip Fracture Anaesthesia Network. *Anaesthesia*, 2010;**65**(3):243–248. doi:10.1111/j.1365-2044.2009.06208.x

10. Grocott MP. Improving outcomes after surgery. *BMJ*, 2009;**339**:b5173. doi:10.1136/bmj.b5173

11. Grocott MP, Pearse RM. Perioperative medicine: the future of anaesthesia? *British Journal of Anaesthesia*, 2012;**108**(5):723–726. doi:10.1093/bja/aes124

The role of the preadmission clinic

James Tomlinson

The Alfred Hospital, Australia

Patient evaluation before anaesthesia for surgical and non-surgical procedures is essential. It is the responsibility of the anaesthetist to ensure it is completed adequately. Traditionally, patients were admitted to hospital several days before surgery for assessment, placing significant demands on hospital resources. Many hospitals now operate an outpatient preadmission clinic (PAC) for elective admissions where patients can be assessed in a timely fashion prior to their hospital procedure. The PAC fulfils multiple important roles (Video 2.1).

1. Patient assessment
2. Risk factor identification and management, and patient optimisation
3. Improved safety and quality of care
4. Improved hospital efficiency
5. Patient support, education and awareness
6. Record keeping and research
7. Staff development

Patient assessment

Information is gathered from multiple sources including patient questionnaires, medical records, patient interview, physical examination and medical investigations.

Information collation

Basic patient health and demographic information should be gathered prior to the PAC to inform risk stratification and appropriate patient triage. Triage helps avoid unnecessary assessment of low-risk patients and improves clinic efficiency [1]. This information can be gathered by institution-specific surveys electronically, via paper questionnaires or by telephone. Many institutions employ nursing staff to collect this information and make the initial risk assessment.

Perioperative Medicine for the Junior Clinician, First Edition. Edited by Joel Symons, Paul Myles, Rishi Mehra and Christine Ball.
© 2015 John Wiley & Sons, Ltd. Published 2015 by John Wiley & Sons, Ltd.
Companion website: www.wiley.com/go/perioperativemed

www.wiley.com/go/perioperativemed

VIDEO 2.1 **Roles of the preadmission clinic.** The modern preadmission clinic fulfils a vital role in the perioperative management of patients.

Assessment by the anaesthetist

Patients triaged as moderate to high risk should attend the PAC for assessment by an anaesthetist. Assessment should include a patient interview and a physical examination of the airway, respiratory and cardiovascular systems. The aim of this assessment is to identify and quantify patient-specific risk factors.

It should be noted that in larger institutions, the anaesthetist assessing the patient in the PAC is commonly not the same anaesthetist providing care on the day of the procedure. It is important that the procedural anaesthetist also assesses the patient independently prior to the commencement of the procedure.

Investigations

Routine investigations (i.e. tests ordered without a clinical indication) should not be ordered preoperatively. Disadvantages to routine testing include cost, time delays and patient discomfort. If routine tests are abnormal, there is then additional cost and time required to determine the clinical relevance of such results. Many studies demonstrate that routine testing does not improve patient care [2]. More importantly, there is evidence that abnormal test results may lead to further investigations that can potentially be harmful to patients [3].

Investigations should therefore only be ordered when clinically indicated. Standardised guidelines for preoperative investigations should be developed by each PAC. They should be specific for the institution, patient population and surgical procedure. These guidelines should be available online to ensure easy access by all clinic staff. Examples of such guidelines are freely available (www.ncbi.nlm.nih.gov/books/NBK48489/) [4].

Multidisciplinary team assessment

The multidisciplinary preoperative team may include the anaesthetist, surgeons, preoperative nurses, pharmacists, physiotherapists, physicians and general practitioners. Depending on the results of the information gathered, the anaesthetist may choose to involve any or all of these healthcare professionals to further investigate, advise on and assist patient optimisation.

Risk factor identification and management, and patient optimisation

Patient risk factors should be assessed and appropriate management plans implemented. Risk factors may be anaesthetic specific (e.g. difficult airway), or pertain to medical co-morbidities and surgical factors. Risk assessment can be useful in planning the patient's perioperative care.

Nine variables provide independent prognostic information.

- Age
- Sex
- Socioeconomic status
- Aerobic capacity
- Coronary artery disease
- Heart failure
- Ischaemic brain disease
- Renal failure
- Peripheral arterial disease

Preoperative patient optimisation should be guided by protocols developed for each institution [5]. They should cover issues such as:

- chronic disease management, e.g. diabetes, anaemia, cardiorespiratory illness
- anticoagulants
- venous thromboprophylaxis
- smoking cessation
- obesity and nutrition
- physiotherapy and inactivity.

A multidisciplinary team is useful to achieve this. Clear lines of communication should be established with the patient's GP so they can assist in preoptimisation.

Improve safety and quality of patient care

Data from the Australian Incident Monitoring Study indicated that more than 10% of reported critical events were linked to inadequate preanaesthetic assessment [6]. These events were considered preventable in over 50% of cases. Many other studies have demonstrated that preoperative patient optimisation results in reduced morbidity and mortality, and a reduction in cancellations and delays [7].

Improve hospital efficiency

Patient assessment allows the multidisciplinary team to establish a clear care plan for the patient.

* Preoperative care and admission requirements
* Hospital suitability depending on patient and surgical complexity
* Day surgery versus postoperative ward care
* High-dependency and intensive care unit support
* Discharge and rehabilitation planning

This aims to reduce cancellations and improve the efficient use of hospital resources, with lower patient bed occupancy and a reduction in length of stay. Many studies have demonstrated a significantly lower cancellation rate amongst patients receiving preassessment [8].

Patient support, education and awareness

The PAC is an ideal opportunity to fully inform patients about all aspects of their care. The information should be specific for the patient and procedure, and ideally should be both verbal and written. Written instructions allow the patients to reference them when convenient. They can also be made available to patients online to improve accessibility. Verbal and written information should include:

* preoperative fasting guidelines
* anaesthetic options including advantages, disadvantages and risks
* options for pain relief
* instructions for patient medication, especially anticoagulants, diabetic and cardiac medication.

It is important not to miss this opportunity for discussion with the patient as improved patient education and awareness reduce fear and anxiety.

Record keeping and research

Many institutions are now adopting electronic medical records. This allows for the standardisation of patient information, avoids redundancy, can enhance quality improvement and can provide a database for research (1).

References

1. Bader AM, Sweitzer B, Kumar A. Nuts and bolts of preoperative clinics: the view from three institutions. *Cleveland Clinic Journal of Medicine*, 2009;**76**(Suppl 4):S104–111. doi:10.3949/ccjm.76.s4.17

2. Schein OD, Katz J, Bass EB, et al. The value of routine preoperative medical testing before cataract surgery. *New England Journal of Medicine*, 2000;**342**(3):168–175. doi:10.1056/Nejm200001203420304

3. Tape TG, Mushlin AI. How useful are routine chest x-rays of preoperative patients at risk for postoperative chest disease? *Journal of General Internal Medicine*, 1988;**3**(1):15–20. doi:10.1007/Bf02595750

4. National Collaborating Centre for Acute Care. *Preoperative Tests: The Use of Routine Preoperative Tests for Elective Surgery*. NICE Clinical Guideline No. 3. London: National Collaborating Centre for Acute Care, 2003.

5. Jones K, Swart M. Anaesthesia services for pre-operative assessment and preparation. In: *Guidelines for the Provision of Anaesthetic Services*. London: Royal College of Anaesthetists, 2013.

6. Kluger MT, Tham EJ, Coleman NA, Runciman WB, Bullock MFM. Inadequate pre-operative evaluation and preparation: a review of 197 reports from the Australian Incident Monitoring Study. *Anaesthesia*, 2000;**55**(12):1173–1178. doi:10.1046/J.1365-2044.2000.01725.x

7. Yen C, Tsai M, Macario A. Preoperative evaluation clinics. *Current Opinion in Anesthesiology*, 2010;**23**(2):167–172. doi:10.1097/Aco.0b013e328336f4b9

8. Ferschi MD, Swoitzer BJ, Huo D, Glick DB. Preoperative clinic visits reduce operating room cancellations and delays. *Anesthesiology*, 2005;**103**(4):855–859. doi:10.1097/00000542-20051 0000-00025

Consent

The Alfred Hospital, Australia

Medical consent is the voluntary agreement by a competent and informed patient to undergo a medical examination or treatment.

Ethical and legal basis of consent

Doctors have an ethical and legal obligation to obtain patient consent prior to medical procedures. A doctor who touches a patient without explicit or implied consent is liable to a claim of *battery*. A doctor who fails to provide adequate information about the risks of a procedure is liable to a claim of *negligence*. Inadequate consent is a common source of patient complaints and disciplinary action by medical boards.

Elements of a valid consent

Patient must have capacity

Adults are presumed to have legal capacity to consent. Capacity may be lost:

- permanently (e.g. dementia)
- temporarily (e.g. sedatives)

or:

- completely (no treatment decisions possible)
- partially (some decisions, not others).

To assess capacity, doctors should ask: does this patient understand the general nature and consequences of the treatment, and are they able to communicate a decision? If the patient has cognitive impairment *and* is unable to understand, retain or weigh up the information needed to make a decision at that time, then this is evidence of incapacity.

Perioperative Medicine for the Junior Clinician, First Edition. Edited by Joel Symons, Paul Myles, Rishi Mehra and Christine Ball.
© 2015 John Wiley & Sons, Ltd. Published 2015 by John Wiley & Sons, Ltd.
Companion website: www.wiley.com/go/perioperativemed

Minors generally require guardians to consent on their behalf. The Common Law does, however, recognise *competent minors* who are able to consent to medical procedures independently [1]. The doctor must be satisfied that the minor has the maturity and understanding to evaluate the treatment and consider the consequences of treatment or non-treatment. The more serious the intervention and consequences, the greater the maturity required.

Patient must be informed

The patient must be informed of the nature and benefits of the proposed treatment, the inherent risks, the alternative treatment options and the likely outcome of no treatment at all. Use plain language and avoid medical jargon. Models, diagrams and written information can be useful aids to understanding. If necessary, use an interpreter service.

In Australia, doctors are legally obliged to disclose all *material risks* to the patient [2]. This means explaining risks that a reasonable person in the circumstances would consider significant, and also the risks that your particular patient may consider significant. This requires doctors to assess the patient's individual circumstances carefully, including temperament, desire for information and general health. Doctors who explain risks using strict protocols may miss this important step.

When explaining the magnitude of a risk, be careful using phrases such as 'low risk' or 'very uncommon' because the patient's perception of these terms may differ from your own. If using numerical data, it is better to explain risks as proportions with a constant denominator (1 in 1000; 25 in 1000) rather than percentages. Using visual aids is one of the most effective means of improving the communication of risk [3].

At the end of any discussion about consent, the patient should be given the opportunity to consider the information and ask questions.

Consent must be voluntary

Consent must be given freely without coercion or induced by fraud or deceit. Undue influence may be exerted by family members, community representatives or medical staff. Doctors should be careful not to coerce patients by withholding important information or overstating benefits.

Consent by junior doctors

> Guidelines recommend that the doctor consenting should be capable of performing the procedure himself or herself, or be specifically trained in advising patients about the procedure [4].

Documenting consent

Health services have mandated standard consent forms for many medical treatments. These do not assure proper consent process. Documenting the discussion, including the risks discussed and questions asked by the patient, provides a more useful record.

Special circumstances

Patient lacks capacity

In Australia, consent can be obtained from this patient's legal guardian or next of kin. If there are no next of kin, or they are unavailable, consent should be sought from a public guardian or court.

In the UK, only legally appointed Lasting Powers of Attorney or court-appointed deputies may consent for these patients, but the patient's family or carers should be consulted to help assess the patient's wishes, beliefs and values. After considering all the circumstances, the treating doctor is required to make a decision based on the best interests of the patient [5].

Emergency treatment

Consent is not required for treatment believed necessary to save a patient's life or to prevent serious mental or physical injury. This is strictly interpreted and should not be used by doctors for convenience.

Patient refuses treatment

Patients have the right to refuse medical treatment generally, or refuse specific procedures. Some jurisdictions have criminal penalties for performing a procedure on a patient who has refused (e.g. s. 6 Medical Treatment Act (Victoria) 1988) [6].

A competent patient has a right to refuse treatment for any reason, rational or irrational, even where the consequence may be serious injury or death [7]. However, the courts are generally reluctant to allow minors to refuse life-saving treatments [8].

An incompetent patient who refuses treatment is a special case. In an emergency, it is reasonable to commence life-saving treatment; for non-emergency care, a court order may be required if treatment is thought to be in the patient's best interests.

Waiver and therapeutic privilege

Occasionally a patient will waive their right to information about a medical treatment ('Please don't tell me, Doctor'). It is important they understand the general nature of the proposed treatment in order to consent but if they request no discussion of risk, then respect their wishes and document.

In rare circumstances, 'therapeutic privilege' can be exercised when a doctor *reasonably* believes disclosing information to a patient may *seriously harm* the patient's health or well-being.

Summary

- Doctors have ethical and legal obligations to obtain patient consent.
- The patient must have legal capacity, be informed and give consent voluntarily.
- Explanation of risk requires an assessment of what the individual patient might consider significant.
- The most common exception to consent is emergency treatment.

References

1. *Gillick v West Norfolk and Wisbech Area Health Authority* [1985] 3 All ER 402

2. *Rogers v Whitaker* [1992] 109 ALR 625 (HCA)

3. Paling J. Strategies to help patients understand risks. *BMJ*, 2003;**327**:745–748. doi:10.1136/Bmj.327.7417.745

4. Department of Health (UK). *Reference Guide for Consent to Examination or Treatment*, 2nd edn. London: Department of Health, 2009. www.gov.uk/government/publications

5. Mental Capacity Act (2005). Code of Practice. Chapter 4. www.publicguardian.gov.uk/mca/code-of-practice

6. Medical Treatment Act (Victoria) (1988). www.legislation.vic.gov.au

7. *Re: MB (Adult, medical treatment)* [1997] 38 BMLR 175 CA

8. *Re: E (a minor)* [1993] 1 FLR 386

4

The early postoperative round

Debra Devonshire[1] and Paul Myles[2]

[1] Monash Health, Australia
[2] The Alfred Hospital and Monash University, Australia

The first 24 hours after major surgery are often complex, with significant physiological, physical and emotional challenges. The physician conducting the early postoperative ward round is important in facilitating a smooth transition to recovery by maximising the patient's ability to overcome these challenges.

Postoperative review should not be limited to surgical problems (or the surgical wound), but includes surveillance for patient delirium, subclinical complications such as myocardial infarction and acute kidney injury, and assessment of deviation from care pathways (refer to Chapter 90 Postoperative delirium and postoperative cognitive dysfunction, Chapter 88 Myocardial injury after non-cardiac surgery and Chapter 47 Acute kidney injury) [1].

Establish rapport

The early round may often be the first time the physician and patient have met. It is important to quickly establish rapport. Mehrabian's studies in non-verbal communication during the late 1960s and early 1970s identified smiles, head nods, eye contact, orientation of body and head towards the person in conversation, and touch (such as a warm handshake) as factors which enhance verbal communication. This may sound obvious but many physicians are often distracted from positive communication as they teach junior trainees, answer staff requests and balance time management so that the round proceeds efficiently. Examining and asking personal questions of patients requires tact and respect. Receiving honest, useful answers requires establishing a rapid empathic connection.

Scan the record

It is essential to briefly become familiar with the patient's history prior to consultation. Specifically check the drug chart, surgical notes, anaesthesia chart and basic investigation results relevant to early management. For example, is the estimated glomerular filtration rate adequate or impaired? The answer may affect how analgesia is prescribed. Check how the patient responded in the recovery room. For example, were they slow to leave recovery due to hypotension or excessive drowsiness? Do they have tolerance or are they sensitive to opioids? Was there the common and distressing problem of postoperative nausea and vomiting (PONV)? Reviewing the surgical notes may reveal that the lower abdominal scar following caesarean section does not simply indicate the delivery of a live infant but also a long history of endometriosis resulting in extra dissection and tissue trauma impacting on pain management.

Take a history

A brief targeted history yields the best results and allows efficient use of time.

Unlike other patient interactions, the early postoperative round often needs a tight focus. Ask the nursing staff and/or relatives, if present, for information.

Open-ended questions are optimal, i.e. how are you this morning? However, it may be necessary to ask some direct questions. For example, do you have a sore throat? Have you passed urine yet?

Specifically ask the patient if they have anything they wish to discuss about the anaesthesia or surgical experience. For example, it would be important to discover if the patient had been aware during the procedure.

Examine the patient

Objectively review the patient after obtaining clues from the subjective history. Target the areas where you will gain maximum yield for benefit. For example:

- remove the covers and look at the surgical site. Consider number and size of incisions/port sites and possible impact on factors such as mobility, respiration, mentation and oral intake
- ask the patient to move, take a deep breath, cough and then auscultate the lungs. Optimising factors which improve respiratory function may reduce hypoxaemia. Can the obese patient sit at 45°?
- gently palpate the abdomen or move limbs, trunk, neck or joints depending on the patient's surgical experience. Consider if analgesia is adequate or could be improved.

Troubleshoot the basics

The early postoperative round is an opportunity to ensure the basics have been met in the patient's management. For example:

- are adequate intravenous fluids charted?
- are appropriate antiemetics charted?
- does the patient have adequate blood pressure, heart rate and peripheral perfusion?
- if a regional block was performed, is there still numbness? How dense is the motor block? Are dermatome levels appropriate and charted? What is the trend? A dense motor block requires special attention. If a continuous epidural or intrathecal infusion is connected, it usually requires cessation until motor function returns before recommencing at a lower rate for ongoing analgesia. It is important to detect possible nerve injury early! Radiological imaging and neurosurgical intervention may be required for a compressing haematoma.

Manage pain effectively

Optimising analgesia and minimising side effects is essential in the early postoperative period. Ask the patient to rate their pain intensity using a 0–10 verbal rating scale. Pain is a continuum and well-managed acute pain places the patient at lower risk for developing chronic pain. The follow-on effects of improved analgesia include earlier mobilisation with less risk of deep vein thrombosis (DVT), pulmonary embolism (PE) and other respiratory complications. Multimodal analgesia is the mainstay of effective postoperative pain relief (refer to Chapter 93 Acute pain).

Detecting deterioration

Postoperative review by the junior doctor can overlap with specialised units such as the acute pain service and critical care outreach teams. Any or all of these clinicians can enhance early recognition of deteriorating patients and facilitate rapid and appropriate management [2]. Beware of hypotension, unexplained tachycardia or dyspnoea and poorly controlled pain – the latter is the fifth vital sign.

Opportunities exist for combined postoperative review teams, for which success has been reported [3]. For example, a group in Australia utilised the expertise of an acute pain service providing critical care outreach and found that the rate of serious adverse postoperative events decreased from 23 events per 100 patients to 16 events per 100 patients, and mortality decreased from 9% to 3% (p = 0.004). Such co-ordinated care is likely to be very cost-effective [4].

Communicate with other staff and formulate an early postoperative plan

4

Once assessment is complete and areas for improvement are identified, any alterations in management should be communicated to the ward nursing staff and parent surgical unit; pharmacy and other allied health staff should be included. For example, if changes in analgesia medication are charted, a referral is requested for intensive chest physiotherapy or a blood test is ordered for liver function, then it is important to ensure a smooth transition to care or follow-up by other disciplines. Co-ordinated communication facilitates early intervention on the postoperative round.

References

1. Lemmens L, van Zelm R, Vanhaecht K, Kerkkamp H. Systematic review: indicators to evaluate effectiveness of clinical pathways for gastrointestinal surgery. *Journal of Evaluation in Clinical Practice*, 2008;**14**(5):880–887. doi:10.1111/j.1365-2753.2008.01079.x

2. Jones DA, Dunbar NJ, Bellomo R. Clinical deterioration in hospital inpatients: the need for another paradigm shift. *Medical Journal of Australia*, 2012;**196**:97–100. doi:10.5694/mja11.10865

3. Story DA, Shelton AC, Poustie SJ, Colin-Thome NJ, McIntyre RE, McNicol PL. Effect of an anaesthesia department led critical care outreach and acute pain service on postoperative serious adverse events. *Anaesthesia*, 2006;**61**(1):24–28. doi:10.1111/j.1365-2044.2005.04435.x

4. Lee A, Chan SK, Chen PP, Gin T, Lau AS, Chiu CH. The costs and benefits of extending the role of the acute pain service on clinical outcomes after major elective surgery. *Anesthesia and Analgesia*, 2010;**111**(4):1042–1050. doi:10.1213/ANE.0b013e3181ed1317

5 Quality improvement and patient safety

Stuart Marshall

Monash University, Australia

Introduction

> Safety and quality are influenced by factors from the micro-level, such as individual decisions and equipment design, all the way up to the macro-level of governmental funding and regulatory frameworks. In a practical sense, all healthcare workers and their patients are responsible for safety and quality. Maintenance of safety only occurs if ongoing monitoring and corrective actions are undertaken.

Healthcare is arguably the most complex of human endeavours. This complexity comes from the rapidly progressing knowledge in medical science, increasing specialisation, the multiprofessional nature of care and, of course, the treatment of an ageing population with more co-morbidities. Despite this, healthcare is safer now than it ever has been. For these improvements to have occurred in health delivery, including perioperative care, safety and quality must be measured and assessed, and appropriate changes implemented.

The terms 'quality and 'patient safety' are difficult to define. The World Health Organization defines six 'dimensions' of quality care. Quality care is care which is effective, efficient, accessible, acceptable (patient centred), equitable and safe [1]. When relating these ideas to perioperative care, it is important to recognise that these dimensions can be influenced at individual, team, unit, organisation and broader cultural and regulatory levels. Put another way, the delivery of safe, high-quality care is not just due to each individual patient–clinician interaction, but also the context in which the interaction occurs.

Perioperative Medicine for the Junior Clinician, First Edition. Edited by Joel Symons, Paul Myles, Rishi Mehra and Christine Ball.
© 2015 John Wiley & Sons, Ltd. Published 2015 by John Wiley & Sons, Ltd.
Companion website: www.wiley.com/go/perioperativemed

The individual and the system

All humans make errors. It might be forgetting to lock the front door, putting salt in your tea rather than sugar or misreading a headline in the newspaper. An error is simply doing the wrong thing when meaning to do the right thing.

Making errors in a clinical situation is no different to any other, except that the consequences can be very different. Forgetting to perform a clinical task, accidentally swapping one drug for another or misreading a pathology report can have profound consequences for a patient's safety.

When something goes wrong in healthcare, the tendency is to attribute blame. However, if other factors such as equipment design, staffing levels and time pressure are taken into account, clearly events are rarely due to the failure of a sole clinician. Patient and doctor interactions do not occur in a vacuum and many other factors, from local policies to government funding, have an influence. Patients can help by keeping themselves informed and asking questions about their care. Patient safety has been said to be everybody's business, 'from patient to politician' [2].

Safety of the perioperative patient

Common threats to patient safety in the perioperative period are primarily related to the disease and the surgery. In most cases, serious threats related to anaesthesia are one or more orders of magnitude less than that of the related surgery. For instance, the risk of significant bleeding following an elective thyroidectomy is approximately 1 in 100 cases, but the chance of a failed intubation is likely to be no more than 1 in 2000 cases [3].

Advances in intraoperative equipment, processes and training in the last three decades have led to safer anaesthesia. Routine preoperative risk identification, pulse oximetry and other monitoring have reduced mortality from anaesthesia as the primary cause from approximately 1 in 10,000 before 1980 to less than 1 in 100,000 today [4].

Postoperatively, the risks are common and minor, such as nausea and vomiting, or rare and severe such as pulmonary thromboembolism. Identification of those patients at risk and implemention of preventive measures occur in more reliable institutions.

Quality improvement

Deming described a four-phase cycle of 'Plan, Do, Study, Act' to iteratively improve the quality and safety of a system [5]. As perioperative mortality is now rare, indices of quality such as rates of readmission or infection are commonly used to track performance. A good example of how interventions and tracking event rates can enhance safety and quality is with the implementation of central line insertion 'bundles' to reduce infection rates. Infections of central venous catheters occurred in approximately 10% of patients with central venous catheters on the intensive care unit, with an associated mortality of 4–25%. Berenholtz and colleagues introduced a suite of five interventions to improve aseptic technique and line utilisation and effectively eliminated infections in one unit [6]. This was estimated to save eight lives and over $2 million in the first year.

Individual factors

Human performance is modified by many factors. Fatigue, worry, illness, medications and alcohol all contribute to poorer functioning and an increased risk of errors. Positive factors that improve practitioners' performance include maintaining currency and adequate training for tasks that they perform. Safe standards can be further ensured through regulation, ongoing credentialling, opportunities for education and self-care.

Team training

The effectiveness of operating theatre teams has been shown to have a significant effect on patient safety. Associations between good team behaviours, such as communication, and patient outcomes have been observed in many settings [7]. Team training has been shown to improve these same indices of team performance [8]. One of the key recommendations from the US Institute for Health Improvement's landmark paper 'To Err is Human' [9] was that those who work in teams should also train as teams.

Organisational and regulatory factors

Every health service should have a structure that monitors safety and quality; standards exist to ensure these are effective. When adverse events occur in healthcare, they may not be immediately apparent, unlike some other industries such as nuclear power generation or commercial aviation. In order to develop a culture of learning and safety, reporting of these adverse events must occur. This is the case even if the patient does not come to any harm as potential hazards may be identified and remedied before injury occurs. Local 'morbidity and mortality' meetings help individuals learn from events in their own institution. National reporting systems may identify rare problems or help estimate the incidences of potential hazards. National bodies may use such data to effect change at a higher, governmental level.

References

1. World Health Organization (WHO). *Quality of Care: A Process for Making Strategic Choices in Health Systems*. Geneva, Switzerland: World Health Organization, 2006.

2. Berwick DM. Improvement, trust, and the healthcare workforce. *Quality and Safety in Health Care*, 2003;**12**(6):448–652. doi:10.1136/qhc.12.suppl_1.i2

3. Cook TM, Woodall N, Harper J, Benger J. Major complications of airway management in the UK: results of the Fourth National Audit Project of the Royal College of Anaesthetists and the Difficult Airway Society. Part 2: intensive care and emergency departments. *British Journal of Anaesthesia*, 2011;**106**(5):632–542. doi:10.1093/bja/aer059

4. Aitkenhead AR. Injuries associated with anaesthesia. A global perspective. *British Journal of Anaesthesia*, 2005;**95**(1):95–109. doi:10.1093/bja/aei132

5. Deming WE. *The New Economics*. Cambridge, MA: MIT Press, 1993, p.135.

6. Berenholtz SM, Pronovost PJ, Lipsett PA, et al. Eliminating catheter-related bloodstream infections in the intensive care unit. *Critical Care Medicine*, 2004;**32**(10):2014–2020. doi:10.1097/01.ccm.0000142399.70913.2f

7. Schraagen JM, Schouten T, Smit M, et al. A prospective study of paediatric cardiac surgical microsystems: assessing the relationships between non-routine events, teamwork

and patient outcomes. *BMJ Quality and Safety*, 2011;**20**(7):599–603. doi:10.1136/Bmjqs.2010.048983

8. Schmutz J, Manser T. Do team processes really have an effect on clinical performance? A systematic literature review. *British Journal of Anaesthesia*, 2013;**110**(4):529–544. doi:10.1093/Bja/Aes513

9. Kohn LT, Corrigan JM, Donaldson MS. *To Err is Human: Building a Safer Health Care System*. Washington, DC: National Academies Press, 1999.

6 Intraoperative and postoperative monitoring

Philip Peyton

Austin Hospital and University of Melbourne, Australia

Patient monitoring is a critical component of perioperative care, when physiological instability is common. Alerting clinicians and carers in real time allows them to intervene early to prevent deterioration and anticipate complications [1].

> Optimal set-up of monitors includes selection and activation of appropriate alarm settings to alert carers promptly to changes and to avoid alarming unnecessarily in response to minor fluctuations in monitored variables.

Intensive monitoring of the circulatory and respiratory systems is now standard practice in major surgery. However, development of reliable technologies for routine monitoring of many vital organs and systems remains an ongoing challenge. Table 6.1 summarises the typical regimens for intra- and postoperative monitoring for patients undergoing general anaesthesia for major and minor surgery.

Cardiovascular system

Routine monitoring

Routine cardiovascular monitoring during surgery includes the electrocardiogram (ECG) which displays heart rate (HR) and rhythm, and arterial blood pressure measurement. Arterial blood pressure measurement can be non-invasive (using an automated oscillotonometric cuff) or invasive (Video 6.1).

Invasive arterial cannulation is essential where sudden cardiovascular changes or significant blood loss are likely. It allows real-time, beat-to-beat blood pressure monitoring. The radial artery at the wrist is usually used but the brachial or femoral arteries may be used if necessary. It also allows ready sampling of arterial blood for repeated blood gas analysis, and measurement of electrolytes and haemoglobin concentration.

Perioperative Medicine for the Junior Clinician, First Edition. Edited by Joel Symons, Paul Myles, Rishi Mehra and Christine Ball.
© 2015 John Wiley & Sons, Ltd. Published 2015 by John Wiley & Sons, Ltd.
Companion website: www.wiley.com/go/perioperativemed

TABLE 6.1 **Typical regimes for intra- and postoperative monitoring for patients undergoing general anaesthesia for major and minor surgery**

Minor surgery	System	Intraoperative	Postoperative HDU/ICU	Postoperative ward
	Oxygenation	SpO_2		SpO_2
		FiO_2		
	Ventilation	Capnograph: RR		RR
	Cardiovascular	ECG: HR, rhythm		HR
		Non-invasive BP		Non-invasive BP
	Metabolic	?Temperature		Temperature
	Conscious state	Anaesthetic agent		GCS/sedation
Major surgery	Oxygenation	SpO_2	SpO_2	SpO_2
		FiO_2	FiO_2	
	Ventilation	Capnograph, RR	?Capnograph, RR	RR
	Cardiovascular	ECG: HR, rhythm	ECG: HR, rhythm	HR
		Invasive BP	Invasive BP	Non-invasive BP
		SPV/PPV	SPV/PPV	
		?CVP	?CVP	?CVP
		+/− Cardiac output	+/− Cardiac output	
	Metabolic	Temperature	Temperature	Temperature
		Blood gas, acid–base	Blood gas, acid–base	
		Haemoglobin	Haemoglobin	Haemoglobin
	Renal	Electrolytes	Electrolytes	Electrolytes
		Urine output	Creatinine	Creatinine
	Conscious state	BIS/entropy	Urine output	Urine output
		Anaesthetic agent	GCS/sedation	GCS/sedation

Anaesthetic agent, expired anaesthetic agent concentration; BIS/entropy, bispectral or entropy index; BP, blood pressure; CVP, central venous pressure; ECG, electrocardiogram; FiO_2, inspired oxygen concentration; GCS/sedation, coma or sedation score; HDU/ICU, high dependency unit/intensive care unit; HR, heart rate; RR, respiratory rate; SpO_2, pulse oximetry oxygen saturation; SPV/PPV, systolic or pulse pressure variation.

www.wiley.com/go/perioperativemed

VIDEO 6.1 **Invasive arterial pressure monitoring can provide real-time information where blood pressure may fluctuate rapidly in a beat-to-beat fashion. Additionally, serial sampling for blood gas analysis can occur with invasive arterial monitoring.**

After discharge from the recovery room, ongoing ECG or invasive arterial pressure monitoring generally requires high-dependency or critical care.

Circulatory volume status

Monitoring of the arterial pressure waveform also allows assessment of blood volume status in patients undergoing controlled ventilation. Cyclic changes in intrathoracic pressure induced by positive pressure ventilation cause breath-to-breath variations in left ventricular preload, and stroke volume and pulse pressure.

Systolic pressure variation (SPV) or pulse pressure variation (PPV) has been shown to be a better predictor than central venous pressure (CVP) of fluid responsiveness; that is, of an increase in cardiac output after administering an intravenous fluid challenge [2]. Fluid responsiveness is frequently used as an indicator of hypovolaemia. These indices are also sensitive to other factors affecting ventricular preload, such as vasomotor tone or patient position.

Direct monitoring of CVP via a central venous cannula is still often done in major surgery, as it provides robust intravenous access for multiple infusions and can be used postoperatively in the ward.

Advanced haemodynamic assessment

Measurement of stroke volume (SV) or cardiac output (SV × HR) allows a much more comprehensive assessment of the circulation than is achieved from arterial blood pressure measurement alone. Systemic vascular resistance (SVR) can be calculated from mean arterial pressure, CVP and cardiac output (CO). Estimation of fluid responsiveness and SVR helps guide the most appropriate choice of fluid and volume resuscitation and/or vasopressor therapy to optimise the circulation (Figure 6.1).

The standard method for estimation of SV or CO in clinical practice has been right heart thermodilution with a pulmonary artery (Swann–Ganz) catheter. This is generally reserved for monitoring in cardiac surgery or critically ill patients in intensive care [3].

A number of less invasive devices are available, using a range of technologies, including:

- measurement of blood flow velocities in the descending aorta by oesophageal doppler probes
- estimation of blood flow and stroke volume from the arterial pulse pressure waveform
- partial carbon dioxide rebreathing
- transthoracic electrical bioimpedance.

These devices have broadened the range of surgery in which advanced haemodynamic monitoring can be employed to guide fluid and vasopressor therapy [4].

$$CO = \frac{MAP-CVP}{SVR}$$

Fluids +/– inotropes   Vasopressors

FIGURE 6.1 **The components of haemodynamic assessment.** Measurement of cardiac output (CO), mean arterial pressure (MAP) and central venous pressure (CVP) allows calculation of systemic vascular resistance (SVR). These can be manipulated with appropriate combinations of fluid and volume resuscitation, or use of vasoactive drugs. Source: Reproduced with permission of Wolters Kluwer Health.

Respiratory system

Pulse oximetry

Oxygen delivery to the brain, heart and other vital organs rapidly deteriorates when lung ventilation is depressed or obstructed. Real-time monitoring of arterial oxygenation saturation using pulse oximetry is mandatory during anaesthesia or procedural sedation and in recovery, where respiration is often depressed by drugs and airway obstruction is common in the presence of reduced conscious state (Video 6.2).

Pulse oximetry monitoring may need to continue in the ward in patients requiring opioid analgesia, oxygen supplementation or with significant co-morbidities.

Newer pulse oximetry technology also provides non-invasive estimation of haemoglobin concentration.

Capnography

Breath-by-breath monitoring of expired carbon dioxide concentration (capnography) is mandatory in anaesthetised or ventilated patients. It indicates the presence and adequacy of lung ventilation and provides a sensitive and prompt patient apnoea alarm. It helps optimise artificial ventilation settings such as respiratory rate and tidal volume.

Deviations from a regular 'square wave' capnogram can indicate disturbances of ventilation due to disconnection or leaks in the breathing system, or a patient 'fighting the ventilator' (Video 6.3).

End-expired (end-tidal) carbon dioxide concentration changes reflect changes in arterial carbon dioxide partial pressures, although an arterial blood gas sample is more accurate.

www.wiley.com/go/perioperativemed

VIDEO 6.2 **Pulse oximetry.**

www.wiley.com/go/perioperativemed

VIDEO 6.3 **Capnography allows monitoring of the ventilation, cardiac output and metabolic state of a patient.**

www.wiley.com/go/perioperativemed

VIDEO 6.4 **Awareness monitoring by processed electroencephalography allows** monitoring of the amounts of anaesthesia agents as well as minimising intraoperative awareness.

Cerebral monitoring

Continuous monitoring of expired concentrations of inhaled anaesthetic agents is mandatory in patients under general anaesthesia. In addition, monitoring of depth of anaesthesia, using processed electroencephalography devices such as bispectral index [5] or entropy, is common practice in general anaesthesia for major surgery when the patient is at increased risk of awareness or neuromuscular blocking agents are used (Video 6.4).

Postoperatively, clinical signs are relied upon to assess conscious state, such as sedation score in patients receiving systemic opioid analgesia.

Cerebral oximetry non-invasively measures cerebral tissue oxygen saturation as an index of cerebral perfusion. It is used mainly during complex cardiac surgery such as that involving the thoracic aorta, where blood flow to the cerebral circulation can be compromised [6].

Major organ function

Renal dysfunction is a common and potentially serious complication of major surgery. Monitoring of urine output via an indwelling catheter is standard in major surgery. Low urine output can be an unreliable indicator of renal perfusion (refer to Chapter 46 Oliguria). A measured change in serum creatinine is the most readily available clinical tool to indicate deteriorating renal function.

Similarly, there are few non-invasive monitors of the function of other major organs such as the liver, pancreas or bowel. Metabolic acidosis and rising serum lactic acid may indicate splanchnic or visceral hypoperfusion. Monitoring of gastric pH has been advocated in intensive care as a continuous, minimally invasive indicator of splanchnic perfusion.

References

1. American Society of Anesthesiologists. *Standards for Basic Anesthetic Monitoring*. www.asahq.org

2. Cannesson M, Le Manach Y, Hofer CK, et al. Assessing the diagnostic accuracy of pulse pressure variations for the prediction of fluid responsiveness: a 'gray zone' approach. *Anesthesiology*, 2011;**115**(2):231–241. doi:10.1097/ALN.0b013e318225b80a

3. ASA Task Force. Practice guidelines for pulmonary artery catheterization: an updated report by the American Society of Anesthesiologists Task Force on Pulmonary Artery Catheterization. *Anesthesiology*, 2003;**99**(4):988–1014. doi:10.1097/00000542-200310000-00036

4. Funk DJ, Moretti EW, Gan TJ. Minimally invasive cardiac output monitoring in the perioperative setting. *Anesthesia and Analgesia*, 2009;**108**(3):887–897. doi:10.1213/ane.0b013e31818ffd99

5. Rampil IJ. A primer for EEG signal processing in anesthesia. *Anesthesiology*, 1998;**89**(4): 980–1002. doi:10.1097/00000542-199810000-00023

6. Murkin J, Arango M, Deschamps A, Denault A. Near-infrared spectroscopy monitoring in cardiac surgery: theory, pactice and utility. In: Bonser RS, editor. *Brain Protection in Cardiac Surgery*. London: Springer-Verlag, 2011. doi:10.1007/978-1-84996-293-3_11

Drugs used for anaesthesia and sedation

Alex Konstantatos

The Alfred Hospital and Monash University, Australia

Definitions

Anaesthesia involves the systemic, inhaled or localised administration of one or more medications to facilitate a surgical or medical procedure. These medications include inhalational agents, known as *volatile agents* and *nitrous oxide*, injectable drugs known as *hypnotics* or *intravenous induction agents,* and locally active agents known as *local anaesthetics.* These medications act to suppress consciousness and pain. Drug-induced unconsciousness is, in essence, *general anaesthesia.*

Conscious sedation is where the patient has reduced consciousness but is able to respond appropriately to verbal or tactile stimuli, but may not remember doing so. An example of conscious sedation is where a painful nerve block is performed but the patient remains comfortable, able to follow instructions and remain in optimal position to facilitate the nerve block. *Procedural sedation* describes a deeper plane of sedation where the patient is able to tolerate a potentially painful event which they are less likely to recall. An example of procedural sedation involves a patient having a colonoscopy.

Dissociative anaesthesia is a condition where a patient may appear awake but is unaware of their surroundings and lacks recall.

Mechanism of action of anaesthetic and sedative drugs

Current knowledge of the mechanism of action of anaesthetic and sedative drugs is limited. Mechanisms of anaesthesia mostly involve potentiation of inhibitory neuronal signals through enhanced chloride ion movement across gamma-aminobutyric acid (GABA) transmembrane channels in areas of the central nervous system. This is not as simple as enhanced inhibition of the reticular activating

Perioperative Medicine for the Junior Clinician, First Edition. Edited by Joel Symons, Paul Myles, Rishi Mehra and Christine Ball.
© 2015 John Wiley & Sons, Ltd. Published 2015 by John Wiley & Sons, Ltd.
Companion website: www.wiley.com/go/perioperativemed

system [1] but may involve additional processes, including inhibition of thalamic communication with cortical areas [1] and reduction in spinal processing of sensory and motor function [2].

Basic pharmacological concepts

All anaesthetics and sedatives are highly lipid soluble and have large volumes of distribution, meaning they achieve significant concentration in the central nervous system, the primary site of action. Most also have a relatively short duration of action after single intravenous injection influenced by redistribution, a process whereby the drug moves out of high blood flow, low-volume compartments, such as the brain, to lower blood flow, high-volume compartments such as subcutaneous fat. This means that the drug can remain in the body for a period of time, acting as a depot or reservoir. Many anaesthetic drugs, such as propofol and midazolam, can be infused to maintain therapeutic levels and so maintain anaesthesia or sedation in settings such as intensive care. Infusions which are rapidly titratable rely on short drug context-sensitive half-times, a property which means that the resultant concentration is, in part, dependent on infusion duration [3].

Medications used as sole anaesthetic agents

Alkylphenols: propofol (sedative, hypnotic)

Propofol is formulated in a white solution as a lipid emulsion and is used to provide sedation, initiate, or initiate and maintain general anaesthesia. Propofol can be administered as a single bolus or infused using programmable syringe drivers to acquire and maintain a desired blood level. Propofol is metabolised at multiple sites and commonly produces pain on injection, myoclonus, fall in blood pressure (about 25%), apnoea, and very rarely causes lipid emulsion overload following prolonged high-dose infusions. Typical induction dose 1–2 mg/kg.

Barbiturates: thiopental (hypnotic)

Presented as a sodium salt requiring reconstitution with water/saline, thiopental can be sedative or hypnotic. Thiopental has a high context-sensitive half-time owing to slowed metabolism with increasing dose, so is rarely infused for maintenance of anaesthesia but has been used for cerebral protection. Common effects of single-dose thiopental include a fall in blood pressure (about 20%), apnoea and, more rarely, porphyria in susceptible individuals. Typical induction dose 3–5 mg/kg.

Imidazolines: etomidate (hypnotic)

Etomidate is presented in propylene glycol (and intralipid in Europe) and is almost solely used for induction of anaesthesia. Favourable attributes include greater cardiovascular stability than propofol and thiopental. Less favourable attributes include pain on injection, thrombophlebitis, nausea and vomiting, and myoclonus. Infusions of etomidate have been associated with adrenocortical suppression. Typical induction dose 0.2–0.6 mg/kg.

Phencyclidines: ketamine (dissociative agent, analgesic)

Ketamine is formulated with benzathonium chloride. Mechanisms of action of ketamine are multiple and differ from those of other agents. A non-competitive inhibitor of N-methyl-D-aspartate (NMDA) receptors, ketamine inhibits the excitatory effects of neurotransmitter glutamate, as well as stimulating opioid receptors and increasing sympathetic drive. Indications for ketamine include sedation, intense analgesia and dissociative anaesthesia. Dissociative anaesthetic doses produce relative cardiovascular stability, preservation of respiration and bronchodilation, but may raise intracranial pressure, and produce strange dreams and delusions on emergence. Typical induction dose 0.5–2 mg/kg.

Sedative agents

Benzodiazepines: midazolam (sedative)

Midazolam is a short-acting, water-soluble benzodiazepine (at low pH) but able to increase its lipid solubility at physiological pH. More commonly used for anxiolysis, amnesia or sedation, midazolam unreliably produces general anaesthesia alone. Usually midazolam is administered as a co-induction agent with agents such as propofol and thiopental to provide general anaesthesia with enhanced amnesia and minimal cardiovascular depression. Problems with use of midazolam include slow offset of effect, particularly in the setting of infusions, post-use amnesia and rarely respiratory depression. Typical dose for anaesthetic co-induction 0.5–2 mg.

Alpha-2 agonists: dexmedetomidine (sedative)

Dexmedetomidine decreases presynaptic release of noradrenaline at alpha-2 receptors, producing sedation with relative preservation of breathing, and reduction in heart rate, cardiac output and blood pressure. It is typically used for short-term sedation after cardiac surgery. Problems with dexmedetomidine include bradycardia and dry mouth. Typical infusion dose is 0.2–1.0 mcg/kg/hr.

Opioids: fentanyl, alfentanil, remifentanil (analgesic sedatives)

Opioids are used for analgesia as a means of reducing sedative and anaesthetic requirements for intravenous anaesthetic agents as they do not reliably produce general anaesthesia alone. Pharmacodynamic effects of opioids are the same, and side effects many, the most important of which are respiratory depression, nausea and vomiting.

> **Sedation is the earliest sign of opioid overdose and occurs prior to respiratory depression.**

Table 7.1 gives examples of the different scenarios in which anaesthetic agents and sedatives are used.

TABLE 7.1 **Use of different sedative/anaesthetics by anaesthetists (full operations, endoscopies)**

Clinical scenario	Example of anaesthetic or sedative agent	Appropriate person administering anaesthetic agent	Reasoning
A patient aged 45 having a laparoscopic cholecystectomy	Propofol used in a dose of 2 mg/kg for induction of general anaesthesia	Anaesthetist	Patient is likely to experience apnoea so practitioner should have skill in managing airway
A male aged 64 who is having a liver biopsy for a solitary mass with normal liver function tests	Midazolam 1 mg plus local anaesthetic infiltration of skin	Anaesthetist or non-anaesthetist sedationist	Small dose of midazolam likely to only be anxiolytic/sedative, therefore safe for non-anaesthetist to manage
A male aged 64 with clinical acute liver impairment and normal clotting having a liver biopsy who becomes uncompliant after midazolam	Midazolam 0.5 mg plus propofol 20 mg plus local anaesthetic infiltration	Anaesthetist	Patient may be unusually susceptible to sedatives, and has become uncompliant and therefore may need doses that may create need for airway support to facilitate procedure
A fit and well male aged 58 who is happy to undergo colonoscopy under conscious sedation	Midazolam 2 mg plus 1 mg every 15 min thereafter	Non-anaesthetist sedationist	Patient will receive enough sedation to be able to comply with instructions which usually means that respiratory depression is minimal so can support his own airway
A male aged 23 involved in a multi-trauma with likely bleeding from his spleen and hypotension and tachycardia about to have an emergency laparotomy	Ketamine 1 mg/kg intravenously or etomidate 0.3 mg/kg intravenously (two drugs with least inhibition of cardiovascular parameters)	Anaesthetist	As well as need for experience in airway support, there may be significant cardiovascular effects accompanying induction which are best managed by an experienced anaesthetist. Note that even ketamine can cause hypotension since its myocardial suppressant effect may be unmasked in a setting such as this where there is maximal sympathetic drive

References

1. Angel A. Central neuronal pathways and the process of anaesthesia. *British Journal of Anaesthesia*, 1993;**71**(1):148–163. doi:10.1093/bja/71.1.148

2. Kendig JJ. In vitro networks: subcortical mechanisms of anaesthetic action. *British Journal of Anaesthesia*, 2002;**89**(1):91–101. doi:10.1093/Bja/Aef158

3. Hughes MA, Glass PSA, Jacobs JR. Context-sensitive half-time in multicompartment pharmacokinetic models for intravenous anesthetic drugs. *Anesthesiology*, 1992;**76**(3): 334–341. doi:10.1097/00000542-199203000-00003

The recovery room

Arvinder Grover

The Alfred Hospital and Monash University, Australia

What is the recovery room?

The recovery room, also known as the postanaesthesia care unit (PACU) or postanaesthesia recovery unit (PARU), is a specifically designed and designated area essential for the safe early management of patients who have recently undergone a surgical or other procedure, regardless of the type of anaesthesia.

Major guidelines recommend that every patient undergoing general or regional anaesthesia for surgical procedures be transferred to the recovery room following their surgical procedure.

Recovery rooms have become considerably more advanced to cope with the increasing complexity of patients and surgical procedures; they have the ability to manage complex patients to a standard similar to that of a critical care unit.

Design of the recovery room [1]

The recovery room (Figure 8.1) is usually located in close proximity to the operating suites, with separate access for transfer of patients to the ward.

Design requirements of a recovery room

- Sufficient bed/trolley spaces for the expected peak loads of the particular hospital.
- Bed layout that allows staff to have an uninterrupted view of several patients at once.
- Bed spaces big enough to allow open access for trolleys, X-ray equipment, resuscitation trolleys and staff members.
- Bed spaces should also include appropriate lighting, scavenging for anaesthetic gases, electrical socket outlets and an emergency system to alert staff to an emergency in the recovery room.
- Dirty utility room, storage areas for equipment and drugs, and areas for staff to access computers.

Perioperative Medicine for the Junior Clinician, First Edition. Edited by Joel Symons, Paul Myles, Rishi Mehra and Christine Ball.
© 2015 John Wiley & Sons, Ltd. Published 2015 by John Wiley & Sons, Ltd.
Companion website: www.wiley.com/go/perioperativemed

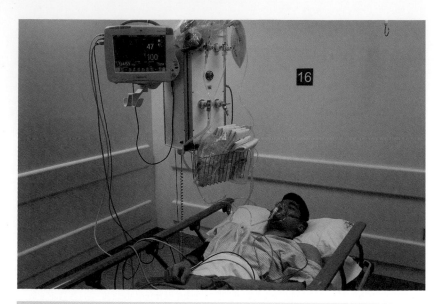

FIGURE 8.1 **Modern recovery rooms provide a location for monitoring of the patient in the immediate postoperative period.**

Monitoring, equipment and drugs

An appropriate standard of monitoring should be maintained until the patient has fully recovered from anaesthesia. Clinical observation should be supplemented by a minimum of pulse oximetry, non-invasive blood pressure (NIBP) monitoring and electrocardiogram (ECG) [2].

Following their anaesthetic, most patients are brought to the recovery room with a patent airway. If the patient has had a supraglottic airway (e.g. laryngeal mask airway [LMA] device) inserted, they are sometimes transported to the recovery with this *in situ*.

Some hospitals will have the facility to manage one or two patients with a tracheal tube in place after their anaesthetic. This requires facilities for mechanical ventilation and staff with a critical care background.

Recovery room staff

Staff trained in the care of patients recovering from anaesthesia must be present at all times. The ratio of registered nurses to patients needs to be flexible so as to provide no less than one nurse to three patients, and one nurse to each patient who has not recovered protective reflexes or consciousness. It is also a requirement that there is a registered nurse in charge of the recovery room. There will be a designated anaesthetist to support recovery room staff.

All staff members working in the recovery room are usually trained in advanced life support (ALS) or advanced paediatric life support (APLS).

Handover of care to the recovery room staff

At the conclusion of anaesthesia, patients should only be transferred to the recovery room when they are physiologically safe. They will be transferred with supplemental oxygen (via Hudson mask or nasal prongs) and monitoring for transfer at the discretion of the anaesthetist. Once the patient has safely arrived in the recovery room, the anaesthetist will provide a detailed verbal handover of the patient to the recovery room staff.

Key components of safe patient handover are covered by the acronym **ISOBAR** [3].

- Patient **I**dentification: name, age, diagnosis, allergies and procedure performed.
- **S**ituation: current clinical status.
- **O**bservations: clinical observation including the surgical site information.
- **B**ackground: medical and surgical history, type of anaesthesia, intraoperative medication and details of fluids and blood loss.
- **A**ssessment and management plan: anticipated recovery and potential problems. Postoperative plan detailing fluids, analgesia, antibiotics and monitoring of physiological variables (e.g. heart rate, blood pressure and SpO_2).
- **R**esponsibility: handover of responsibility should only occur at a time when the clinical status of the patient is stable and no foreseeable adverse events are likely to occur.

Management of patients in the recovery room

Patients must be observed on a one-to-one basis by an anaesthetist or registered member of staff until they have regained airway control, respiratory and cardiovascular stability, and are able to communicate [2].

The recovery of a patient from anaesthesia is a period during which complications can occur. During this time, it is important that all patients are appropriately monitored. The frequency of observations will depend on the stage of recovery, nature of surgery and surgical condition of the patient [2] (Box 8.1).

BOX 8.1 Minimum information recorded for patients in the recovery room

- Level of consciousness
- Patency of the airway
- Respiratory rate and adequacy
- Oxygen saturation and administration
- Blood pressure
- Heart rate and rhythm
- Pain intensity as per an objective scale
- Nausea and vomiting
- Intravenous infusions
- Drugs administered
- Core temperature
- Other: urine output, central venous pressure, expired CO_2, surgical drain volume

Source: Adapted from Whitaker et al. [2]. Reproduced with permission of John Wiley and Sons.

Common management issues in the recovery room

Airway devices

Many patients will be handed over to the recovery room nurse with an LMA device or oropharyngeal airway *in situ*. Recovery room nurses are specifically trained in the management and removal of the airway device. The removal of tracheal tubes is generally the responsibility of the anaesthetist.

Pain and postoperative nausea and vomiting (PONV)

Prior to discharge to the ward, all patients should have adequate control of pain and PONV. Recovery room staff are specifically trained in the management of patients with patient-controlled analgesia (PCA), epidurals, spinals and peripheral nerve blockade [3]. Anaesthetists prescribe analgesics and medications for PONV as per hospital protocols; these allow nurses to administer intravenous analgesics and antiemetics in the recovery room.

Regional anaesthesia

Patients transferred to the recovery room following a spinal, epidural or any regional technique should have the following noted.

- Time and dosing of drugs administered
- Level of sensory and motor block
- Rates of any continuous infusions

Discharge of patients from the recovery room

All recovery rooms have strict criteria for patient discharge – to the ward, critical care environments or home (for those patients having day stay surgery) (Box 8.2).

BOX 8.2 Discharge criteria for patients from the recovery room

- Airway: the patient is fully conscious and able to protect their airway
- Breathing: respiration and oxygenation are satisfactory (e.g. SpO_2 >92% and RR 10–18 bpm)
- Circulation: stable HR and BP, within normal preoperative values for the patient
- Written orders for fluid therapy and oral intake
- Normothermia
- Pain and PONV should be appropriately controlled
- Appropriate analgesia and antiemetic regimens are prescribed for the patient whilst managed on the ward
- Surgical drains: checked and appropriately placed
- Documentation: specific postoperative treatment or prophylaxis (e.g. antibiotics and thromboprophylaxis)

Source: Adapted from Whitaker et al. [2].

If a patient does not meet the criteria in Box 8.2, the anaesthetist will be asked to review the patient. If after medical review the patient is unstable or does not meet the above criteria for discharge, they may have an extended stay in the recovery room or be transferred to the high-dependency unit or intensive care unit.

References

1. Australian and New Zealand College of Anaesthetists (ANZCA). *Recommendation for the Post-Anaesthesia Recovery Room*. Professional Document 6. Melbourne, Australia: Australia and New Zealand College of Anaesthetists, 2006.

2. Whitaker DK, Booth H, Clyburn P, et al. Immediate post-anaesthesia recovery 2013. Association of Anaesthetists of Great Britain and Ireland. Anaesthesia, 2013;**68**(3):288–297. doi:10.1111/Anae.12146

3. Australian Commission on Safety and Quality Health Care. *Implementation Toolkit for Clinical Handover Improvement and Resource*. www.safetyandquality.gov.au/our-work/clinical-communications/clinical-handover/implementation-toolkit-for-clinical-handover-improvement-and-resource-portal/

∞

Perioperative genomics

Christopher Bain[1] and Andrew Shaw[2]

[1] The Alfred Hospital and Monash University, Australia
[2] Vanderbilt University Medical Center, United States of America

Perioperative genomics is the science of human genome interaction with the perioperative environment and how this affects outcomes in perioperative medicine.

The completion of the Human Genome Project in 2001 heralded a new era in medical science, seeking to understand how the function of the entire genome affects the body's response to different environments [1]. The human genome is a sequence of 3 billion deoxyribonucleic acid (DNA) base pairs, and contains approximately 25,000 functional units (genes). Perioperative genomic investigations relate variation in the inherited DNA sequence and non-sequence variation in DNA, known as *epi*genetic factors, to normal (recovery) and abnormal (complications, morbidity) perioperative responses.

Perioperative genomic investigations

The most familiar gene-based testing in hospitalised patients is the polymerase chain reaction (PCR) for infectious and other medical conditions. This test utilises a specific enzyme (DNA polymerase) to amplify specific regions of the genome for further DNA sequence analysis. By cycling the temperature, a chain reaction occurs that exponentially replicates the DNA in the reaction mixture (Video 9.1).

Genome-wide association studies (GWAS) analyse the relationship between DNA sequence variation within the entire genome and complex perioperative events like atrial fibrillation or postoperative nausea and vomiting (PONV) [2,3]. These discovery investigations reveal regions within the genome where genetic variation directly or indirectly affects the body's response to surgery.

In contrast to GWAS, investigations that focus on specific genes, known as candidate genes, are conducted when the encoded proteins are likely to be important in the body's response to surgical stress or medical therapy. This includes the field of pharmacogenomics, which investigates how genetic variation may directly alter drug absorption, distribution, metabolism and elimination. Examples include altered opioid responses due to variation in the *OPRM1* gene and altered sensitivity to beta-blockers due to variation in the structure and function of beta-adrenergic receptors.

Perioperative Medicine for the Junior Clinician, First Edition. Edited by Joel Symons, Paul Myles, Rishi Mehra and Christine Ball.
© 2015 John Wiley & Sons, Ltd. Published 2015 by John Wiley & Sons, Ltd.
Companion website: www.wiley.com/go/perioperativemed

www.wiley.com/go/perioperativemed

VIDEO 9.1 **Polymerase chain reaction (PCR) and microkit analysis provide a way of rapidly identifying genetic sequences that can be of use in perioperative genomics.**

Perioperative transcriptomics investigates patterns of gene *expression* (RNA production) in specific organs or systems during the perioperative period, to reveal genes whose actions may underpin normal and abnormal responses to surgical stress. Initial investigations have focused on the inflammatory response to cardiopulmonary bypass.

Perioperative epigenetic studies assess the impact of epigenetic mechanisms, such as DNA methylation, histone acetylation and non-coding RNA, during the perioperative period (Figure 9.1). This new area of investigation explores how these modifications alter the activity of the genome, by modifying gene expression, during the stress response.

Importantly, unlike the static DNA sequence variants, these modifications are tissue specific and dynamic in nature; they are able to change in response to different environmental exposures throughout life. This means they represent potentially novel drug targets. Initial investigations have focused on perioperative pain, specifically the development of persistent postsurgical pain (PPSP) [4].

Pharmacogenomics and altered drug response (clopidogrel)

Clopidogrel requires bioactivation to its active thiol metabolite to irreversibly bind the P2Y12 receptor on the platelet membrane. Several cytochrome (CYP) P450 isoenzymes exist that affect the biotransformation process. The CYP2C19*1 genotype results in normal metabolic function, but the *2 genotype results in loss of enzymatic function and poor metabolism. This information can now be used to personalise clopidogrel administration. For example, in a patient with a new percutaneous coronary stent, it is now recommended that either dose-adjusting clopidogrel therapy or switching to an alternative antiplatelet drug (prasugrel) be considered when the isoenzyme genotype is indicative of poor bioactivation (refer to Chapter 25 Anticoagulants and antiplatelet agents) [5,6].

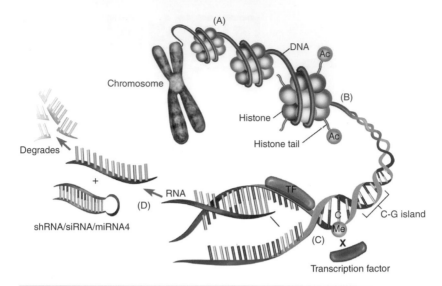

FIGURE 9.1 **Epigenetic mechanisms. (A)** Chromatin is made up of DNA wrapped around histone proteins. **(B)** Histone proteins may be modified through several processes including acetylation (Ac). This generally opens or relaxes the chromatin structure and facilitates transcription factor (TrF) binding enhancing gene expression (RNA). **(C)** DNA methylation (Me) of cytosine nucleotides prevents the binding of transcription factors, reducing or silencing gene expression. **(D)** Post-transcriptional regulation by micro-RNA (miRNA), short interfering RNA (siRNA) and short hairpin RNA (shRNA) that bind RNA to induce its degradation.

Epigenomics and chronic pain

The epigenome is the complete collection of cell-specific patterns of histone modifications, DNA methylation and other non-sequence related DNA variations in a particular tissue at a given point in time. These modifications are epigenetic mechanisms (Figure 9.1) that are critical to the function of the genome in any individual cell type.

Chronic pain is common following certain surgeries (amputation, hernia repair, thoracotomy and mastectomy) (refer to Chapter 95 The chronic pain patient) [7]. Monozygotic twins have been shown to exhibit different chronic pain phenotypes, indicating that chronic pain is not intrinsically related to the inherited DNA sequence. Just as epigenetic modifications have been shown to play an important role in cognition and memory formation, it is now thought that the chronic pain response to surgical injury may reflect modified neural plasticity caused by acquired epigenetic variation in the central nervous system (CNS) during development [4,8]. The neural epigenome has modified gene expression in response to neural injury, essentially priming the spinal neuronal networks to central sensitisation and chronic pain.

Perioperative biobanks

Perioperative biobanks contain tissue from tens of thousands of surgical patients. High-throughput DNA sequencing technologies (next-generation sequencing and microarrays) make it possible to analyse DNA sequence variants, gene expression patterns and epigenetic markers in large numbers of patients at the same time.

When combined with detailed clinical bioinformatics, these data can be related to clinical outcomes. This research has the potential to reveal novel biological mechanisms that significantly impact on clinical outcomes in association with co-existing disease states, ultimately forming the basis for personalised perioperative medicine.

References

1. Lander ES, Linton LM, Birren B, et al. Initial sequencing and analysis of the human genome. *Nature*, 2001;**409**(6822):860–921. doi:10.1038/35057062

2. Body SC, Collard CD, Shernan SK, et al. Variation in the 4q25 chromosomal locus predicts atrial fibrillation after coronary artery bypass graft surgery. *Circulation Cardiovascular Genetics*, 2009;**2**(5):499–506. doi:10.1161/CIRCGENETICS.109.849075

3. Janicki PK, Vealey R, Liu J, Escajeda J, Postula M, Welker K. Genome-wide association study using pooled DNA to identify candidate markers mediating susceptibility to postoperative nausea and vomiting. *Anesthesiology*, 2011;**115**(1):54–64. doi:10.1097/ALN.0b013e31821810c7

4. Doehring A, Geisslinger G, Lotsch J. Epigenetics in pain and analgesia: an imminent research field. *European Journal of Pain*, 2011;**15**(1):11–16. doi:10.1016/j.ejpain.2010.06.004

5. Simon T, Verstuyft C, Mary-Krause M, et al. Genetic determinants of response to clopidogrel and cardiovascular events. *New England Journal of Medicine*, 2009;**360**(4):363–375. doi:10.1056/NEJMoa0808227

6. Pulley JM, Denny JC, Peterson JF, et al. Operational implementation of prospective genotyping for personalized medicine: the design of the Vanderbilt PREDICT project. *Clinical Pharmacology and Therapeutics*, 2012;**92**(1):87–95. doi:10.1038/clpt.2011.371

7. Niraj G, Rowbotham DJ. Persistent postoperative pain: where are we now? *British Journal of Anaesthesia*, 2011;**107**(1):25–29. doi:10.1093/bja/aer116

8. Buchheit T, van de Ven T, Shaw A. Epigenetics and the transition from acute to chronic pain. *Pain Medicine*, 2012;**13**(11):1474–1490. doi:10.1111/j.1526-4637.2012.01488.x

Part II
Preoperative risk assessment

Perioperative medication management

Paul Myles

The Alfred Hospital and Monash University, Australia

A complete medication history, including herbal and other non-prescription medicines, is essential for safe perioperative care [1]. Most patients undergoing surgery take one or more medications, the most common being for underlying cardiovascular conditions [2].

Unfortunately, many patients fail to receive essential medications. Common reasons for this include preoperative fasting, failure to prescribe and unwarranted withholding of prescribed medications. In contrast, some patients continue to receive medications that have adverse interactions with anaesthetic and other perioperative medications, or that increase the risk of bleeding, excessive sedation or physiological derangement after surgery. Preadmission or inpatient medication prescribing by a pharmacist can reduce the incidence of clinically significant omissions and prescribing errors [3].

Decisions about commencing, stopping or continuing medications perioperatively should be based on an individual clinical assessment of the patient and the planned operation [4]. Some also require direct consultation with the patient's usual treating doctor, especially those with a cardiovascular, endocrine, neurological or psychiatric condition. Some recommendations are provided in Table 10.1.

Nearly all patients can be given their routine medications with sips of water up to two hours before anaesthesia. For patients who are nil orally, alternative formulations are available: parenteral (IM, IV), transdermal, inhalational or dissolvable tablet formulations. This may involve a change in dose due to differing bioavailability of the active drug. In addition, an alternative drug from another class can be used to bridge treatment.

Key aspects of perioperative medication management

- Accurate charting of preoperative medications.
- Local guidelines for stopping or bridging medications before and after surgery.
- Consider alternative formulations or drug class for essential treatments.
- Review of discharge medications to ensure discontinuation of surgery-specific drugs (e.g. analgesics, anticoagulants, diuretics, hypnotics).

Perioperative Medicine for the Junior Clinician, First Edition. Edited by Joel Symons, Paul Myles, Rishi Mehra and Christine Ball.
© 2015 John Wiley & Sons, Ltd. Published 2015 by John Wiley & Sons, Ltd.
Companion website: www.wiley.com/go/perioperativemed

TABLE 10.1 Recommendations for perioperative medication management

System/Drug class (examples)	Recommendation
Cardiovascular	
ACE inhibitors (lisonopril)	Omit morning dose on day of surgery
Angiotensin II receptor blockers (irbesarten)	Omit morning dose on day of surgery
Beta-blockers (metoprolol, atenolol)	Continue
Calcium channel blockers (diltiazem)	Continue
Statins (atorvastatin)	Continue
Diuretics (hydrochlorothiazide, furosomide)	Omit morning dose on day of surgery
Digoxin	Continue
Nitrates (nitroglycerin, isosorbide)	Continue
Antiplatelet/anticoagulant	
Aspirin	Withhold 3–5 days before surgery (unless minor surgery or coronary stent)
Warfarin	Withhold 1 week before surgery
Clopidogrel, prasugrel	Withhold 5 days before surgery
Ticlopidine	Withhold 2 weeks before surgery
Novel oral anticoagulants (dabigatran, rivaroxaban, apixaban)	Withhold 1 week before surgery
Analgesics	
Opioids (codeine, oxycodone, buprenorphine, methadone)	Continue, including day of surgery
Paracetamol	Continue, including day of surgery
Antiretroviral agents	
Nucleoside reverse transcriptase inhibitors (zidovudine, tenofovir)	Continue
Non-nucleoside reverse transcriptase inhibitors (nevirapine)	Continue
Protease inhibitors (ritonavir, saquinavir)	Continue, but avoid midazolam
Musculoskeletal	
NSAIDs (naproxen, ibuprofen, diclofenac)	Withhold on the day before surgery
COX-2 inhibitors (celecoxib)	Continue
Allopurinol, probenecid, colchicine	Continue
Hydroxychloroquine	Continue
Immunomodulators/disease modifiers	
Methotrexate	Continue
Azathioprine, leflunomide, etanercept, infliximab, rituximab, adalimumab, certolizumab, golimumab, abatacept, tocilizumab, anakinra	Withhold 2 weeks prior to surgery
Psychiatry	
MAOIs (pargyline, phenelzine, tranylcypromine)	Withhold 2 weeks prior to surgery, consider bridging with a TCA or SSRI or avoid pethidine and indirect sympathomimetics
Tricyclics (imipramine, sertraline)	Continue
Selective serotonin reuptake inhibitors (sertraline, fluoxetine)	Continue, use caution if using tramadol
Selective noradrenaline reuptake inhibitors (duloxetine, venlafaxine)	Continue, use caution if using tramadol
Antipsychotics and mood stabilisers (clozapine, olanzapine)	Continue
Anxiolytics (alprazolam, lorazepam, tofisopam)	Continue
Psychostimulants (methylphenidate, amphetamine)	Omit morning dose on day of surgery
Lithium	Withhold 2 days prior to major surgery (only)

TABLE 10.1 (Continued)

System/Drug class (examples)	Recommendation
Neurology	
Anticonvulsants (carbamazepine, lamotrigine, topiramate)	Continue; use an IV alternative if nil orally after surgery
Antiparkinsonian drugs (levodopa, carbidopa, pramipexole)	Continue, but monitor for hypotension
Endocrinology	
Oral hypoglycaemics (glibenclamide, glimepiride, metformin)	Omit morning dose, consider insulin regimen in major surgery
Insulin	Give half normal morning dose of long-acting insulin
Corticosteroids (prednisone, hydrocortisone)	Continue; consider additional perioperative coverage (see text)
Thyroxine	Continue; if nil orally for >3 days use IV formulation at reduced dose
Propylthiouracil	Continue
Hormone therapies (oral contraceptives, oestrogen, tamoxifen and raloxifene)	Continue in minor surgery; consider discontinuing for four weeks if major surgery (risk of DVT), or include strict thromboprophylaxis
Respiratory	
Inhaled bronchodilators and steroids	Continue
Pulmonary vasodilators (bosentan, sildenafil)	Continue
Leukotriene receptor antagonists (zafirlukast, montelukast)	Continue
Gastrointestinal	
H2-blockers (ranitidine)	Continue
Proton pump inhibitors (omeprazole, pantoprazole)	Continue
Sulfasalazine, azulfidine	Withhold 1 week prior to surgery
Herbal medications	
Ephedra, garlic, ginkgo, ginseng, kava, St John's wort	Withhold at least 1 week before surgery
Echinacea, valerian, most others	Withhold day before surgery

ACE, angiotensin converting enzyme; COX, cyclo-oxygenase; DVT, deep vein thrombosis; IV, intravenous; MAOI, monoamine oxidase inhibitor; NSAID, non-steroidal anti-inflammatory drug; SSRI, selective serotonin reuptake inhibitor; TCA, tricyclic antidepressant.

There are many drugs that pose additional risks in the perioperative period. Some drugs rely upon or inhibit CYP2D6 and/or CYP3A4 drug metabolism and so interact with other drugs used perioperatively (e.g. protease inhibitors, rifampicin, midazolam). Others prolong the QT interval (e.g. clozapine, some antiemetics) or interact with some perioperative medications and induce a serotonin syndrome (e.g. many antidepressants).

Cardiovascular medications

In general, beta-blockers (e.g. metoprolol, atenolol), calcium channel blockers (e.g. diltiazem) and statins should be continued until and including the day of surgery (refer to Chapter 11 The cardiac patient for non-cardiac surgery). Initiation of beta-blockers on the day of surgery is not recommended. An IV formulation of beta-blockade (e.g. metoprolol) can be given if the patient cannot take oral medications.

Angiotensin converting enzyme (ACE) inhibitors and angiotensin receptor blockers (ARBs) should be stopped before the day of surgery if the patient has well-controlled blood pressure (BP) or can be treated with an alternative drug, and is undergoing major surgery with significant anticipated blood loss or fluid shifts. This should reduce the risk of intraoperative and postoperative hypotension. ACE inhibitors or ARBs should be resumed postoperatively if the patient is not hypotensive and has normal renal function. For those undergoing less extensive surgery, ACE inhibitors and ARBs do not need to be stopped.

Aspirin and other antiplatelet drugs

For many patients receiving aspirin therapy, there is a competing risk of thrombotic complications and excessive surgical bleeding (including a greater need for blood transfusion). In general, it is reasonable to continue aspirin unless the risk of bleeding is substantial. This includes for vascular surgery or cataract surgery. However, aspirin should *not* be stopped in patients who have a coronary stent – for at least 12 months if they have a drug-eluting stent and six weeks for bare metal stents (refer to Chapter 31 Coronary artery disease and coronary stents). Patients at low risk for cardiovascular events undergoing major surgery should stop aspirin three to five days before surgery. Aspirin can generally be restarted on the day after surgery when there is adequate haemostasis.

Clopidogrel and other potent antiplatelet drugs may or may not be stopped, according to the bleeding risks of the surgery, stent location and type, and timing since insertion – advice should be sought from the patient's cardiologist and in consultation with the surgeon. The consequences of in-stent thrombosis are dire, with perioperative mortality approaching 50%.

Warfarin and other anticoagulants

Patients undergoing elective major surgery should have their warfarin therapy substituted with low molecular weight heparin to maintain anticoagulation until the time of surgery. The international normalised ratio (INR) should be checked on the morning of surgery. If elevated, and in those undergoing non-elective surgery, factor concentrates and vitamin K may be required (refer to Chapter 24 Thromboprophylaxis, and Chapter 25 Anticoagulants and antiplatelet agents). Heparin bridging therapy is mostly necessary for those with a prosthetic heart valve.

For those undergoing minor surgery (e.g. cataract surgery) and some vascular surgery, warfarin does not need to be stopped. Patients receiving warfarin for atrial fibrillation can have their therapy stopped without bridging of anticoagulation, unless they are deemed to be at high risk (e.g. prior stroke, known atrial thrombus).

Newer oral anticoagulants such as dabigatran, rivaroxaban and apixaban can be managed in a similar fashion to warfarin, but the timing of cessation varies, their effects are not easily monitored and there is no specific antidote to reverse their anticoagulant effect.

Corticosteroids

Patients on longer-term corticosteroid therapy have an increased perioperative risk of hyperglycaemia, wound infection and wound dehiscence. If the patient is taking more than 10 mg/day of prednisolone (or equivalent), some adrenocortical suppression is likely and supplemental hydrocortisone is required during and after surgery. The required dose should be adjusted according to the patient's steroid intake, the duration of such therapy (if longer than one month) and the expected physiological stress response of surgery (refer to Chapter 27 Steroid medication).

In general, a single IV dose of hydrocortisone 50–100 mg after induction of anaesthesia is sufficient for minor surgery. For major surgery, repeat IV doses of hydrocortisone 50 mg every eight hours should be used until the patient is recovered and is eating normally.

Antidepressants

Monoamine oxidase inhibitors (MAOIs) are not commonly used to treat depression but are used in patients with refractory mood disorders. Concomitant administration of sympathomimetic drugs such as phenylephrine and ephedrine can result in a severe hypertensive crisis.

Antiepileptics

Antiepileptic drugs should be continued perioperatively in patients with epilepsy. Some of these drugs have a narrow therapeutic index and changing organ function and drug interactions may result in loss of seizure control or drug toxicity. Perioperative plasma drug monitoring is probably unhelpful (refer to Chapter 56 Epilepsy).

Antiparkinson medications

Abrupt withdrawal of antiparkinson therapy will worsen Parkinson symptoms and may induce the neuroleptic malignant syndrome. Carbidopa-levodopa has a short duration of action and so should be given on the morning of surgery and continued through the perioperative period (refer to Chapter 18 Central nervous system risk assessment).

Chronic opioid therapy

Abrupt discontinuation of chronic opioid therapy may result in withdrawal symptoms, sympathetic activation and possibly a greater risk of hyperalgesia. Patients on oral opioid maintenance for drug dependency or chronic pain should receive their usual daily dose preoperatively, and have their postoperative analgesic requirements covered with additional opioids as required, plus a multimodal regimen of opioid-sparing drugs such as non-steroidal anti-inflammatory drugs (NSAIDs), paracetamol and ketamine (refer to Chapter 28 Opioids and opioid addiction).

Herbal medications

Herbal medications can be dangerous in the perioperative period [1]. Some ostensibly natural therapies are associated with bleeding complications and others have interactions with anaesthetic drugs [5]. For example, the 'three Gs' (garlic, gingko and ginseng) increase bleeding risk, ephedra and guarana are CNS stimulants that may lead to excessive agitation and hypertensive crisis, and St John's wort induces cytochrome P450 enzymes and so may impair drug metabolism.

References

1. Braun LA, Cohen M. Use of complementary medicines by cardiac surgery patients: undisclosed and undetected. *Heart Lung Circulation*, 2011;**20**(5):305–311. doi:10.1016/J.Hlc.2011.01.013

2. Kluger MT, Gale S, Plummer JL, Owen H. Peri-operative drug prescribing pattern and manufacturers' guidelines. An audit. *Anaesthesia*, 1991;**46**(6):456–459. doi:10.1111/j.1365-2044.1991.tb11682.x

3. Hale AR, Coombes ID, Stokes J, et al. Perioperative medication management: expanding the role of the preadmission clinic pharmacist in a single centre, randomised controlled trial of collaborative prescribing. *BMJ Open*, 2013;**3**(7). doi:10.1136/bmjopen-2013-003027

4. Castanheira L, Fresco P, Macedo AF. Guidelines for the management of chronic medication in the perioperative period: systematic review and formal consensus. *Journal of Clinical Pharmacy and Therapeutics*, 2011;**36**(4):446–467. doi:10.1111/j.1365-2710.2010.01202.x

5. Ang-Lee MK, Moss J, Yuan CS. Herbal medicines and perioperative care. *JAMA*, 2001;**286**(2):208–216. doi:10.1001/jama.286.2.208

The cardiac patient for non-cardiac surgery

Howard Machlin

The Alfred Hospital and Monash University, Australia

Cardiovascular complications are among the most significant risks to patients undergoing non-cardiac surgery. The level of risk for each individual depends upon patient factors, the surgery planned and the circumstances under which the surgery will occur.

A 'cardiac' patient has one or more of the following problems: coronary artery disease, heart failure, significant valvular heart disease, significant cardiac rhythm disturbances and/or a history of cardiac transplantation.

Not all patients are aware that they have a cardiovascular problem so it is important to take a consistent perioperative approach including:

1. initial preoperative evaluation
2. further investigation if required
3. considering consultation with other medical personnel involved in the patient's care (time and situation permitting)
4. risk stratification of the patient
5. an open discussion with the patient regarding the risks of the procedure and the expected outcome(s)
6. consideration of preoperative strategies to modify/prevent perioperative complications
7. determining the most suitable intraoperative technique
8. planning postoperative analgesia
9. planning postoperative care (e.g. recovery room, HDU, general ward, etc.).

Preoperative assessment

Guidelines for the assessment and management of these patients have been published in both North America [1] and Europe [2]. History is critical to determine the presence/absence/severity of symptoms and the clinical course of any problem.

Perioperative Medicine for the Junior Clinician, First Edition. Edited by Joel Symons, Paul Myles, Rishi Mehra and Christine Ball.
© 2015 John Wiley & Sons, Ltd. Published 2015 by John Wiley & Sons, Ltd.
Companion website: www.wiley.com/go/perioperativemed

Cardiac functional status (in metabolic equivalents – METs) [3] should be assessed as perioperative cardiac and long-term risk is increased in patients unable to meet a 4-MET demand during most normal daily activities (refer to Chapter 33 Arrhythmias). Cardiopulmonary exercise testing can be used in an elective surgery setting to more objectively determine functional capacity (refer to Chapter 16 Preoperative cardiopulmonary exercise testing).

A detailed physical examination should be performed looking for any signs that relate to the cardiac conditions, e.g. heart failure, murmur.

In certain situations the history and examination will be limited, e.g. in the unconscious or acutely confused patient.

It is **not** appropriate to defer immediate life-saving surgery to further evaluate the patient's underlying cardiac status.

The Revised Goldman Cardiac Risk Index (RCRI) [4,5] can be used to simplify the prediction of postoperative risk of complications (Box 11.1). When a 'major' risk factor is identified (Box 11.2), intensive management of this should be considered. This may result in delay or cancellation of proposed elective surgery. The proposed surgery (low risk or high risk) (Table 11.1), its timing (i.e. elective or emergency), expected duration and all the physiological consequences of the surgery and anaesthesia will influence the risk of complications postoperatively. Various

---

BOX 11.1 Revised Goldman Cardiac Risk Index [4,5].

Six independent predictors of major cardiac complications

High-risk type of surgery (examples include vascular surgery and any open intraperitoneal or intrathoracic procedures)
History of ischaemic heart disease (history of MI or a positive exercise test, current complaint of chest pain considered to be secondary to myocardial ischaemia, use of nitrate therapy, or ECG with pathological Q waves; do not count prior coronary revascularisation procedure unless one of the other criteria for ischemic heart disease is present)
History of heart failure
History of cerebrovascular disease
Diabetes mellitus requiring treatment with insulin
Preoperative serum creatinine > 2.0 mg/dL (177 µmol/L)

Rate of cardiac death, non-fatal myocardial infarction and non-fatal cardiac arrest according to the number of predictors

No risk factors – 0.4% (95% CI: 0.1–0.8)
One risk factor – 1.0% (95% CI: 0.5–1.4)
Two risk factors – 2.4% (95% CI: 1.3–3.5)
Three or more risk factors – 5.4% (95% CI: 2.8–7.9)

Source: Reproduced with permission of Wolters Kluwer Health. CI, confidence interval; ECG, electrocardiogram; MI, myocardial infarction.

BOX 11.2 Clinical predictors of increased perioperative cardiovascular risk (myocardial infarction, heart failure, death)

Major predictors that require intensive management and may lead to delay in or cancellation of the operative procedure unless emergency

- Unstable coronary syndromes including unstable or severe angina or recent MI
- Decompensated heart failure including NYHA functional class IV or worsening or new-onset HF
- Significant arrhythmias including high-grade AV block, symptomatic ventricular arrhythmias, supraventricular arrhythmias with ventricular rate >100 beats per minute at rest, symptomatic bradycardia, and newly recognised ventricular tachycardia
- Severe heart valve disease including severe aortic stenosis or symptomatic mitral stenosis
- Cardiomyopathy
- Pulmonary vascular disease (pulmonary arterial hypertension, pulmonary artery systolic pressures >70 mmHg)

Other clinical risk factors that warrant careful assessment of current status

- History of ischaemic heart disease
- History of cerebrovascular disease
- History of compensated heart failure or prior heart failure
- Diabetes mellitus
- Renal insufficiency

Source: Adapted from Fleisher et al. [1]. AV, atrioventricular; HF, heart failure; IV, intravenous; MI, myocardial infarction; NYHA, New York Heart Association.

TABLE 11.1 **Surgical risk estimate. Risk of myocardial infarction and cardiac death within 30 days after surgery**

Low risk (<1%)	Elevated risk (>1%)
Breast	Abdominal
Dental	Carotid
Endocrine	Peripheral vascular surgery
Ophthalmology	Peripheral arterial angioplasty
Gynaecology	Aortic and major vascular surgery
Reconstructive	Endovascular aneurysm repair
Orthopaedic – minor (knee surgery)	Head and neck surgery
Urological – minor	Neurological
	Orthopaedic – major (hip and spine surgery)
	Pulmonary, renal, liver transplant
	Urological – major

Source: Modified from Boersma et al. [7].

calculators have been developed to allow more precise calculation of surgical risk [6], e.g. http://riskcalculator.facs.org.

Routine use of investigations is unlikely to change patient management, is costly, inefficient and potentially delays surgery. An investigation should only be considered if the result is likely to influence, or change, patient management in some way.

The patient's regular medical practitioners may need to be contacted to inform decision making and avoid duplication of investigations.

If the surgical condition is likely to cause more issues for the patient than the identified patient cardiovascular risk factors, in almost all cases it is prudent to proceed to surgery without undue delay.

Further investigations will depend upon patient- and surgery-specific risk factors and what information is required; low-risk surgical procedures generally only require a clinical preoperative evaluation.

1. To investigate for coronary artery disease consider:
   - exercise stress testing (not always appropriate, e.g. intermittent claudication, orthopaedic degenerative joint disease)
   - pharmacological stress testing* (based upon local experience, availability and patient factors):
     ○ dipyridamole thallium radionuclide myocardial perfusion imaging
     ○ dobutamine echocardiography
   - multislice computed tomography (CT)
   - magnetic resonance imaging (MRI)
   - coronary angiography.

*Note: negative results may provide greater clinical utility than positive results.

2. To investigate for heart failure, valvular heart disease or to assess heart transplant recipients, a resting transthoracic echocardiogram. Other methods include:
   - radionuclide ventriculography
   - gated single photon emission computed tomography (SPECT) imaging
   - cardiac MRI
   - multislice CT.

3. To investigate for cardiac rhythm disturbances:
   - resting 12-lead ECG
   - 24-hour Holter monitor may be required.

Once all the information is available, the risks of surgery and anaesthesia, and the likelihood of postoperative cardiovascular complications can be discussed with the patient.

If the patient consents to proceed with the planned procedure then consideration should be given to risk modification strategies, in addition to ensuring medical optimisation of all co-existing medical conditions, e.g. chronic obstructive pulmonary disease (COPD), diabetes mellitus.

Currently all preoperative cardiac risk modification strategies are pharmacological and include:

- beta-blockers
- statins
- nitrates
- ACE inhibitors
- calcium channel blockers
- alpha-2 agonists
- anticoagulant therapy.

> For patients with stable coronary artery disease scheduled to undergo non-cardiac surgery, the current evidence suggests that most such patients do not benefit from prophylactic revascularisation, unless they have current indications for revascularisation.

Careful consideration should be given to how to best manage patients with coronary stents who are taking antiplatelet therapy as cessation of these agents to minimise the risk of perioperative haemorrhage has to be balanced against the risk of acute in-stent thrombosis.

Intraoperative management

Anaesthetic choices include, but are not limited to, general anaesthesia, neuraxial techniques and regional anaesthesia, the choice being determined by factors such as duration of surgery, fluid loss and each patient's capacity to tolerate the technique. In addition, patient preference should be addressed.

In high-risk patients, intraoperative monitoring will be increased. The use of invasive techniques such as an arterial line, a central venous catheter, a pulmonary artery catheter and/or transoesophageal echocardiography may be considered. Depth of anaesthesia monitoring and cerebral oximetry may be useful in certain settings.

As always, good-quality postoperative analgesia is important. In the cardiac patient, there is a need to prevent sympathetic activation postoperatively to avoid tachycardia and hypertension. The choice of technique/regimen to provide postoperative analgesia will include all commonly described techniques including multimodal oral regimens, intravenous techniques, regional techniques (including catheter-based techniques) and neuraxial techniques.

Postoperative care

The range of options varies from discharge home on day of surgery, up to admission to a HDU/ICU. This will be determined by the age and risk profile of the patient, the extent and duration of the surgery, the fluid shifts occurring intraoperatively, intraoperative complications (including hypotension, hypoxia or tachycardia) and the anticipated postoperative analgesia requirements.

An appropriate plan should be tailored for each patient.

References

1. Fleisher LA, Fleischmann KE, Auerbach AD, et al. 2014 ACC/AHA Guideline on Perioperative Cardiovascular Evaluation and Management of Patients Undergoing Noncardiac Surgery: a report of the American College of Cardiology/American Heart Association Task Force on Practice Guidelines. *Journal of the American College of Cardiology*, 2014. doi:10 1016/ j.jacc.2014.07.945

2. Poldermans D, Bax JJ, Boersma E, et al. Guidelines for pre-operative cardiac risk assessment and perioperative cardiac management in non-cardiac surgery. *European Heart Journal*, 2009;**30**(22):2769–2812. doi:10.1093/Eurheartj/Ehp337

3. Jette M, Sidney K, Blumchen G. Metabolic equivalents (METS) in exercise testing, exercise prescription, and evaluation of functional capacity. *Clinical Cardiology*, 1990;**13**(8):555–565. doi:10.1002/clc.4960130809

4. Lee TH, Marcantonio ER, Mangione CM, et al. Derivation and prospective validation of a simple index for prediction of cardiac risk of major noncardiac surgery. *Circulation*, 1999;**100**(10):1043–1049. doi:10.1161/01.cir.100.10.1043

5. Devereaux PJ, Goldman L, Cook DJ, Gilbert K, Leslie K, Guyatt GH. Perioperative cardiac events in patients undergoing noncardiac surgery: a review of the magnitude of the problem, the pathophysiology of the events and methods to estimate and communicate risk. *Canadian Medical Association Journal*, 2005;**173**(6):627–634. doi:10.1503/cmaj.050011

6. Bilimoria KY, Liu Y, Paruch JL, et al. Development and evaluation of the universal ACS NSQIP surgical risk calculator: a decision aid and informed consent tool for patients and surgeons. *Journal of the American College of Surgeons*, 2013;**217**(5):833–842 e1-3. doi:10.1016/ j.jamcollsurg.2013.07.385

7. Boersma E, Kertai MD, Schouten O, et al. Perioperative cardiovascular mortality in noncardiac surgery: validation of the Lee cardiac risk index. *American Journal of Medicine*, 2005;**118**(10):1134–1141. doi:10.1016/j.amjmed.2005.01.064

Cardiovascular risk assessment in cardiac surgery

Christopher Duffy

The Alfred Hospital, Australia

Patients presenting for cardiac surgery are becoming increasingly complex, in terms of both age and co-morbidities. Whilst outcomes in even these more complex patients are generally excellent, any cardiac surgical procedure will carry a finite risk of death or serious adverse outcome. Understanding the factors which negatively impact on patient outcomes is vital to the physician managing these patients in the perioperative period because some of these are modifiable and all can be used to guide appropriate postoperative care.

Scoring systems

Cardiac surgical patients are amongst the most studied of all surgical disciplines in terms of risk factors and outcomes. These data have allowed the development of sophisticated scoring systems that can be used to facilitate predictions of death or adverse outcome after cardiac surgery. The first such scoring system was developed by Parsonnet [1] and was used extensively during the 1990s. Of the many other scoring systems developed at that time, probably the most widely adopted was the European System for Cardiac Operative Risk Evaluation (EuroSCORE) [2] developed in 1999. This was shown to be predictive of death or adverse outcome for patients undergoing cardiac surgical procedures, and was validated in the UK, Europe, North America and Australia. The main limitation of this simple additive scoring system was its tendency to underpredict mortality in high-risk patients, and in 2003, a more complex and advanced 'logistic' EuroSCORE [3] was developed. The simple and logistic EuroSCORE was updated and relaunched in 2011 as EuroSCORE II, now the most widely used scoring system for predicting outcome from cardiac surgery.

The EuroSCORE was developed after studying nearly 20,000 consecutive patients from 128 hospitals in eight European countries. Information on 97 risk factors was collected and related to outcome (survival or death). The risk factors which were shown to have impact on patient outcomes are shown in Box 12.1.

The way that each of these factors affects outcome is based on complex calculations requiring a free online calculator, available at www.euroscore.org.

Perioperative Medicine for the Junior Clinician, First Edition. Edited by Joel Symons, Paul Myles, Rishi Mehra and Christine Ball.
© 2015 John Wiley & Sons, Ltd. Published 2015 by John Wiley & Sons, Ltd.
Companion website: www.wiley.com/go/perioperativemed

BOX 12.1 Risk factors affecting patient outcomes in cardiac surgery

Patient-related factors
Age
Gender
Renal impairment
Extracardiac arteriopathy
Poor mobility
Previous cardiac surgery
Chronic lung disease
Active endocarditis
Critical preoperative state
Diabetes on insulin

Cardiac-related factors
NYHA
CCS class 4 angina
LV function
Recent MI
Pulmonary hypertension

Operation-related factors
Urgency
Type of surgery
Surgery on the thoracic aorta

CCS, Canadian Cardiovascular Society; LV, left ventricular; MI, myocardial infarction; NYHA, New York Heart Association.

Practical application

When assessing a cardiac surgical patient preoperatively, the conventional approach of thorough history, full physical examination and review of relevant investigations is crucial. In addition, an understanding of the risk factors which have been shown to impact on patient outcomes (Box 12.1) will allow a more targeted history and examination to facilitate an accurate assessment of the patient's surgical risk. In conducting this assessment, particular focus should be placed upon the following.

Functional assessment

Documenting the patient's functional capacity is an important step in understanding the severity of the disease process and its impact on the patient's lifestyle. Many patients presenting for cardiac surgery are likely to have their exercise capacity limited by symptoms such as shortness of breath, chest pain/heaviness, syncope or general fatigue. The level of workload at which these symptoms appear has an important impact on their risk assessment. Patients should be classified using the New York Heart Association (NYHA) classification of functional capacity, where NYHA Class I refers to a patient with cardiac disease

TABLE 12.1 Canadian Cardiovascular Society angina scale [5]

Grade	Activity
I	Ordinary physical activity does not cause angina, e.g. walking or climbing stairs. Angina occurs with strenuous/rapid/prolonged exertion at work/recreation
II	Slight limitation of ordinary activity; for example, angina occurs walking/climbing stairs after meals, in cold, in wind, under emotional stress or only during the few hours after awakening, walking > two blocks on the level or climbing > one flight of stairs at a normal pace and in normal conditions
III	Marked limitation of ordinary physical activity, e.g. angina occurs walking one to two blocks on the level and climbing one flight of stairs at a normal pace and in normal conditions
IV	Inability to carry on any physical activity without discomfort – angina syndrome may be present at rest

Source: Reproduced with permission of Wolters Kluwer Health.

but no limitation of physical activity, fatigue, palpitations, dyspnoea or angina, Class II refers to a patient with cardiac disease resulting in slight limitation of physical activity, with ordinary physical activity resulting in fatigue, palpitations, dyspnoea or angina, Class III refers to patients with cardiac disease that results in marked limitation of physical activity with less than ordinary activity resulting in fatigue, palpitations, dyspnoea or angina. Finally, Class IV refers to patients with cardiac disease who are unable to carry out any physical activity without experiencing discomfort and symptoms of heart failure or angina at rest [4]. An alternative is to use the Canadian Cardiovascular Society (CCS) angina scale as shown in Table 12.1 [5].

Renal function

Patients should be placed into one of three categories based on creatinine clearance, as calculated using the Cockcroft–Gault formula:

- on dialysis (regardless of serum creatinine)
- moderately impaired renal function (50–85 mL/min)
- severely impaired renal function (<50 mL/min).

The following formula can be used to calculate creatinine clearance:

$$\text{Creatinine clearance (mL / min)} = \frac{(140 - \text{age}) \times \text{weight (kg)} \times (0.85 \text{ if female})}{(72 \times \text{serum creatinine (mg /dL)})}$$

Renal function should always be checked preoperatively and monitored postoperatively in cardiac surgical patients. Wherever possible, avoid nephrotoxic agents (NSAIDs, contrast dyes, etc.) and maintain appropriate levels of hydration to limit renal injury in the perioperative period.

Left ventricular function

Assessing left ventricular (LV) function, both systolic and diastolic, is crucial due to its profound impact on the perioperative management of cardiac surgical patients. Patients with severe LV failure have a significantly higher risk of mortality, are more likely to have prolonged ICU admissions requiring ventilation and higher use of inotropes, and are more likely to develop multiorgan dysfunction. LV function should be assessed by:

- *History*: exertional dyspnoea, orthopnoea, paroxysmal nocturnal dyspnoea, fatigue.
- *Examination*: protodiastolic (S3) gallop, accentuation of P2 heart sound is a cardinal sign of increased pulmonary pressure, cardiomegaly (displaced apex beat), pulsus alternans, crepitations heard over lung bases.
- *Investigations*: carefully review any recent echocardiogram for an estimate of LV ejection fraction (e.g. from Simpson's biplane, fractional area change, fractional shortening) as an indication of systolic function. Diastolic function should also be noted, as measured by tissue doppler or transmitral inflow doppler. The diastolic function can be graded as normal, impaired relaxation, pseudonormal or restrictive physiology.

Pulmonary hypertension

The presence of severe pulmonary hypertension (pulmonary artery [PA] systolic >55 mmHg) is an ominous sign in patients presenting for cardiac surgery. This group of patients are at significantly higher risk, particularly at the induction of anaesthesia due to the cardiodepressant and vasodilatory effect of the induction agents, combined with the impact on pulmonary pressures of instituting positive pressure ventilation. These patients are prone to developing acute right heart failure in the perioperative period (refer to Chapter 37 Pulmonary hypertension).

Many patients presenting for cardiac surgery may have a degree of pulmonary hypertension secondary to impaired LV function. This group of patients may be expected to improve postoperatively as the surgical intervention aims to improve LV function (e.g. revascularisation, aortic or mitral valve repair/replacements). However, those with pulmonary hypertension in the setting of normal LV function due to intrinsic lung or pulmonary vascular pathology can be significantly more challenging to manage perioperatively. Primary pulmonary hypertension is typically more resistant to treatment and unlikely to be improved after cardiac surgical intervention.

Conclusion

It is vital that the perioperative physician understands the factors that are likely to affect the patient's outcome or survival. An informed, comprehensive discussion of risks with the patient is important in the consent process and when considering appropriateness of treatment. It also guides the perioperative physician in risk factor management both pre- and post-operatively with the aim of improving surgical outcomes.

References

1. Parsonnet V, Dean D, Bernstein AD. A method of uniform stratification of risk for evaluating the results of surgery in acquired adult heart disease. *Circulation*, 1989;**79**(6 Pt 2):I3–12.
2. Nashef SA, Roques F, Michel P, Gauducheau E, Lemeshow S, Salamon R. European System for Cardiac Operative Risk Evaluation (EuroSCORE). *European Journal of Cardio-Thoracic Surgery*, 1999;**16**(1):9–13. doi:10.1016/s1010-7940(99)00134-7
3. Roques F, Michel P, Goldstone AR, Nashef SA. The logistic EuroSCORE. *European Heart Journal*, 2003;**24**(9):881–882.
4. AHA medical/scientific statement. 1994 Revisions to classification of functional capacity and objective assessment of patients with diseases of the heart. *Circulation*, 1994;**90**:644–645.
5. Campeau L. Letter: Grading of angina pectoris. *Circulation*, 1976;**54**(3):522–523.

13

Preoperative cardiac testing

Joshua Martin[1] and Peter Bergin[2]

[1] The Alfred Hospital, Australia
[2] The Alfred Hospital and Monash University, Australia

Cardiovascular complications remain the leading cause of death after non-cardiac surgery. Identification of patients at risk of such events is an essential component of preoperative assessment [1].

Preoperative cardiac testing should supplement a comprehensive clinical assessment. It should provide an objective measure of functional capacity, detect myocardial ischaemia or cardiac arrhythmias, assess cardiac structure and function, and assist in estimating perioperative cardiac risk and long-term prognosis (refer to Chapter 11 The cardiac patient for non-cardiac surgery and Chapter 12 Cardiovascular risk assessment in cardiac surgery).

Which patients require preoperative cardiac testing?

Routine use of preoperative cardiac testing in low-risk asymptomatic patients is not recommended. The use of both non-invasive and invasive preoperative testing should be limited to those circumstances in which the results of such tests will clearly affect patient management.

Patients at high risk for cardiac events can be considered for preoperative cardiac investigation for further risk stratification and management prior to surgery. The recently published AHA/ACC Guidelines on Perioperative Cardiovascular Evaluation and Management of Patients Undergoing Noncardiac Surgery provide a stepwise approach to preoperative cardiac testing (Figure 13.1) [2].

Functional capacity

The patient's exercise tolerance in METs is a good measure of functional capacity. Patients with good functional capacity have an excellent prognosis, even in the presence of stable coronary artery disease (CAD) or risk factors; their perioperative management is unlikely to be changed as a result of further cardiac testing.

Perioperative Medicine for the Junior Clinician, First Edition. Edited by Joel Symons, Paul Myles, Rishi Mehra and Christine Ball.
© 2015 John Wiley & Sons, Ltd. Published 2015 by John Wiley & Sons, Ltd.
Companion website: www.wiley.com/go/perioperativemed

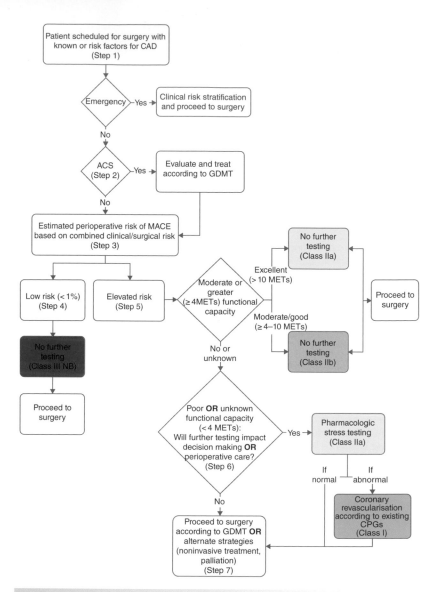

FIGURE 13.1 **Proposed algorithm for preoperative cardiac testing.** ACS, acute coronary syndrome; CAD, coronary artery disease; CPG, clinical practice guidelines; GDMT, guideline-directed medical therapy; MACE, major adverse cardiac event; MET, metabolic equivalent. Source: Adapted from Fleisher et al. [2]. Reproduced with permission from Elsevier.

Assessment of cardiac structure and function

Identification of patients with poor cardiac function remains a priority given the added haemodynamic demands of surgery and anaesthesia. Patients with left ventricular ejection fraction (LVEF) <35% have a higher risk of postoperative heart failure, perioperative myocardial infarction and mortality in both the immediate and longer term.

Stress echocardiography studies indicate that those with reduced EF and inducible ischaemia or scar tissue are at particularly high risk for cardiac events [3].

Routine assessment of left ventricular function is not recommended unless patients have worsening symptoms of heart failure, unexplained dyspnoea or a known cardiomyopathy that is unquantified.

Resting LV function can be assessed using a number of modalities, including echocardiography, myocardial perfusion imaging, MRI, multislice CT and contrast ventriculography.

Echocardiography

Echocardiography remains the most widely available investigation for assessing ventricular function. It can also provide additional structural and haemodynamic information, such as the severity of valvular lesions and estimation of pulmonary artery pressures.

Patients whose body habitus limits accuracy can be considered for contrast echocardiography or an alternative imaging modality.

Cardiac MRI

Cardiac MRI (CMR) is the current reference standard for non-invasive assessment of LVEF as it does not depend on geometric assumptions and is operator independent. CMR is not widely available and cost may be prohibitive. It may not be appropriate in patients with implanted devices such as defibrillators.

Myocardial perfusion scintigraphy

Myocardial perfusion scintigraphy (MPS) can assess myocardial perfusion as well as LV volumes and function. The drawback of MPS is radiation exposure and it would only routinely be recommended if other modalities were unavailable or non-diagnostic, or if the patient were also undergoing stress perfusion imaging to assess for ischaemia.

Gated cardiac CT

Radiation exposure and intravenous contrast preclude this from being a recommended first-line investigation.

Note that a measure of LVEF may have already been obtained from previous investigations such as MPS, ventriculography during invasive coronary angiography or cardiac CT, reducing the need for further testing and delays in surgery.

Assessment of coronary artery disease and myocardial ischaemia

Non-invasive cardiac imaging has become important in the diagnosis and management of patients with known or suspected CAD.

Stress ECG, stress myocardial perfusion scintigraphy with SPECT and stress echocardiography are well established in the role of assessing for inducible ischaemia. More recently, cardiac CT and CMR have played important and emerging roles in patients with CAD.

Exercise stress testing

> Where possible, exercise stress testing is the preferred method for assessment of ischaemia as it provides a measure of functional capacity and haemodynamic response as well as detection of inducible myocardial ischaemia (refer to Chapter 16 Preoperative Cardiopulmonary Exercise Testing).

Stress-induced myocardial ischaemia is an important risk factor for perioperative cardiac events.

Patients in whom exercise testing induces ischaemia at low-level exercise (<5 METs or heart rate <100/min) are a high-risk group, whereas those able to achieve more than 7 METs (or heart rate >130 beats per minute) are a low-risk group. Vascular patients who are able to exercise to 85% of their maximal heart rate are at lower risk of perioperative cardiac events [4].

Individuals with impaired mobility or poor functional ability may not be able to exercise to a level to adequately raise heart rate and blood pressure. In these patients, pharmacological stress testing should be considered, using vasodilators or adrenergic stimulation in conjunction with radionuclide or echocardiographic cardiac imaging. These tests are similarly predictive of perioperative cardiac events in patients scheduled for non-cardiac surgery [5].

The most appropriate modality for stress testing will largely be determined by individual patient factors (such as body habitus and mobility) and the availability of a particular test.

Myocardial perfusion scintigraphy

Stress MPS is superior to standard stress ECG. The test is usually performed using a standardised treadmill or stationary cycling exercise protocol. At peak exertion the patient is injected with a radionuclide tracer agent such as technetium, thallium or tetrofosmin which is absorbed by viable myocardium. A second set of resting images is taken hours later, allowing comparison.

In patients who are unable to exercise, a pharmacological stress test can be performed using either dobutamine or vasodilatory agents such as adenosine or dipyridamole (Figures 13.2 and 13.3) (Video 13.1). Vasodilator testing is preferred in those with left bundle branch block (LBBB) to reduce the effects of false septal ischaemia.

Stress echocardiography

Stress echocardiography provides information on LV function at rest and valvular abnormalities and detects ischaemia by inducing wall motion abnormality. Images are taken at rest and then using either an incremental treadmill test, where images are

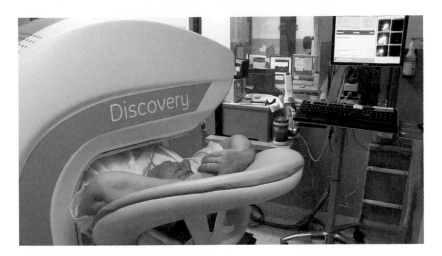

FIGURE 13.2 Vasodilator therapy such as dypyridamole (Persantin) is often combined with radionuclide tracer agents such as thallium for cardiac testing. A rotating gamma camera is subsequently used to image the heart and evaluate for the presence of cardiac disease.

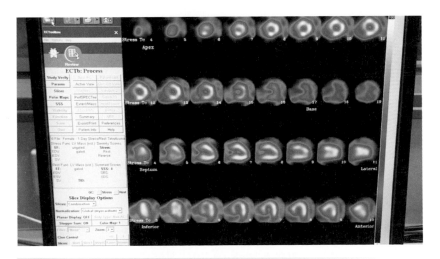

FIGURE 13.3 Imaging of the myocardium produced by scintigraphy.

taken immediately post exercise, or during peak exertion on a supine bicycle protocol. Postexercise images are then compared to those obtained at baseline, assessing for regional wall motion abnormality. Image quality can be affected by high respiratory rates at peak exertion but technological improvements have reduced this effect.

Patients who are unable to exercise can be considered for dobutamine stress echocardiography (Figure 13.4) (Video 13.2). This technique can also be used in patients with suspected low-flow aortic stenosis.

www.wiley.com/go/perioperativemed

VIDEO 13.1 Dipyridamole (Persantin) thallium scan.

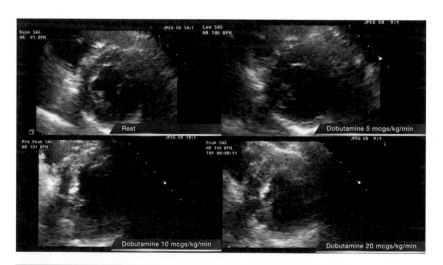

FIGURE 13.4 Dobutamine can be infused at varying doses with simultaneous imaging via transthoracic echocardiography. This allows evaluation of cardiac disease.

Perioperative cardiac risk has been directly associated with the extent of jeopardised viable myocardium identified by stress cardiac imaging. Patients with a moderate-to-large perfusion defect detected by either stress echocardiography or nuclear perfusion study have greater risk for postoperative MI and death [5].

Patients with extensive stress-induced ischaemia represent a high-risk population in whom standard medical therapy appears to be insufficient to prevent perioperative cardiac events [6].

www.wiley.com/go/perioperativemed

VIDEO 13.2 **Dobutamine stress echocardiography.**

Computed tomography coronary angiography

Computed tomography coronary angiography (CTCA) has become the leading non-invasive imaging modality to assess coronary artery anatomy. Newer multislice CT scanners have up to 320 slices and excellent temporal resolution. CTCA has an excellent negative predictive value but there are no data yet around preoperative evaluation risk stratification using CTCA.

13

References

1. Devereaux PJ, Goldman L, Cook DJ, Gilbert K, Leslie K, Guyatt GH. Perioperative cardiac events in patients undergoing noncardiac surgery: a review of the magnitude of the problem, the pathophysiology of the events and methods to estimate and communicate risk. *Canadian Medical Association Journal*, 2005;**173**(6):627–634. doi:10.1503/cmaj.050011

2. Fleisher LA, Fleischmann KE, Auerbach AD, et al. 2014 ACC/AHA Guideline on Perioperative Cardiovascular Evaluation and Management of Patients Undergoing Noncardiac Surgery: a report of the American College of Cardiology/American Heart Association Task Force on Practice Guidelines. *Journal of the American College of Cardiology*, 2014;**64**(22):2373–2405. doi:10.1016/j.jacc.2014.07.945

3. Karagiannis SE, Feringa HH, Vidakovic R, et al. Value of myocardial viability estimation using dobutamine stress echocardiography in assessing risk preoperatively before noncardiac vascular surgery in patients with left ventricular ejection fraction <35%. *American Journal of Cardiology*, 2007;**99**(11):1555–1559. doi:10.1016/j.amjcard.2007.01.033

4. Weiner DA, Ryan TJ, McCabe CH, et al. Prognostic importance of a clinical profile and exercise test in medically treated patients with coronary artery disease. *Journal of the American College of Cardiology*, 1984;**3**(3):772–779. doi:10.1016/s0735-1097(84)80254-5

5. Beattie WS, Abdelnaem E, Wijeysundera DN, Buckley DN. A meta-analytic comparison of preoperative stress echocardiography and nuclear scintigraphy imaging. *Anesthesia and Analgesia*, 2006;**102**(1):8–16. doi:10.1213/01.ane.0000189614.98906.43

6. Boersma E, Poldermans D, Bax JJ, et al. Predictors of cardiac events after major vascular surgery: role of clinical characteristics, dobutamine echocardiography, and beta-blocker therapy. *JAMA*, 2001;**285**(14):1865–1873. doi:10.1097/00132586-200112000-00039

Airway assessment and planning

Pierre Bradley and Joel Symons

The Alfred Hospital and Monash University, Australia

Airway assessment is an essential step in the patient's work-up prior to anaesthesia. Its aim is to ensure appropriate oxygenation and ventilation and minimise the aspiration risk to the patient. Difficulties with airway management can be life-threatening and can cause significant perioperative morbidity and mortality. Airway assessment follows the traditional model of assessment: history, physical examination and investigations. It aims to identify patient, surgical and anaesthetic issues that may suggest a difficulty with airway management. Core elements of airway assessment are listed in Table 14.1.

The information obtained from assessment will help the clinician plan a well-formulated strategy for managing the patient's anaesthetic. Particular attention should be paid to alternative or rescue approaches in case the primary plan is unsuccessful. It also allows for appropriate resource and time planning.

Specific questions that have to be answered are as follows.

- Is there a previously documented history of a difficult airway? This is probably the single most important question you can ask.
- Is there a previous anaesthetic chart with a modified Cormack-Lehane Classification for Direct Laryngscopy documented (Table 14.2)?
- How does the presenting complaint affect the airway or alter the cardiorespiratory reserves?
- Does the patient smoke? If so, how much and when was the last time they had a cigarette?
- Is there any aspiration risk? Can it be minimised?
- Is there any condition that places the patient in a high-risk group (Table 14.3)?

Physical assessment

The cardiorespiratory reserve assessment is done by performing a standard cardiorespiratory examination. The remainder of the assessment is tailored to the core elements of airway assessment: bag mask, supraglottic, intubation and infraglottic approaches.

Perioperative Medicine for the Junior Clinician, First Edition. Edited by Joel Symons, Paul Myles, Rishi Mehra and Christine Ball.
© 2015 John Wiley & Sons, Ltd. Published 2015 by John Wiley & Sons, Ltd.
Companion website: www.wiley.com/go/perioperativemed

TABLE 14.1 Core elements of airway assessment

No.	Core element
1	Is there a previous history of difficult intubation?
2	How does the surgery affect the airway?
3	How easy is it to bag and mask oxygenate?
4	How easy is it to place a supraglottic airway device?
5	How easy is it to intubate the patient?
6	How easy is it to achieve an infraglottic airway?
7	What is the aspiration risk?
8	Is there any altered cardiorespiratory physiology?
9	How easy will the patient be to extubate?

TABLE 14.2 Modified Cormack and Lehane Classification of Direct Laryngoscopy [7]

Classification	Description
Grade 1	Full view of the glottis
Grade 2a	Partial view of the glottis
Grade 2b	Only posterior portion of glottis or arytenoid cartilages
Grade 3a	Epiglottis *can* be lifted from the posterior pharyngeal wall
Grade 3b	Epiglottis *cannot* be lifted from the posterior pharyngeal wall
Grade 4	Neither glottis or epiglottis can be seen

TABLE 14.3 High-risk factors for airway management

Patient	Surgical	Anaesthetic
OSA	Head and neck surgery	PMHx of difficult airway
Degenerative spine conditions: rheumatoid arthritis, ankylosing spondylitis	Trauma	Previous tracheostomy
Endocrine: acromegaly, diabetes mellitus	Malignancy	
Obesity	Neck and dental abscesses	
Infection: epiglottitis, tetanus	Airway burns	
Congenital: Down's, Pierre-Robin, Treacher Collins, Goldenhar	Neck haematomas: postoperative complication of CEA, thyroidectomy	

CEA, carotid endarterectomy; OSA, obstructive sleep apnoea; PMHx, past medical history.

Unfortunately, the traditional components of the physical assessment used as a single marker of difficulty have a low sensitivity and specificity [1], so it is best to use a combination of the following.

A general assessment of:

- respiratory rate
- airway noises, wheeze, stridor

- body habitus
- Body Mass Index (BMI)
- pregnancy
- burns or radiation therapy
- previous surgical scars
- any head or neck masses.

Specific airway components assessed:

- interincisor gap (mouth opening) [2]
- Mallampati score (Figure 14.1) [3,4]
- jaw protrusion. This is graded on a simple ABC scale.
  - Grade A: the patient can protrude their lower incisors in front of their upper incisors.
  - Grade B: the lower incisors are in line with the upper incisors.
  - Grade C: the lower incisors cannot be protruded.

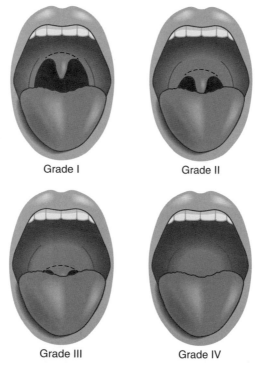

Grade I Grade II

Grade III Grade IV

Grade	Pharyngeal structures visible
I	Faucial pillars, soft palate and uvula visible.
II	Faucial pillars and soft palate visible. Uvula obscured by tongue.
III	Only the soft palate is visible.
IV	Soft palate not visible.

FIGURE 14.1 **The Mallampati scoring system [3].**

- sternomental distance [5]. The head is placed in full extension and the mouth closed prior to the measurement being performed
- thyromental distance [6]. The neck is fully extended prior to the mental hyoid distance being measured
- cervical spine movement
- teeth or denture.

Airway anatomy and assessment are shown in Video 14.1.

Figure 14.2 illustrates a patient with a normal airway (on the left), and a difficult airway (on the right). The factors that suggest a greater incidence of difficulty for individual airway management strategies are shown in Table 14.4.

www.wiley.com/go/perioperativemed

VIDEO 14.1 **Airway assessment.** This video demonstrates some of the features of airway assessment that should be undertaken in the preoperative planning of patient perioperative care.

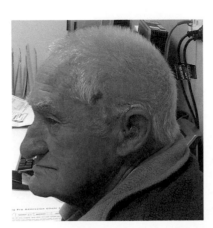 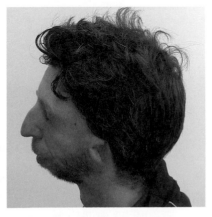

FIGURE 14.2 **Airway assessment in patients with an easy (on the left) and potentially difficult (on the right) airway.**

TABLE 14.4 Factors that may indicate increased difficulty with different airway management strategies

Strategy	Factor
Bag mask [8]	Age >55 years Body Mass Index >26 kg/m² Mallampati 3 or 4 Facial hair Radiation of neck Lack of dentition History of snoring Mandibular protrusion
Supraglottic [9]	Interincisor gap <2.5 cm Thyromental distance Large neck circumference Poor dentition Distorted airway anatomy Airway obstruction Obstructive sleep apnoea
Intubation [10]	Sternomental distance <12.5 cm Mallampati 3 or 4 Thyromental distance <6 cm Interincisor gap <3.8 cm Jaw protrusion test Grade C (an underbite) Anterior posterior flexion of cervical spine <80%
Infraglottic	Previous surgery on the neck Mass effect from infection, haematoma, tumour Radiation Obesity

Specific investigations are rarely required but can provide some useful information.

- Nasoendoscopy will provide an assessment of the laryngeal inlet.
- CT/MRI scan provides information about the anatomical airway position relating to the surrounding tissues and any tracheal narrowing or compression.
- Ultrasound can be used to locate the trachea in the infraglottic approach and masses in the neck.
- Lateral cervical spine X-ray may provide some limited airway information about mandibular–hyoid distance, atlanto-occipital gap, air spaces and soft tissues.

> Careful airway assessment and planning are an essential part of preoperative assessment. The junior clinician should become familiar with basic airway skills such as bag mask ventilation as a temporising measure prior to the arrival of an airway specialist.

References

1. Yentis SM. Predicting difficult intubation – worthwhile exercise or pointless ritual? *Anaesthesia*, 2002;57(2):105–109. doi:10.1046/j.1365-2044.2002.02913_22.x

2. Khan ZH, Mohammadi M, Rasouli MR, Farrokhnia F, Khan RH. The diagnostic value of the upper lip bite test combined with sternomental distance, thyromental distance,

and interincisor distance for prediction of easy laryngoscopy and intubation: a prospective study. *Anesthesia and Analgesia*, 2009;**109**(3):822–824. doi:10.1213/ane.0b013e3181af7f0d

3. Mallampati SR, Gatt SP, Gugino LD, et al. A clinical sign to predict difficult tracheal intubation: a prospective study. *Canadian Anaesthetists' Society Journal*, 1985;**32**(4): 429–434. doi:10.1007/bf03011357

4. Samsoon GL, Young JR. Difficult tracheal intubation: a retrospective study. *Anaesthesia*, 1987;**42**(5):487–490. doi:10.1097/00006534-199001000-00091

5. Al Ramadhani S, Mohamed LA, Rocke DA, Gouws E. Sternomental distance as the sole predictor of difficult laryngoscopy in obstetric anaesthesia. *British Journal of Anaesthesia*, 1996;**77**(5):701. doi:10.1097/00132586-199706000-00025

6. Patil VU, Stehling LC, Zauder HL. Predicting the difficulty of intubation utilizing an intubation guide. *Anesthesiology*, 1983;**10**:32–33.

7. Kheterpal S, Martin L, Shanks AM, Tremper KK. Prediction and outcomes of impossible mask ventilation: a review of 50,000 anesthetics. *Anesthesiology*, 2009;**110**(4):891–897. doi:10.1097/ALN.0b013e31819b5b87

8. Ramachandran SK, Mathis MR, Tremper KK, Shanks AM, Kheterpal S. Predictors and clinical outcomes from failed Laryngeal Mask Airway Unique: a study of 15,795 patients. *Anesthesiology*, 2012;**116**(6):1217–1226. doi:10.1097/ALN.0b013e318255e6ab

9. Williamson JA, Webb RK, Szekely S, Gillies ER, Dreosti AV. The Australian Incident Monitoring Study. Difficult intubation: an analysis of 2000 incident reports. *Anaesthesia and Intensive Care*, 1993;**21**(5):602–607. doi:10.1046/J.1365-2044.2000.01725.x

10. Yentis SM, Lee DJ. Evaluation of an improved scoring system for the grading of direct laryngoscopy. *Anaesthesia*, 1998;**53**(11):1041–1044. doi:10.1046/j.1365-2044.1998.00605.x

14

Pulmonary risk assessment

David Daly

The Alfred Hospital and Monash University, Australia

Pulmonary risk assessment is complicated by inconsistent definitions of postoperative pulmonary complications (PPC). Important postoperative pulmonary problems are those that are associated with mortality, longer hospital and ICU admission, unexpected ICU admission and morbidity related to other organ systems.

The most important postoperative pulmonary complications are [1]:

- atelectasis
- pneumonia
- respiratory failure
- exacerbation of underlying chronic lung disease.

Clinical features associated with PPC

Pulmonary risk assessment begins with the patient history. Patients should be asked about breathlessness, exercise tolerance, current or previous smoking, cough, wheeze, home oxygen and respiratory infections.

Clinical signs include tachypnoea, decreased breath sounds, wheeze, prolonged expiration, rhonchi and/or a positive cough test – the patient is asked to take a deep breath and cough once. If the patient coughs more than once the test is positive. The results of this simple test have been linked to PPC risk.

Pulse oximetry has become an extension of the clinical examination for the perioperative physician. Preoperative SpO_2 breathing room air in the supine position is a very strong patient-related PPC risk factor. One large study found that 3%, 10% and 29% of patients with a preoperative SpO_2 ≥96%, 91–95% and ≤90%, respectively, developed a PPC [2].

Patient-related factors

The ARISCAT study was a prospective, multicentre, randomised study that evaluated and validated risk factors for PPC in patients undergoing surgery (n = 2464).

The incidence of PPC is higher in patients aged more than 50 years. Even healthy older patients carry an increased risk of PPC. There is an inflection point (80 years) at which the PPC rate increases markedly (Box 15.1).

Perioperative Medicine for the Junior Clinician, First Edition. Edited by Joel Symons, Paul Myles, Rishi Mehra and Christine Ball.
© 2015 John Wiley & Sons, Ltd. Published 2015 by John Wiley & Sons, Ltd.
Companion website: www.wiley.com/go/perioperativemed

Asthmatics with a peak flow of >80% predicted have near-normal surgical PPC risk.

At least four weeks of smoking cessation preoperatively is associated with a reduced risk of many postoperative complications. Each extra week of cessation increases the magnitude of this effect. Observational studies demonstrate that smoking cessation reduces the risk of PPC by about 20% (relative risk [RR] 0.81, 95% confidence interval [CI] 0.70–0.93) [3].

Obesity *per se* does not seem to be an independent predictor of PPC.

Since the American College of Physicians guidelines were compiled [1], several new studies have found obstructive sleep apnoea (OSA) to be associated with PPC ranging from hypoxaemia to acute respiratory distress syndrome.

The risk of PPC appears to be higher in patients with heart failure than in patients with COPD (Box 15.1).

Whenever possible, surgery should be deferred if the patient has had a recent upper airway infection.

Both preoperative anaemia (haemoglobin concentration <10 g/dL) and intraoperative transfusion are independent risk factors for PPC.

Two metabolic risk factors for PPC have been identified [4]. Low serum albumin (<30 g/L) is associated with the risk of postoperative respiratory failure (PRF) (odds ratio [OR] 2.53, 95% CI 2.28–2.80). Elevated blood urea nitrogen (>30 mg/dL or >10.7 mmol/L) is associated with the risk of postoperative pneumonia (OR 1.41, 95% CI 1.22–1.64) and respiratory failure (OR 2.29, 95% CI 2.04–2.56).

Utility of laboratory investigations in non-thoracic surgery

Chest X-ray

A meta-analysis of more than 14,000 patients was conducted to estimate the frequency with which routine preoperative chest X-rays lead to clinically relevant new information [5]. The authors found abnormalities in 10% of routine chest X-rays. In 1.3% of the films, the abnormalities were unexpected. In only 0.1% of routine X-rays did the findings lead to changes in patient management. A multicentre European study found age >60 years, ASA physical status ≥3 and the presence of respiratory disease to be significantly related to the probability of a useful preoperative chest X-ray (i.e. a preoperative chest X-ray that altered anaesthetic management) [6].

Lung function tests

Most patients with abnormal respiratory function can be identified using clinical symptoms and signs. It is uncertain whether spirometry adds incrementally to risk estimates based on clinical assessment. A study of patients undergoing abdominal surgery matched smokers with severe airway obstruction and a forced expiratory volume in one second (FEV1) <40% (predicted) with similar smokers with a normal FEV1 and concluded that preoperative airway obstruction predicted the occurrence of bronchospasm, but not prolonged ventilation, pneumonia, prolonged ICU stay or death [7].

It is probably reasonable to perform preoperative lung function tests (Video 15.1) in the following circumstances:

- in a patient with airway obstruction where clinical evaluation cannot determine that the degree of airway obstruction is optimised for that patient
- in a patient with dyspnoea that is unexplained following clinical assessment.

www.wiley.com/go/perioperativemed

VIDEO 15.1 Lung function testing can provide useful information to help predict respiratory risk in certain high-risk groups.

Arterial blood gases

Several studies have found that the detection of hypercapnia with arterial blood gas assessment does not improve the identification of high-risk patients that would not have been identified on clinical grounds.

Functional testing

The 6-minute walking test (6MWT) and cardiopulmonary exercise test (CPET) are sometimes useful for preoperative evaluation. CPET has an established place in determining the suitability of candidates for lung resection. Although popular in some places, as with lung function tests, it is uncertain whether functional testing adds incrementally to risk estimates based on clinical assessment.

Surgery-related factors

Surgical site remains the single most important predictor of PPC. The incidence of PPC is inversely proportional to the distance of the surgical incision from the diaphragm [1]. Thus, those undergoing thoracic and upper abdominal surgery are at greatest risk (between four- and seven-fold) whilst those undergoing neurosurgery, head and neck surgery and vascular surgery are at a two-fold increased risk. Emergency surgery, prolonged surgery and general anaesthesia increase the risk of PPC two-fold.

Scoring systems to predict PPC

Several scoring systems (risk scales) for predicting PPC have been developed and are recommended reading for those who wish to develop a deeper understanding of this issue.

- PRF risk index [4]
- Pneumonia risk index [8]
- ARISCAT PPC score [2]
- PRF risk calculator [9]

Several risk calculators have been made available online; interested readers should visit www.surgicalriskcalculator.com.

Conclusion

Postoperative pulmonary complications are common. The incidence of PPC is probably higher than the incidence of postoperative cardiac complications. PPC are associated with increased length of ICU stay and hospital stay, increased morbidity and mortality, and healthcare costs. Respiratory failure is a marker of poor health and predicts other complications. Laboratory investigations such as chest X-ray, lung function studies and arterial blood gas analysis infrequently add useful information to facilitate pulmonary risk assessment. The most powerful predictor of PPC is the proximity of the surgical procedure to the diaphragm.

References

1. Smetana GW, Lawrence VA, Cornell JE. Preoperative pulmonary risk stratification for noncardiothoracic surgery: systematic review for the American College of Physicians. *Annals of Internal Medicine*, 2006;**144**(8):581–595. doi:10.7326/0003-4819-144-8-200604180-00009

2. Canet J, Gallart L, Gomar C, et al. Prediction of postoperative pulmonary complications in a population-based surgical cohort. *Anesthesiology*, 2010;**113**(6):1338–1350. doi:10.1097/ALN.0b013e3181fc6e0a

3. Mills E, Eyawo O, Lockhart I, Kelly S, Wu P, Ebbert JO. Smoking cessation reduces postoperative complications: a systematic review and meta-analysis. *American Journal of Medicine*, 2011;**124**(2):144–154 e8. doi:10.1016/j.amjmed.2010.09.013

4. Arozullah AM, Daley J, Henderson WG, Khuri SF. Multifactorial risk index for predicting postoperative respiratory failure in men after major noncardiac surgery. The National Veterans Administration Surgical Quality Improvement Program. *Annals of Surgery*, 2000;**232**(2):242–253. doi:10.1097/00000658-200008000-00015

5. Archer C, Levy AR, McGregor M. Value of routine preoperative chest x-rays: a meta-analysis. *Canadian Journal of Anaesthesia*, 1993;**40**(11):1022–1027. doi:10.1007/BF03009471

6. Silvestri L, Maffessanti M, Gregori D, Berlot G, Gullo A. Usefulness of routine pre-operative chest radiography for anaesthetic management: a prospective multicentre pilot study. *European Journal of Anaesthesiology*, 1999;**16**(11):749–760. doi:10.1046/j.1365-2346.1999.00577.x

7. Warner DO, Warner MA, Offord KP, Schroeder DR, Maxson P, Scanlon PD. Airway obstruction and perioperative complications in smokers undergoing abdominal surgery. *Anesthesiology*, 1999;**90**(2):372–379. doi:10.1097/00132586-199912000-00041

8. Arozullah AM, Khuri SF, Henderson WG, Daley J, Participants in the National Veterans Affairs Surgical Quality Improvement Program. Development and validation of a multifactorial risk index for predicting postoperative pneumonia after major noncardiac surgery. *Annals of Internal Medicine*, 2001;**135**(10):847–857.

9. Gupta H, Gupta PK, Fang X, et al. Development and validation of a risk calculator predicting postoperative respiratory failure. *Chest*, 2011;**140**(5):1207–1215. doi:10.1378/chest.11-0466

16 Preoperative cardiopulmonary exercise testing

Chris Snowden[1] and Serina Salins[2]

[1]Newcastle Hospitals NHS Trust and Newcastle upon Tyne University, United Kingdom
[2]Christian Medical College, India

Cardiopulmonary exercise testing (CPET) is a non-invasive technique that measures the simultaneous cardiovascular and respiratory response to exercise stress. Increasingly preoperative CPET is being used for risk assessment [1,2].

> Cardiorespiratory function is an independent predictor of perioperative morbidity and mortality [1,3–5].

History

Cardiopulmonary exercise testing has been used in the objective assessment of both healthy individuals (especially sports medicine) and those with medical conditions such as heart failure [6,7], respiratory disease [8], and those being evaluated for heart-lung transplantation [9].

> Recent CPET development acknowledges that improved perioperative outcome is related to the ability to increase oxygen consumption in response to surgical stress.

Preoperative rationale

The American College of Cardiology (ACC) and the American Heart Association (AHA) joint guidelines on risk stratification for non-cardiac surgery [10] identify three areas for assessment:

Perioperative Medicine for the Junior Clinician, First Edition. Edited by Joel Symons, Paul Myles, Rishi Mehra and Christine Ball.
© 2015 John Wiley & Sons, Ltd. Published 2015 by John Wiley & Sons, Ltd.
Companion website: www.wiley.com/go/perioperativemed

- surgery-specific risk
- patient-specific risk
- exercise capacity.

Exercise capacity may be assessed indirectly through clinical history, targeted questionnaires and semi-objective assessments (e.g. 6-minute walking test). Objective assessment of functional capacity must incorporate the direct measurement of oxygen consumption for which CPET is considered as the gold standard.

Advanced analysis of a preoperative CPET may also uncover asymptomatic disease or specific functional reserve limitations that allow intervention strategies.

Physiological background

Global oxygen uptake (VO_2 in mL/min):

$$VO_2 = \text{Cardiac output} \times \text{oxygen extraction}$$

$$\left(\text{oxygen extraction} = \text{arterial oxygen content} - \text{venous (central) oxygen content}\right)$$

Thus, VO_2 is directly proportional to cardiac output. Increasing oxygen consumption during exercise requires an increase in oxygen delivery and tissue extraction, resulting in an increase in minute volume ventilation and cardiac output.

During early exercise, oxygen delivery keeps up with the increasing demands, thus ensuring aerobic metabolism. As exercise continues to increase, the oxygen supply is unable to keep up with demand and continued production of adenosine triphosphate (ATP) relies more on anaerobic metabolism. H^+ ions produced require buffering:

$$\left[H^+\right] + \left[HCO_3^-\right] < -> [H_2CO_3] < -> [CO_2] + [H_2O]$$

This excess CO_2 alters the equivalence of oxygen utilisation and CO_2 production so that more CO_2 is exhaled than oxygen consumed. This disparity objectively determines the cardiorespiratory reserve and is known as the anaerobic threshold obtained from CPET. Prolonged exercise overwhelms the person's ability to further increase oxygen consumption, leading to ultimate cessation of the test.

Conduct of the CPET test

Preoperative CPET involves the measuring of respiratory gases (oxygen consumption and carbon dioxide production) continuously, throughout a period of increasing resistance (ramped) exercise on a treadmill or cycle ergometer. Preoperatively, cycle ergometry is the method of choice. Communication and encouragement take place throughout and the test may be stopped by the patient (symptom limited) or the clinician (e.g. cardiac ischaemia) (Video 16.1).

Protocol

Usually preoperative CPET consists of four phases.

- *Rest*: 2–5-minute period remaining stationary on the cycle to determine resting gaseous exchange parameters and to avoid hyperventilation.
- *Unloaded cycling (freewheel)*: 3-minute period of cycling against no resistance, allows stabilisation of baseline measurements during exercise.

www.wiley.com/go/perioperativemed

VIDEO 16.1 **Cardiopulmonary exercise testing.**

- *Ramped exercise*: continual increase in resistance (watts) to pedalling. Protocols are designed to produce a maximum predicted work for an individual in approximately 10 minutes. The speed at which resistance is increased will depend on patient's age, sex and co-morbidities.
- Recovery phase.

Test output

Multiple combination graphs of measured haemodynamic and ventilatory variables can be produced from the test. The most common summary of the combined data is the nine panel plot [11]. In the context of preoperative risk, the important outcomes of the test relate to markers of reduced functional reserve and measures that may implicate specific system dysfunction.

Markers of functional reserve

These common markers relate to postoperative outcome in several populations including abdominal, colorectal, vascular, hepatobiliary, oesophageal and liver transplantation.

Peak and maximal oxygen uptake (Figure 16.1)

If oxygen uptake is plotted against work, the VO_2 will increase in a consistently linear fashion (10 mL/min/watt), ultimately plateauing (VO_{2max}) as one of the system variables, such as cardiac output or ventilation, reaches its limit. In the perioperative setting, fatigue or symptoms usually limit the test and the plateau is rarely reached; VO_{2peak} (last value of VO_2 before stopping the test) is then used instead. VO_{2peak} represents overall cardiorespiratory reserve. Unfortunately, maximal or peak oxygen parameters are subject to an individual's motivation, introducing a source of repeat test variation.

Anaerobic threshold (AT) (Figure 16.2)

The AT measured by gaseous exchange (sometimes called the ventilatory anaerobic threshold) represents the measured oxygen consumption at the point where anaerobic metabolism supplements aerobic metabolism. AT is usually determined by

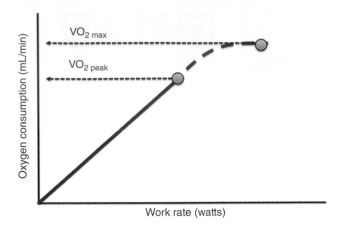

FIGURE 16.1 **Graphic representation of peak and maximal oxygen uptake.**

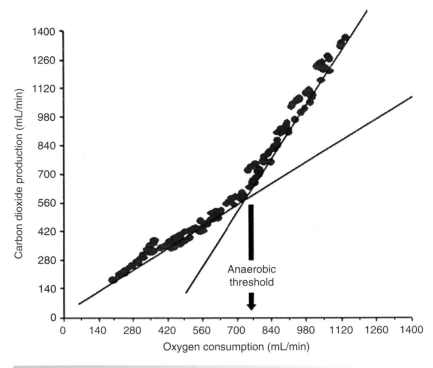

FIGURE 16.2 **Graphic demonstration of the anaerobic threshold.**

analysis of the slope achieved when VO_2 is plotted against VCO_2. It is reached as the gradient of the VCO_2/VO_2 line moves away from unity. Further simultaneous changes in CPET measured variables (including VE/VCO_2, VE/VO_2 and end-tidal PO_2) can assist in confirming the value of the AT. AT is an objective, non-volitional end-point that is an independent predictor of postoperative complications [1,5] and an indicator of surgical mortality risk in the elderly population [3,4]. AT may vary depending on the modality and muscle groups used for exercise (e.g. AT is lower when performed on a cycle ergometer than on a treadmill).

Markers of specific system dysfunction
Ventilatory equivalents
Ventilatory equivalents are the ratio of VE (minute volume) to either O_2 consumed or CO_2 produced and change throughout exercise. The ratio values represent the degree of pulmonary physiological dead space; normal value of VE/VCO_2 is less than 34 at AT. It is raised in disease states such as cardiac failure or respiratory disease, including pulmonary hypertension. It correlates with 30-day survival after abdominal aortic aneurysm repair [1] and, in combination with AT, is a predictor of early death in chronic heart failure [12].

Oxygen pulse
The oxygen pulse is the VO_2/HR ratio or the oxygen consumed per heartbeat. This should increase as the stroke volume and oxygen extraction increase during incremental exercise, until it levels at peak function. Abnormality can be seen in a flattened response (reflecting pulmonary disease, poor stroke volume or poor oxygen uptake, e.g. peripheral vascular disease) or a downturning response consistent with cardiac ischaemia.

References

1. Carlisle J, Swart M. Mid-term survival after abdominal aortic aneurysm surgery predicted by cardiopulmonary exercise testing. *British Journal of Surgery*, 2007;**94**(8):966–969. doi:10.1016/j.jvs.2007.10.026

2. Huddart S, Young EL, Smith R, Holt PJE, Prabhu PK. Preoperative cardiopulmonary exercise testing in England – a national survey. *Perioperative Medicine*, 2013;**2**(4):Open access. doi:10.1186/2047-0525-2-4

3. Older P, Hall A, Hader R. Cardiopulmonary exercise testing as a screening test for perioperative management of major surgery in the elderly. *Chest*, 1999;**116**(2):355–362. doi:10.1378/Chest.116.2.355

4. Snowden CP, Prentis J, Jacques B, et al. Cardiorespiratory fitness predicts mortality and hospital length of stay after major elective surgery in older people. *Annals of Surgery*, 2013;**257**(6):999–1004. doi:10.1097/SLA.0b013e31828dbac2

5. Wilson RJT, Davies S, Yates D, Redman J, Stone M. Impaired functional capacity is associated with all-cause mortality after major elective intra-abdominal surgery. *British Journal of Anaesthesia*, 2010;**105**(3):297–303. doi:10.1093/Bja/Aeq128

6. Myers J, Gullestad L, Vagelos R, et al. Cardiopulmonary exercise testing and prognosis in severe heart failure: 14 mL/kg/min revisited. *American Heart Journal*, 2000;**139**(1):78–84. doi:10.1016/S0002-8703(00)90312-0

7. Guazzi M, Myers J, Arena R. Cardiopulmonary exercise testing in the clinical and prognostic assessment of diastolic heart failure. *Journal of the American College of Cardiology*, 2005;**46**(10):1883–1890. doi:10.1016/J.Jacc.2005.07.051

8. Arena R, Sietsema KE. Cardiopulmonary exercise testing in the clinical evaluation of patients with heart and lung disease. *Circulation*, 2011;**123**(6):668–680. doi:10.1161/Circulationaha.109.914788

9. ATS. ATS/ACCP statement on cardiopulmonary exercise testing. *American Journal of Respiratory and Critical Care Medicine*, 2003;**167**(2):211–277. doi:10.1164/Rccm.167.2.211

10. Fleisher LA, Fleischmann KE, Auerbach AD, et al. 2014 ACC/AHA Guideline on Perioperative Cardiovascular Evaluation and Management of Patients Undergoing Noncardiac Surgery:

A Report of the American College of Cardiology/American Heart Association Task Force on Practice Guidelines. *Journal of the American College of Cardiology*, 2014;**64**(22):e77–e137. doi:10.1016/j.jacc.2014.07.944

11. Hansen JE, Sue DY. *Principles of Exercise Testing and Interpretation*. Philadelphia, PA: Lippincott Williams and Wilkins, 2011.

12. Gitt AK, Wasserman K, Kilkowski C, et al. Exercise anaerobic threshold and ventilatory efficiency identify heart failure patients for high risk of early death. *Circulation*, 2002;**106**(24):3079–3084. doi:10.1161/01.cir.0000041428.99427.06

Anaemia

Amanda Davis[1] and Angus Wong[2]

[1]The Alfred Hospital and Monash University, Australia
[2]The Alfred Hospital, Australia

A significant proportion of surgical patients are anaemic prior to surgery. Perioperative anaemia has been associated with increased morbidity and mortality in surgical patients, therefore its management is necessary to optimise patient outcomes.

Patient blood management

The National Health and Medical Research Council (NHMRC) has recently published patient blood management guidelines for the use of blood components. This chapter will expand on module 2 of the guidelines, which addresses the management of perioperative anaemia [1] (Figure 17.1). These guidelines aim to improve clinical outcomes by reducing the risk of anaemia and avoiding unnecessary exposure to blood.

Preoperative optimisation of anaemia

Preoperative anaemia, even if mild, is associated with increased perioperative morbidity and mortality [2]. Furthermore, it has a negative impact on functional recovery, length of stay and quality of life. This evidence suggests that preoperative treatment of anaemia should be instituted where clinically allowable.

Patients should have their haemoglobin (Hb) optimised prior to any elective surgery. A thorough history and examination should be undertaken to evaluate for symptoms of bleeding, symptoms of anaemia, past history and medications. Investigations for anaemia should be performed at least 28 days prior to surgery to allow sufficient time for management.

The most common causes of anaemia are iron deficiency and chronic disease. Treatment of the underlying cause of the anaemia should be instituted, particularly through supplementation of iron, vitamin B12 and folic acid.

An informative review for the management of iron deficiency was recently published [3]. Currently, there is a lack of evidence to support the routine use of erythropoietin-stimulating agents. The evidence behind the therapies is constantly evolving. If the cause of anaemia is unclear or there is uncertainty about the management, the patient should be referred to a haematologist.

A target haemoglobin level within the normal range is desired but there is no strong evidence to support the preoperative use of blood transfusions.

Perioperative Medicine for the Junior Clinician, First Edition. Edited by Joel Symons, Paul Myles, Rishi Mehra and Christine Ball.
© 2015 John Wiley & Sons, Ltd. Published 2015 by John Wiley & Sons, Ltd.
Companion website: www.wiley.com/go/perioperativemed

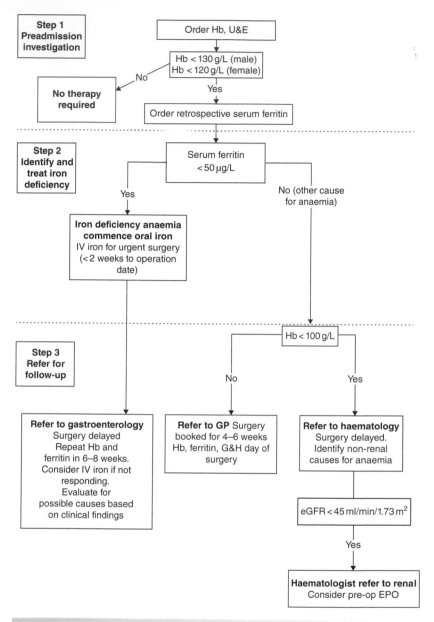

FIGURE 17.1 **Algorithm for the investigation and management of anaemia prior to elective surgery.** This template is for patients undergoing procedures in which substantial blood loss is anticipated such as cardiac surgery, major orthopaedic, vascular and general surgery. Specific details including reference ranges and therapies may need adaptation for local needs, expertise or patient groups. eGFR, estimated glomerular filtration rate; EPO, erythropoietin; G&H, group and hold; Hb, haemoglobin; IV, intravenous; U&E, urea and electrolytes. Source: Adapted from NHMRC [1].

Figure 17.1 presents an algorithm for preoperative assessment of anaemia. Similar algorithms have been validated in colorectal surgery, raising perioperative haemoglobin level and reducing perioperative transfusion requirements. More recent retrospective studies demonstrate similar results in orthopaedic surgery [4]. Furthermore, blood supplies are conserved and outcomes improved. Ongoing studies are required to determine the optimal approach for preoperative haemoglobin optimisation.

Intraoperative management of anaemia

There are many ways of optimising haemostasis and reducing blood loss in the intraoperative period [1], which include the following.

- *Anaesthetic techniques*: including preventing hypothermia and applying appropriate transfusion triggers.
- *Surgical techniques*: including meticulous haemostasis.
- *Pharmacological techniques*: including appropriate antithrombotic management and antifibrinolytics.
- *Transfusion techniques*: cell salvage, acute normovolaemic haemodilution and blood products (refer to Chapter 77 Blood transfusion).

Alternatives to transfusion should be considered, including topical therapies to help reduce bleeding. The antifibrinolytic drug tranexamic acid is increasingly used in cardiac surgery and there is evidence to show benefit when used topically for total knee replacement surgery. More studies are needed, however, before its intravenous use is adopted for all joint replacement surgery. Certainly, considering use of this medication seems reasonable in those surgeries where there is a predictable high risk of bleeding and the thrombotic risk is acceptable.

Postoperative optimisation of anaemia

Postoperative anaemia is multifactorial. Optimising a patient's postoperative tolerance to anaemia is a goal of management. Important considerations include optimal volume management, optimisation of erythropoiesis, restricting blood tests and appropriate transfusion use. Iron and/or erythropoietin (EPO) supplementation appear to be ineffective in the postoperative period.

Of particular importance are the appropriate triggers for transfusion. Perioperative transfusion (even just one unit) is associated with increased morbidity and mortality [5]. There are increased perioperative complications associated with transfusion including ischaemic events, infection and transfusion-related adverse effects. Note that causation is not established and the need for transfusion may represent a sicker patient group. Transfusion has never undergone safety and efficacy evaluation by the Food and Drug Administration (FDA) so unnecessary transfusion should be avoided.

The Australian NHMRC guidelines recommend the following (Table 17.1).

- Red cell transfusion should not be dictated by a haemoglobin trigger alone, but should be based on assessment of the patient's clinical status.
- Patients should not receive a transfusion when the haemoglobin level is > 100 g/L.
- In postoperative patients with acute myocardial or cerebrovascular ischaemia and a haemoglobin level of 70–100 g/L, transfusion of a single unit followed by reassessment of clinical efficacy is appropriate.

TABLE 17.1 NHMRC practice guidelines for red cell transfusion

Haemoglobin g/L	Considerations
<70	Lower thresholds may be acceptable in patients without symptoms and/or where specific therapy is available
70–100	Likely to be appropriate during surgery associated with major blood loss or if there are signs or symptoms of impaired oxygen transport
>80	May be appropriate to control anaemia-related symptoms in a patient on a chronic transfusion regimen or during marrow suppressive therapy
>100	Not likely to be appropriate unless there are specific indications

Source: Adapted from NHMRC [1].

There is growing literature questioning the benefits of transfusion and supporting a restrictive transfusion protocol in the absence of cardiac disease. Early studies have shown that in the presence of normal cardiac function, there appears to be little consequence from moderate anaemia [6]. A sentinel randomised controlled trial was performed in ICU patients comparing a restrictive (Hb 70–90 g/L) against a liberal (Hb 100–120 g/L) transfusion strategy. The study findings showed that the restrictive strategy was as effective and possibly superior to a liberal transfusion strategy, except perhaps in those patients with significant cardiac disease. A similar study in elderly patients undergoing hip fracture surgery also demonstrated no difference in outcomes between a restrictive and a liberal transfusion strategy. Furthermore, a recent study demonstrated an improved survival with a restrictive transfusion strategy over a liberal strategy in acute upper gastrointestinal bleeding. Reviews on the subject have recommended further studies involving patients with cardiac disease given the conflicting evidence that has been published [7].

> The perioperative management of anaemia is turning towards preventative approaches aiming to reduce the risk of anaemia and need for transfusion. The ever-escalating costs of transfusion and predicted shortages in supply mean more stringent transfusion use in the future. There is emerging evidence that reduced transfusion use can subsequently improve patient outcomes from surgery.

References

1. National Health and Medical Research Council. *Patient Blood Management Guidelines: Module 2, Perioperative.* Canberra, Australia: National Health and Medical Research Council, 2012.

2. Musallam KM, Tamim HM, Richards T, et al. Preoperative anaemia and postoperative outcomes in non-cardiac surgery: a retrospective cohort study. *Lancet,* 2011;**378**(9800):1396–1407. doi:10.1016/S0140-6736(11)61381-0

3. Pasricha SR, Flecknoe-Brown SC, Allen KJ, et al. Diagnosis and management of iron deficiency anaemia: a clinical update. *Medical Journal of Australia,* 2010;**193**(9):525–532. doi:10.1016/j.beha.2004.08.022

4. Enko D, Wallner F, von-Goedecke A, Hirschmugl C, Auersperg V, Halwachs-Baumann G. The impact of an algorithm-guided management of preoperative anemia in perioperative hemoglobin level and transfusion of major orthopedic surgery patients. *Anemia,* 2013;**2013**:641876. doi:10.1155/2013/641876

5. Glance LG, Dick AW, Mukamel DB, et al. Association between intraoperative blood transfusion and mortality and morbidity in patients undergoing noncardiac surgery. *Anesthesiology*, 2011;**114**(2):283–292. doi:10.1097/Aln.0b013e3182054d06

6. Weiskopf RB, Viele MK, Feiner J, et al. Human cardiovascular and metabolic response to acute, severe isovolemic anemia. *JAMA*, 1998;**279**(3):217–221. doi:10.1001/jama.279.3.217

7. Rao SV, Jollis JG, Harrington RA, et al. Relationship of blood transfusion and clinical outcomes in patients with acute coronary syndromes. *JAMA*, 2004;**292**(13):1555–1562. doi:10.1001/jama.292.13.1555

17

Central nervous system risk assessment

Richard Stark

The Alfred Hospital and Monash University, Australia

Parkinson's disease

The major problem with management of Parkinson's disease in the perioperative period is that very few options are available for parenteral management. Most patients will be on oral L-dopa and some will also be on a dopamine agonist. There is no parenteral form of L-dopa.

Patients vary enormously in their response to missing L-dopa therapy. Some show no effect from missing a dose, while others become immobile. Rarely, missing dopaminergic medication can result in a neuroleptic malignant-like syndrome, associated with fever, confusion, raised creatinine kinase levels and even death.

A retrospective cohort study of 234 people with Parkinson's disease and 40,979 controls undergoing major abdominal surgery found a higher incidence of aspiration pneumonia, bacterial infection and urinary tract infection in the group with Parkinson's disease [1].

Current options are therefore to omit all medication during the time the patient is 'nil by mouth' or to switch to a parenteral dopamine agonist.

L-dopa in serum is rapidly metabolised to dopamine and other compounds, and much is excreted so that little remains after four to six hours, but the biological effect in many patients with Parkinson's disease is much longer as the dopamine is taken up and stored in the target areas of the basal ganglia. Thus, for most patients, many hours or even a day or two without L-dopa therapy should produce no major problem.

The parenteral dopamine agonists to consider are apomorphine and rotigotine. Apomorphine is given subcutaneously. Switching a patient from oral treatment to apomorphine for the duration of surgery has superficial attraction but abrupt introduction of apomorphine usually causes vomiting. If there is time to titrate apomorphine therapy, the emetic effect can be minimised by domperidone. Potential side effects include hallucinations and hypotension.

Perioperative Medicine for the Junior Clinician, First Edition. Edited by Joel Symons, Paul Myles, Rishi Mehra and Christine Ball.
© 2015 John Wiley & Sons, Ltd. Published 2015 by John Wiley & Sons, Ltd.
Companion website: www.wiley.com/go/perioperativemed

Rotigotine is a new agent, delivered by transdermal patch. In an open label study, 14 patients were switched from their usual treatment to rotigotine the day before undergoing surgery. This proved effective. Neuropsychiatric side effects would be the major concern with such an approach but only one patient had transient hallucinations and nausea attributed to the therapy [2].

Suggested formulae for converting oral L-dopa and dopaminergic agent dosages to equivalents of apomorphine and rotigotine are shown in Figure 18.1 [3].

It is important to remember that standard antiemetics and neuroleptics aggravate the features of Parkinson's disease and these should be avoided if possible. Ondansetron is less likely to cause substantial problems.

> Most patients with Parkinson's disease rely on oral medications which do not exist in parenteral form. Perioperative management should aim to minimise the 'nil by mouth' period. Subcutaneous apomorphine and transdermal rotigotine are possible alternatives to oral L-dopa if substitutes are necessary.

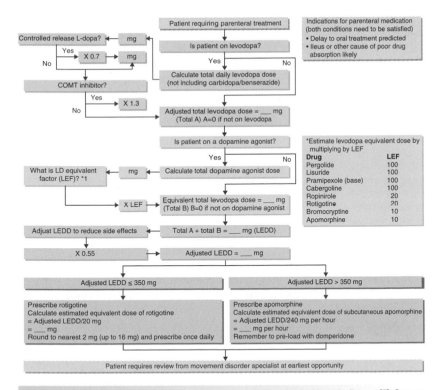

FIGURE 18.1 **Algorithm for estimating parenteral doses of drugs for Parkinson's disease [3].** Source: Reproduced with permission of BMJ Publishing Group Ltd. COMT, catechol-O-methyltransferase; LD, L-dopa; LEDD, L-dopa equivalent daily dose.

Multiple sclerosis

Patients with multiple sclerosis (MS) are sensitive to hyperthermia; this is the basis for Uhthoff's phenomenon in which exercise transiently aggravates symptoms of MS and for 'pseudo-exacerbations' caused by fever. Thus it is important to avoid hyperthermia in the perioperative period.

There are anecdotal reports of true exacerbations of MS apparently triggered by the stress of surgery, but the risk seems low [4]. Some authors have recommended high-dose prophylactic steroids in the perioperative period to reduce the risk of exacerbations [5] but there is no hard evidence or consensus opinion to support this view.

> Hyperthermia should be avoided if possible in multiple sclerosis patients, as symptoms may be aggravated.

Headache

Perioperative headache is common (28% of patients in one study [6]) and may occur for many reasons. Caffeine withdrawal is thought to account for many cases [7] so advising heavy coffee drinkers to cut back well before surgery may be useful. Certain anaesthetic techniques may contribute to postoperative headache. Low-pressure headache after dural puncture for spinal anaesthesia is well known, but sinus headache associated with nitrous oxide anaesthesia has also been reported.

Migraine is common (18% of women and 6% of men) and attacks may occur in the perioperative period. Despite earlier concerns that triptans might provoke coronary events, the risk seems very small [8] and these useful drugs should not be excluded from consideration in surgical patients at risk of coronary artery disease.

Chronic daily headache occurs in about 4% of the population, with chronic migraine accounting for about half of these [9]. High-frequency episodic migraine (8–15 days per month) is common too. Patients with such frequent headache are at high risk of aggravating the headache pattern with medication overuse, especially opioids such as codeine [10]. Hence, it is important to know a patient's headache history, including history of analgesic use, when they present for preoperative assessment; in a patient at high risk of medication overuse headache, the use of opioids should be extremely judicious.

> Perioperative headache is common, occurring because of caffeine withdrawal, certain anaesthetic techniques or aggravation of underlying headache disorder.

References

1. Pepper PV, Goldstein MK. Postoperative complications in Parkinson's disease. *Journal of the American Geriatrics Society*, 1999;**47**(8):967–972.

2. Wullner U, Kassubek J, Odin P, et al. Transdermal rotigotine for the perioperative management of Parkinson's disease. *Journal of Neural Transmission*, 2010;**117**(7):855–859.

3. Brennan KA, Genever RW. Managing Parkinson's disease during surgery. *BMJ*, 2010;**341**:c5718. doi:10.1136/bmj.c5718

4. Ridley A, Schapira K. Influence of surgical procedures on the course of multiple sclerosis. *Neurology*, 1961;**11**:81–82. doi:10.1212/wnl.11.1.81

5. Dickerman RD, Schneider SJ, Stevens QE, Matarese NM, Decker RE. Prophylaxis to avert exacerbation/relapse of multiple sclerosis in affected patients undergoing surgery. *Surgical observations and recommendations. Journal of Neurosurgical Sciences*, 2004;**48**(3):135–137.

6. Gill PS, Guest C, Rabey PG, Buggy DJ. Perioperative headache and day case surgery. *European Journal of Anaesthesiology*, 2003;**20**(5):401–403. doi:10.1017/s0265021503000619

7. Fennelly M, Galletly DC, Purdie GI. Is caffeine withdrawal the mechanism of postoperative headache? *Anesthesia and Analgesia*, 1991;**72**(4):449–453. doi:10.1213/00000539-199104000-00006

8. Dodick DW, Martin VT, Smith T, Silberstein S. Cardiovascular tolerability and safety of triptans: a review of clinical data. *Headache*, 2004;**44**:S20–S30. doi:10.1111/J.1526-4610.2004.04105.x

9. Natoli JL, Manack A, Dean B, et al. Global prevalence of chronic migraine: a systematic review. *Cephalalgia*, 2010;**30**(5):599–609. doi:10.1111/J.1468-2982.2009.01941.x

10. Bigal ME, Serrano D, Buse D, Scher A, Stewart WF, Lipton RB. Acute migraine medications and evolution from episodic to chronic migraine: a longitudinal population-based study. *Headache*, 2008;**48**(8):1157–1168. doi:10.1111/J.1526-4610.2008.01217.x

Risk assessment for perioperative renal dysfunction

David McIlroy

The Alfred Hospital and Monash University, Australia

Acute kidney injury (AKI) is a multifactorial syndrome leading to an acute decline in renal function. In the absence of a gold-standard tissue-based diagnosis, it is defined and staged according to clinical consensus definitions by either an increase in serum creatinine or periods of oliguria. A recent Kidney Disease: Improving Global Outcomes work group suggested a hybrid definition incorporating elements of both the RIFLE [1] and AKIN [2] consensus criteria (Table 19.1) [3].

The term AKI replaces older terminology such as acute renal failure, acute tubular necrosis or prerenal azotaemia, reflecting that:

- renal injury is a continuum from mild to severe, and even mild injury is associated with an increased incidence of adverse outcomes
- the aetiology of renal injury is incompletely understood, probably multifactorial and typically not known with certainty on a case-by-case basis.

Aetiology

In the absence of a validated perioperative AKI animal model, the precise aetiology is difficult to establish [4]. It is almost certainly multifactorial and probably represents the end-result of multiple complex and overlapping pathways which culminate in the clinical syndrome of AKI. Contributing factors may include ischaemia-reperfusion, inflammatory activation, sepsis, various nephrotoxins (antibiotics, non-steroidal anti-inflammatory drugs, radio-contrast media, free haemoglobin/myoglobin) and atheroembolism.

Epidemiology

The true incidence of perioperative AKI has been difficult to establish due to large variations in definitions employed in the existing literature. Conservative methodology estimates an incidence around 1% [5] although recent data using a more liberal definition suggest the incidence may be nearer 6% [6]. Perioperative AKI is consistently associated with an increase in perioperative mortality, increased

Perioperative Medicine for the Junior Clinician, First Edition. Edited by Joel Symons, Paul Myles, Rishi Mehra and Christine Ball.
© 2015 John Wiley & Sons, Ltd. Published 2015 by John Wiley & Sons, Ltd.
Companion website: www.wiley.com/go/perioperativemed

TABLE 19.1 Acute kidney injury definition and staging

AKI is defined as any of the following:
Increase in serum creatinine by ≥0.3 mg/dL (≥26.5 μmol/L) within 48 hours; or
Increase in serum creatinine to ≥1.5 times baseline, known or presumed to have occurred
within the prior 7 days; or
Urine volume <0.5 mL/kg/hr for 6 hours [3]

Stage	Serum creatinine	Urine output
1	1.5 × baseline ≤ relative increase in serum creatinine <2 × baseline OR Absolute increase in serum creatinine by ≥0.3 mg/dL (≥26.5 μmol/L)	<0.5 mL/kg/hr (>6 hr)
2	2 × baseline ≤ relative increase in serum creatinine <3 × baseline	<0.5 mL/kg/hr (≥12 hr)
3	Relative increase in serum creatinine ≥3× baseline OR Increase in serum creatinine to ≥4.0 mg/dL (≥353.6 μmol/L) with acute rise ≥0.5 mg/dL OR Initiation of renal replacement therapy	<0.3 mL/kg/hr (≥24 hr) OR Anuria (≥12 hr)

length of stay and increased cost [7–9]. AKI may also be associated with increased risk of subsequent progression to chronic kidney disease and despite apparent biochemical recovery from AKI, long-term mortality remains increased even at 10 years postoperatively.

Risk factors for perioperative AKI

Refer to Chapter 47 Acute kidney injury.

Diagnostic challenges

> While small increases in serum creatinine are powerfully and consistently associated with adverse outcomes, it is an imperfect diagnostic tool for AKI.

The physiology of creatinine is such that glomerular filtration rate needs to decline about 50% before serum creatinine increases above the reference range of many laboratories; it therefore provides only limited sensitivity and specificity for modest changes in renal function. Additionally, the pharmacokinetics of serum creatinine mean it is slow to increase in response to an acute decline in glomerular filtration rate [10]. Consequently, one to two days may elapse after injury before serum creatinine rises sufficiently to diagnose AKI, which makes effective intervention more challenging.

> Although oliguria is a 'stand-alone' diagnostic criterion for AKI, its validity is not well established.

Multiple studies in ICU and cardiac surgery populations confirm that use of the oliguric criteria increases the measured incidence of AKI but an association with adverse outcomes is less certain. Few if any data exist on perioperative oliguria and clinical outcomes (refer to Chapter 46 Oliguria). However, the perioperative activation of numerous neuroendocrine and other 'stress' response pathways, together with fluctuations in renal perfusion pressure, may impact urine flow rate independent of renal injury. Consequently, the relationship between perioperative oliguria and true renal injury remains uncertain.

Early recognition of evolving AKI is likely to represent an essential step toward effective intervention. The use of sophisticated proteomic and other analyses has lead to the identification of numerous molecules in the plasma and urine that may allow highly sensitive and specific recognition of evolving renal injury in real time (e.g. neutrophil gelatinase-associated lipocalin, liver fatty acid-binding protein, kidney injury molecule-1). However, none of these candidate biomarkers is currently ready to replace serum creatinine in the diagnosis of AKI.

Prevention and treatment

Despite numerous clinical trials, there are no established interventions to either prevent or alter the course of established AKI [11].

Previous common interventions, including 'renal-dose' dopamine and furosemide, have not been shown to be effective and may be associated with increased toxicity. Many of the identified risk factors for AKI are non-modifiable and in the absence of clearly identified mechanisms of renal injury, there is no certainty that risk factor modification, where possible, can favourably impact the development of perioperative AKI.

Management of perioperative AKI

In the absence of known preventive or therapeutic interventions, the management of perioperative AKI remains supportive. Additional renal insults should be avoided or minimised. Fluid balance should be optimised, recognising that while overt hypovolaemia probably contributes to renal injury, increased capillary permeability in the perioperative period combined with the non-distensible renal capsule may make excessive intravenous fluid similarly injurious. Renal replacement therapy may be required to assist in the management of fluid overload, uraemia, acidaemia and electrolyte derangements.

A suggested approach to patients at risk for perioperative AKI is to identify at-risk patients, minimising additional renal insults and other factors that likely contribute to AKI throughout the perioperative period by:

- considering correcting preoperative anaemia with iron or other supplements where clinically practicable as part of a perioperative blood management strategy
- maintaining adequate renal perfusion with regard to an individual patient's usual preoperative blood pressure [12]. A shift in the autoregulatory curve for renal blood flow may mean relative hypotension is poorly tolerated
- targeting euvolaemia aggressively rather than treating urine output *per se*
- considering protocol-based haemodynamic and oxygenation algorithms
- avoiding starch-based IV solutions [13]

- considering limiting administration of 0.9% saline and other high chloride-containing solutions that may induce a hyperchloraemic metabolic acidosis [14]
- limiting the use/duration of non-steroidal anti-inflammatory drugs.

References

1. Bellomo R, Ronco C, Kellum JA, Mehta RL, Palevsky P. Acute renal failure – definition, outcome measures, animal models, fluid therapy and information technology needs: the Second International Consensus Conference of the Acute Dialysis Quality Initiative (ADQI) Group. *Critical Care*, 2004;**8**(4):R204–212. doi:10.1186/cc2872

2. Mehta RL, Kellum JA, Shah SV, et al. Acute Kidney Injury Network: report of an initiative to improve outcomes in acute kidney injury. *Critical Care*, 2007;**11**(2):R31. doi:10.1186/cc5713

3. Kidney Disease Improving Global Outcomes Acute Kidney Injury Working Group. KDIGO Clinical Practice Guideline for Acute Kidney Injury. *Kidney International*, 2012;**2**(Suppl):1–138.

4. Heyman SN, Rosenberger C, Rosen S. Experimental ischemia-reperfusion: Biases and myths – the proximal vs. distal hypoxic tubular injury debate revisited. *Kidney International*, 2009;**77**:9–16. doi:10.1038/ki.2009.347

5. Kheterpal S, Tremper KK, Heung M, et al. Development and validation of an acute kidney injury risk index for patients undergoing general surgery: results from a national data set. *Anesthesiology*, 2009;**110**(3):505–515. doi:10.1097/ALN.0b013e3181979440

6. Story DA, Leslie K, Myles PS, et al. Complications and mortality in older surgical patients in Australia and New Zealand (the REASON study): a multicentre, prospective, observational study. *Anaesthesia*, 2010;**65**(10):1022–1030. doi:10.1111/j.1365-2044.2010.06478.x

7. Ricci Z, Cruz D, Ronco C. The RIFLE criteria and mortality in acute kidney injury: a systematic review. *Kidney International*, 2008;**73**(5):538–546. doi:10.1038/sj.ki.5002743

8. Dasta JF, Kane-Gill SL, Durtschi AJ, Pathak DS, Kellum JA. Costs and outcomes of acute kidney injury (AKI) following cardiac surgery. *Nephrology Dialysis Transplantation*, 2008;**23**(6):1970–1974. doi:10.1093/ndt/gfm908

9. Bihorac A, Yavas S, Subbiah S, et al. Long-term risk of mortality and acute kidney injury during hospitalization after major surgery. *Annals of Surgery*, 2009;**249**(5):851–858. doi:10.1097/SLA.0b013e3181a40a0b

10. Waikar SS, Bonventre JV. Creatinine kinetics and the definition of acute kidney injury. *Journal of the American Society of Nephrology*, 2009;**20**(3):672–679. doi:10.1681/ASN.2008070669

11. Shaw A, Swaminathan M, Stafford-Smith M. Cardiac surgery-associated acute kidney injury: putting together the pieces of the puzzle. *Nephron Physiology*, 2008;**109**(4):55–60. doi:10.1159/000142937

12. Joannidis M, Druml W, Forni LG, et al. Prevention of acute kidney injury and protection of renal function in the intensive care unit. Expert opinion of the Working Group for Nephrology, ESICM. *Intensive Care Medicine*, 2010;**36**(3):392–411. doi:10.1007/s00134-009-1678-y

13. Myburgh JA, Finfer S, Bellomo R, et al. Hydroxyethyl starch or saline for fluid resuscitation in intensive care. *New England Journal of Medicine*, 2012;**367**(20):1901–1911. doi:10.1056/NEJMoa1209759

14. Yunos NM, Bellomo R, Hegarty C, Story D, Ho L, Bailey M. Association Between a chloride-liberal vs chloride-restrictive intravenous fluid administration strategy and kidney injury in critically ill adults. *JAMA*, 2012;**308**(15):1566–1572.

19

Medical futility and end-of-life care

Mark Shulman[1] and Matthew Richardson[2]

[1]The Alfred Hospital and Monash University, Australia
[2]The Alfred Hospital, Australia

The aim of this chapter is to highlight some of the important issues around end-of-life care in the perioperative setting, in particular relating to medical futility, decision making and the obligations of the treating doctor. The chapter will also cover some common misconceptions surrounding end-of-life care. These principles are further elucidated in Chapter 104 Case Study 9 Medical futility.

Definitions

It is important to clearly define the terms used in end-of-life care discussions. For the purposes of this chapter, the following definitions will be used.

- *Medical futility*: where balancing effectiveness, potential benefit and potential burden of intervention warrants withdrawing or withholding treatment [1]
- *End of life*: a patient is approaching the end of their life when they are likely to die within the next 12 months. This includes those patients whose death is imminent (likely in days to hours) [2].

Medical futility

Recognising and avoiding medical futility can only be achieved by appreciating how the patient and their medical condition interact. The following questions should be considered.

Question 1. How would you rate your patient's risk of significant morbidity or mortality in the perioperative period?

The REASON Study [3] provides us with good-quality data to help identify which groups of patients are at greatest risk in the perioperative period. Overall, patients aged 70 years and over had a 5% risk of 30-day postoperative mortality and a 20% risk of a major complication, but specific factors increased that risk (Table 20.1). The ability to appraise and report the real risk to the patient for a given intervention is very informative.

Perioperative Medicine for the Junior Clinician, First Edition. Edited by Joel Symons, Paul Myles, Rishi Mehra and Christine Ball.
© 2015 John Wiley & Sons, Ltd. Published 2015 by John Wiley & Sons, Ltd.
Companion website: www.wiley.com/go/perioperativemed

TABLE 20.1 Perioperative factors associated with increased 30-day postoperative mortality (% 30-day mortality)

Preoperative factors	Surgical factors	Postoperative factors
Increasing age >90 (12%)	Non-scheduled surgery (10%)	Unplanned ICU admission (20%)
ASA ≥4 (17%)	Thoracic surgery (14%)	Systemic inflammation (15%)
Male gender (6%)		Acute renal impairment (17%)
Plasma albumin <30 g/L (15%)		
Respiratory disease (11%)		

Source: Story et al. [3].
ASA, American Society of Anesthesiologists; ICU, intensive care unit.

Question 2. What further information do you need to obtain from your patient to decide whether this operation is in their 'best interests'? [4]

A patient's understanding of the diagnosis, operative plan and its consequences is required in order for them to make an informed decision.

- How the patient *feels* about having a major operation, invasive treatments *and* a prolonged hospital stay.
- Their current functional level and things they enjoy in day-to-day life.
- If the patient has chronic illness, have they reached the 'end of the road' with their medical problems or do they consider themselves a 'fighter' and want to 'push on' if there is even a small chance of prolonging life?
- Whether there are particular sorts of treatment that they would not want (such as intensive care, dialysis, prolonged intubation).

Clarifying these issues allows us to better advise the patient with respect to their particular experiences, wishes and concerns.

Question 3. What factors should be considered when deciding which treatment option is best for a patient nearing the end of their life?

When a patient is nearing the end of their life, the best treatment option for that patient should be selected based on several factors.

- *Likelihood of success*: invasive treatment should not be offered to a patient when it is likely to be futile or not in the patient's best interests. Remember that a doctor is not obliged to provide a treatment that a patient demands when he or she feels that treatment is not in the patient's best interests.
- *Risk versus benefit*: the pain, suffering and potential complications associated with a treatment should be weighed against the potential quality of life improvement the treatment may offer.
- *Patient priorities*: some patients may be prepared to accept the potential adverse effects of a treatment for even a small chance that it may prolong their lives. Other patients may choose the treatment that offers the best quality of life with the least pain and suffering possible.

20

Question 4. What options exist for your patient's care and how would you advise them with regard to choosing the best option?

When caring for patients with complex medical issues, the ability to identify treatment options most appropriate for a patient's particular circumstance is a crucial skill for doctors to master. When a patient is approaching the end of their life, recognising when a potential treatment is no longer appropriate for the patient is equally important. Avoiding the pursuit of medically futile treatment of such patients can prevent unnecessary pain, suffering and discomfort.

The following major headings are helpful when considering which treatment course may best suit a particular patient.

- Surgery with curative intent
- Surgery with palliative intent – symptom control
- Medical/radiotherapeutic management
- Medical palliative care
- A combination of any of the above

Before offering advice, a patient's particular situation should be discussed with the consultant physician and/or surgeon responsible for their care. Ideally, this discussion would take place at a multidisciplinary meeting that includes medical, surgical, anaesthetic, nursing and intensive care representatives.

> It is important to provide your patient with clear and consistent advice, as conflicting information can be very distressing to patients and their relatives.

Misconceptions

The decision to transition from treatment with curative intent to palliative care can be a difficult one. Contributing to this difficulty is the fact that there are many misconceptions regarding what constitutes palliative care. Besdine outlined some of the misconceptions regarding attitudes towards palliative care [5].

- 'Palliative care is synonymous with euthanasia'
  - Fact: Euthanasia is illegal in the United Kingdom and not practised by palliative care specialists.
- 'Accepting palliative care means you are giving up'
  - Fact: Engaging palliative care services is focused on actively treating the symptoms most distressing to the patient in order to *improve* quality of life [2].
- 'Accepting palliative care means a shorter life expectancy'
  - Fact: Early palliative care can result in better quality of life, less depression and in some circumstances, a prolonged life expectancy [6].
- 'There is no need for palliative care because my doctor can manage my pain'
  - Fact: Palliative care physicians are experts in managing the symptoms associated with chronic and terminal illnesses.
- 'Accepting palliative care means you must stop treatment'
  - Fact: Many treatments can be considered simultaneously while receiving the benefits of palliative care.

Palliative care is a medical specialty focused on managing pain and other distressing symptoms experienced by patients approaching the end of their life. Palliative care teams are also skilled in providing psychological, social and spiritual support to such patients and those close to them.

Obligations of the treating doctor

The complexities of managing patients approaching the end of their life have some important medico-legal ramifications. Being aware of the obligations of the treating doctor is vital in ensuring appropriate care is available for your patient. The following points are identified in *Treatment and Care Towards the End of Life: Good Practice in Decision Making* [2].

- *Presumption in favour of prolonging life*: while normally the doctor is required to take all reasonable steps to prolong life, there is no absolute obligation to prolong life irrespective of the consequences for the patient and their views.
- *Presumption of capacity*: the doctor must assume the patient has the capacity to make decisions about their treatment. Age, disability, behaviour, beliefs and apparent inability to communicate should *not* lead the doctor to assume the patient lacks capacity to make decisions about their care.
- *Adults who lack capacity*: where a patient lacks capacity to make decisions regarding treatment:
  - consult the patient's medical record to identify any previously documented legally binding advance directive refusing treatment.
  - enquire whether there were any previous appointments of an attorney or other legal proxy who can decide on behalf of the patient.
  - where no attorney or legal proxy exists, the treating doctor must decide which treatment will provide overall benefit to the patient after consulting with those close to the patient and other members of the healthcare team.

Conclusion

In general, an inclusive approach to end-of-life care decision making involving the patient, their loved ones and other members of the healthcare team is the best way to ensure the doctor's obligations are met and patient's wishes are understood.

References

1. Beauchamp T, Childress J. Nonmaleficence. In: *Principles of Biomedical Ethics*, 6th edn. New York: Oxford University Press, 2009, p. 167.
2. General Medical Council. *Treatment and Care Towards the End of Life: Good Practice in Decision Making*. http://www.gmc-uk.org/End_of_life.pdf_32486688.pdf
3. Story DA, Leslie K, Myles PS, et al. Complications and mortality in older surgical patients in Australia and New Zealand (the REASON study): a multicentre, prospective, observational study. *Anaesthesia*, 2010;**65**(10):1022–1030. doi:10.1111/j.1365-2044.2010.06478.x
4. Mental Capacity Act 2005. Chapter 9. www.legislation.gov.uk/ukpga/2005/9/pdfs/ukpga_20050009_en.pdf
5. Besdine R. Why everyone deserves palliative care. http://www.huffingtonpost.com/richard-w-besdine-md/palliative-care_b_3095190.html
6. Temel JS, Greer JA, Muzikansky A, et al. Early palliative care for patients with metastatic non-small-cell lung cancer. *New England Journal of Medicine*, 2010;**363**(8):733–742. doi:10.1056/NEJMoa1000678

The surgical safety checklist

Pedro Guio-Aguilar[1] and Russell Gruen[2]

[1]The Alfred Hospital, Australia
[2]Monash University, Australia

Approximately 1 in 10 hospitalised patients suffers an adverse event, half of which may be avoidable. Among the estimated 234 million patients who undergo anaesthesia for major surgery each year, at least 7 million have a severe complication, from which 1 million die [1].

Inadequate communication is a leading cause of adverse events, and in many countries deaths have been more commonly attributed to communication errors than to other clinical inadequacies. Particularly in the operating room, it has been suggested that communication could be improved through attention to listening, clear accurate speech, courteous behaviours and acknowledging requests.

In 2008, the WHO World Alliance for Patient Safety launched the 'Safe Surgery Saves Lives' campaign and subsequently developed a surgical safety checklist to strengthen communication and improve patient safety [2,3]. This chapter highlights the role of anaesthetic and surgical staff in patient safety, the importance of good communication and teamwork, and the effects of the surgical safety checklist (SSC).

Development of a surgical safety checklist

In complex situations, experts face two main difficulties: the fallibility of human memory and the undue confidence that may lull people into skipping steps [4]. A checklist is a list of actions, items or criteria arranged systematically, helping the user to record the presence or absence of the individual items listed to ensure that all are considered or completed.

Checklists provide memory recall and guidance to users. They are tools for verification of completion, standardisation and regulation of processes. Checklists are an inexpensive approach to preventing human error and promoting best practices in complex and high-intensity work.

Many industries such as the automobile, food and pharmaceutical manufacturing industries have adopted checklists. In the military, checklists have been instrumental, along with briefing and debriefing, in enhancing the safety culture. In aviation,

Perioperative Medicine for the Junior Clinician, First Edition. Edited by Joel Symons, Paul Myles, Rishi Mehra and Christine Ball.
© 2015 John Wiley & Sons, Ltd. Published 2015 by John Wiley & Sons, Ltd.
Companion website: www.wiley.com/go/perioperativemed

checklists were introduced after the crash of Boeing's new 299-model aeroplane in 1935, under control of an experienced pilot. The investigations concluded that 'the plane was too complex for one man's memory' [4].

Interest in checklists in clinical practice began in earnest in 1999. Peter Pronovost, a critical care physician at Johns Hopkins University in Baltimore, aimed to reduce the incidence of catheter-related bloodstream infections in the ICU at Johns Hopkins Hospital by implementing a checklist. He found that in more than one-third of patients, doctors skipped at least one step. He persuaded the hospital administration to authorise nurses to confront doctors if they appeared to be skipping any steps on the checklist. Within the following two years, only two such infections occurred; 43 infections and eight deaths appeared to be prevented, and savings were estimated to approximate $2 million [5].

The WHO checklist

In 2006, as part of its 'Safe Surgery Saves Lives' campaign, the WHO recommended a SSC be developed and used to promote surgical patient safety worldwide. The WHO SSC was the first major international effort to promote use of checklists into everyday practice, and it was highly successful at engaging governments, professional groups and healthcare organisations in many countries.

The SSC (Figure 21.1) comprises a set of core safety checks to be verbally performed by the operation theatre team at three specified stages of a surgical procedure:

- the period before induction of anaesthesia or *Sign In*
- the period after induction and before surgical incision or *Time Out*
- the period during or immediately after wound closure or *Sign Out*.

The implementation of the WHO surgical safety checklist into operating rooms was associated with significant reductions in the in-hospital rates of death, surgical site infection, unplanned reoperation and overall complications among patients 16 years and older undergoing non-cardiac surgery. Its use in urgent operations was also associated with reduced mortality, blood loss and surgical site infections [6].

These results have been replicated in both low- and high-income countries. How the checklist saves lives, even in high-income countries, has spawned considerable debate and further research. Two main hypotheses have been considered. The first is that the SSC improves adherence to important clinical practices such as antibiotic administration and DVT prophylaxis which can reduce avoidable morbidity and mortality. Patients not receiving antibiotics prior to skin incision decreased from 12% to 6% of patients with the use of the checklist.

The second hypothesis is that the SSC enhances teamwork and communication in the operating theatre in a way that improves outcomes. Checklists seem to enhance teamwork by establishing an open dialogue during the whole perioperative period, promoting the flow of information and exposing knowledge gaps, as well as encouraging the articulation of concerns and prompting changes in the care plan. Checklists therefore seem to support interdisciplinary decision making and enhance the 'team feeling' (Video 21.1).

Other important considerations are acceptance of the checklist among practitioners and compliance with its use. The WHO aimed to foster these by publishing a generic checklist (see Figure 21.1) and encouraging professional bodies, health

Surgical safety checklist

World Health Organization | **Patient Safety**
A World Alliance for Safer Health Care

Before induction of anaesthesia

(with at least nurse and anaesthetist)

Has the patient confirmed his/her identity, site, procedure, and consent?
☐ Yes

Is the site marked?
☐ Yes
☐ Not applicable

Is the anaesthesia machine and medication check complete?
☐ Yes

Is the pulse oximeter on the patient and functioning?
☐ Yes

Does the patient have a:

Known allergy?
☐ No
☐ Yes

Difficult airway or aspiration risk?
☐ No
☐ Yes, and equipment/assistance available

Risk of > 500 ml blood loss (7 ml/kg in children)?
☐ No
☐ Yes, and two IVs/central access and fluids planned

Before skin incision

(with nurse, anaesthetist and surgeon)

☐ **Confirm all team members have introduced themselves by name and role.**
☐ **Confirm the patient's name, procedure, and where the incision will be made.**

Has antibiotic prophylaxis been given within the last 60 minutes?
☐ Yes
☐ Not applicable

Anticipated critical events

To Surgeon:
☐ What are the critical or non-routine steps?
☐ How long will the case take?
☐ What is the anticipated blood loss?

To Anaesthetist:
☐ Are there any patient-specific concerns?

To nursing team:
☐ Has sterility (including indicator results) been confirmed?
☐ Are there equipment issues or any concerns?

Is essential imaging displayed?
☐ Yes
☐ Not applicable

Before patient leaves operating room

(with nurse, anaesthetist and surgeon)

Nurse verbally confirms:
☐ The name of the procedure
☐ Completion of instrument, sponge and needle counts
☐ Specimen labelling (read specimen labels aloud, including patient name)
☐ Whether there are any equipment problems to be addressed

To surgeon, anaesthetist and nurse:
☐ What are the key concerns for recovery and management of this patient?

FIGURE 21.1 The WHO surgical safety checklist summarises the more important aspects of safety: correct patient identification, surgical site and side, safe anaesthesia and airway, prevention of infection and successful teamwork [2].

www.wiley.com/go/perioperativemed

VIDEO 21.1 The surgical safety checklist is an important tool that minimises errors as well as promoting team communication in the operating room.

departments and hospitals to tailor it to local circumstances, including use of locally relevant language and logos. In nine prospective observational studies, the overall compliance averaged 75%, but ranged from 12% to 100%. The most frequent reasons for non-compliance with the SSC were having 'forgotten' (66%), 'logistics' (45%), 'lack of time' (34%), 'take a long time to complete' (20%), 'motivation' and 'other' (11%).

21

> The surgical safety checklist has impacted upon the practice of surgery and anaesthesia across the world, and is a truly great global patient safety initiative. It is now standard practice to use a checklist in operating theatres and for good reason – available evidence tells us that teamwork and communication are improved, as are patient outcomes. The exact reasons why are still to be elucidated, and challenges still remain, particularly in promoting uptake and accuracy, and maintaining interest and adherence.

References

1. Haynes AB, Weiser TG, Berry WR, et al. A surgical safety checklist to reduce morbidity and mortality in a global population. *New England Journal of Medicine*, 2009;**360**(5):491–499. doi:10.1056/NEJMsa0810119

2. World Health Organization. *Implementation Manual: WHO Surgical Safety Checklist. Safe Surgery Saves Lives.* Geneva, Switzerland: World Health Organization, 2008.

3. Mahajan RP. The WHO surgical checklist. *Best Practice and Research in Clinical Anaesthesiology*, 2011;**25**(2):161–168. doi:10.1016/j.bpa.2011.02.002

4. Gawande A. *The Check List Manifesto*. London: Profile Books, 2010.

5. Gawande A. The checklist: if something so simple can transform intensive care, what else can it do? *New Yorker*, 2007. www.newyorker.com/magazine/2007/12/10/the-checklist

6. Weiser TG, Haynes AB, Dziekan G, et al. Effect of a 19-item surgical safety checklist during urgent operations in a global patient population. *Annals of Surgery*, 2010;**251**(5):976–980. doi:10.1097/SLA.0b013e3181d970e3

Part III

Perioperative investigations

22 Preoperative investigations (non-cardiac surgery)

Arvinder Grover

The Alfred Hospital and Monash University, Australia

The routine ordering of a range of tests preoperatively was once common practice [1]. This practice has now been comprehensively rejected by credible guidelines and authorities in many countries [2]. Ordering tests without a clear clinical indication will lead to false positives, further delays and potential harm to patients.

> Preoperative testing should be reserved for those situations where it will change overall management. Very few, if any, patients undergoing ambulatory or other minor surgery require any preoperative investigations.

Following a comprehensive history and examination, appropriate preoperative investigations can be used to predict underlying disease or perioperative risk, which can lead to preventative measures to optimise the patient's preoperative condition.

Common preoperative investigations

Bedside tests

Electrocardiogram

The main goal of a preoperative ECG is to detect underlying cardiac disease such as recent myocardial infarction, ischaemia, conduction defects or arrhythmias which have the potential to alter the anaesthesia plan or postpone surgery (Video 22.1).

There is little evidence to support the ordering of 'routine' or baseline ECG, particularly in patients undergoing low-risk surgery [3]. A preoperative ECG is indicated in patients undergoing intermediate or major surgery *and* with a known history of cardiovascular disease or with multiple clinical risk factors (diabetes, renal

Perioperative Medicine for the Junior Clinician, First Edition. Edited by Joel Symons, Paul Myles, Rishi Mehra and Christine Ball.
© 2015 John Wiley & Sons, Ltd. Published 2015 by John Wiley & Sons, Ltd.
Companion website: www.wiley.com/go/perioperativemed

www.wiley.com/go/perioperativemed

VIDEO 22.1 **Electrocardiography.** The ECG provides a cheap, non-invasive and reproducible method of looking at rhythm disturbances, the presence of ischaemia or other electrolyte abnormalities.

impairment, peripheral vascular disease, hypertension, past history, and in those undergoing vascular surgery) (Figure 22.1) [3,4].

All results should be interpreted in the context of the patient's clinical state. If it is thought the patient has underlying cardiac disease, consideration should be given to non-invasive cardiac stress testing or referral to a cardiologist for further review and management (refer to Chapter 11 The cardiac patient for non-cardiac surgery).

Chest X-ray (CXR)
A routine preoperative CXR is not recommended for ambulatory patients unless suggested by the history and/or physical examination findings. Obtaining a CXR is reasonable if acute cardiopulmonary disease is suspected or there is a history of chronic stable cardiopulmonary disease [5].

Laboratory tests

Urinalysis
Routine urine analysis is not recommended in asymptomatic patients. It should be reserved for those patients having urological surgery.

Consider a pregnancy test in all women of child-bearing age presenting for surgery.

Full blood examination (FBE)
An FBE should be ordered if a patient has significant medical co-morbidities, which would indicate a higher preoperative probability of anaemia (e.g. chronic renal failure, chronic liver disease or inflammatory conditions such as vasculitis) or for patients at high risk of significant intraoperative blood loss (Table 22.1).

Urea, electrolytes and creatinine (U&E)
Preoperative U&E will highlight any underlying electrolyte disturbance, renal impairment and potential acid–base disturbance. Significant components of the history and examination which will guide selective U&E testing include diabetes, long-standing hypertension, chronic heart or kidney disease, or

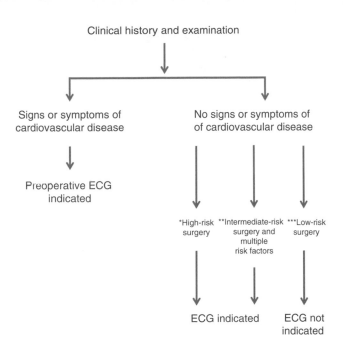

Clinical history and examination

Signs or symptoms of
cardiovascular disease

No signs or symptoms of
of cardiovascular disease

Preoperative ECG
indicated

*High-risk **Intermediate-risk ***Low-risk
surgery   surgery and   surgery
           multiple
           risk factors

ECG indicated   ECG not
                     indicated

* Examples of high-risk surgery: vascular surgery. Thoracic patients are commonly
included as high-risk patients despite not being strictly defined as high risk as per
the AHA/ACC guidelines

** Examples of intermediate-risk surgery: major orthopaedic surgery, colorectal
surgery, ENT, neurosurgery

*** Examples of low-risk surgery: sedation, breast surgery and endoscopy

FIGURE 22.1 **Algorithm for preoperative ECG testing [3,4].**

patients prescribed particular medications (diuretics, non-steroidal
anti-inflammatory agents or ACE inhibitors).

Liver function test (LFT)
Liver function tests include alanine transaminase (ALT), aspartate transaminase
(AST), alkaline phosphatase (ALP), gamma glutamyl transpeptidase (GT), albumin
and total bilirubin. Clinical history and examination should guide ordering of LFTs
(e.g. history of acute or chronic liver disease, heart failure, bleeding disorders, heavy
alcohol intake). The LFTs will highlight underlying liver disease including synthetic
function (albumin and bilirubin), cellular damage (AST, ALT and gamma-GT) and
nutritional state (albumin). Hypoalbuminaemia is associated with increased
perioperative risk.

Coagulation testing
Coagulation tests include activated partial thromboplastin time (APTT), INR and
prothrombin time (PT).

The goal of coagulation testing is to detect patients with bleeding or coagulation
disorders who may be a higher risk of bleeding in the perioperative period.

TABLE 22.1 Components of the FBE, normal range and indication for each

Parameter	Normal range (may vary between institutions)	Indication
Haemoglobin (g/L)	122–170	• Symptoms of anaemia • Polycythaemia • Risk factors for anaemia – chronic disease, CRF, liver failure, heart failure, thyroid disease, immune suppression • Malignancy • Known PR or upper GI tract blood loss • Procedures where large blood loss is expected • Patients who have had multiple surgical procedures
Haematocrit (L/L)	0.36–0.49	• Similar indications to the above
Mean corpuscular volume (f/L)	80–97	To assess the cause of anaemia • Macrocytic • Microcytic • Normocytic
White cell count (10⁹/L)	4.6–10.50	• Inflammation • Infection
Platelet count (10⁹/L)	150–400	• Clinical bleeding risk • Prior to neuraxial blockade

CRF, chronic renal failure; GI, gastrointestinal; PR, per rectum.

Coagulation testing should be reserved for patients with medical conditions associated with impaired haemostasis (e.g. liver disease), patients taking anticoagulants, and those whose history or examination findings suggest an underlying coagulation disorder (e.g. history of spontaneous bruising or excessive surgical bleeding, family history of a known heritable coagulopathy). A history of bleeding should be obtained from all patients, and appropriate coagulation testing should be considered if the history is abnormal [3].

Coagulation tests are useful in patients having a spinal or epidural analgesic technique who also have a history of coagulopathy or are prescribed antiplatelet or anticoagulation medications.

Specific tests

Thyroid function tests (TFTs)

Patients presenting for thyroid surgery should have preoperative TFTs. Patients with thyroid disease do not routinely need preoperative TFTs unless they have symptoms or signs of hypo- or hyperthyroidism.

Haemoglobin A_1c (HbA$_1$c)

HbA$_1$c has an important role in long-term management of patients with either type 1 or type 2 diabetes. HbA$_1$c is a form of haemoglobin that is measured primarily to identify the average plasma glucose concentration over prolonged periods of time. It is an important screening tool for patients before surgery whilst also providing an assessment of perioperative risk. It is a particularly good screening test for the elderly and those presenting for vascular and cardiac surgery. An $HbA_1c < 7\%$ is seen as very good control, while greater than 10% indicates poor control. Patients with poor control should be referred to their endocrinologist or local physician.

Arterial blood gas (ABG)

There are no data to support the use of preoperative arterial blood gas analysis to assess or stratify patient risk for postoperative pulmonary complications.

Transthoracic echocardiography (TTE)

Transthoracic echocardiography is indicated for those patients with new dyspnoea, a history of heart failure and no recent TTE, or a newly diagnosed murmur. It is not recommended as a screening test for coronary artery disease. A focused echocardiogram (TTE done in preadmission clinic or holding bay of theatre) is frequently done to assess volume state, severe valvular pathology and global cardiac function.

Pulmonary function tests

Preoperative lung function testing is indicated in those patients with new-onset dyspnoea, to confirm a diagnosis of asthma, emphysema or COPD, and in those patients with known lung pathology who may not be at their optimal function.

Cardiac testing

Patients with an active cardiac condition or those with new cardiac symptoms (for elective surgery) should be referred for further cardiac testing (refer to Chapter 13 Preoperative cardiac testing).

Invasive cardiac tests (e.g. coronary angiogram or CT angiogram) are reserved for patients with a positive stress test or those with multiple cardiac risk factors and active cardiac conditions.

References

1. Munro J, Booth A, Nicholl J. Routine preoperative testing: a systematic review of the evidence. *Health Technology Assessment*, 1997;**1**(12):i–iv; 1–62. doi:10.3310/hta1120

2. Johansson T, Fritsch G, Flamm M, et al. Effectiveness of non-cardiac preoperative testing in non-cardiac elective surgery: a systematic review. *British Journal of Anaesthesia*, 2013;**110**(6):926–939. doi:10.1093/bja/aet071

3. Feely MA, Collins CS, Daniels PR, Kebede EB, Jatoi A, Mauck KF. Preoperative testing before noncardiac surgery: guidelines and recommendations. *American Family Physician*, 2013;**87**(6):414–418.

4. Fleisher LA, Fleischmann KE, Auerbach AD, et al. 2014 ACC/AHA Guideline on Perioperative Cardiovascular Evaluation and Management of Patients Undergoing Noncardiac Surgery: Executive Summary: A Report of the American College of Cardiology/American Heart Association Task Force on Practice Guidelines. *Journal of the American College of Cardiology*, 2014;**64**(22):e77–e137. doi:10.1016/j.jacc.2014.07.944

5. Cassel CK, Guest JA. Choosing wisely: helping physicians and patients make smart decisions about their care. *JAMA*, 2012;**307**(17):1801–1802. doi:10.1001/Jama.2012.476

23 Postoperative investigations

Arvinder Grover

The Alfred Hospital and Monash University, Australia

Postoperative investigations should be guided by the clinical state of the patient, the surgical procedure and the anaesthetic technique.

- The goal of postoperative testing is to identify and optimise conditions that have the potential to increase perioperative morbidity and mortality.
- Postoperative investigations are usually ordered as a result of a change in the patient's postoperative course.
- Patients having low-risk surgery will not routinely require postoperative investigations.
- Common postoperative investigations include bedside tests, laboratory tests and chest X-ray.
- Routine tests are often required for patients admitted to the ICU in the postoperative period.

All patients will have routine postoperative observations when transferred from theatre to the recovery room. These include assessment of conscious state, blood pressure, heart rate, oxygen saturation and temperature. If the patient has had regional anaesthesia they will also have a detailed assessment of their sensory and motor function.

Any abnormality or deterioration in clinical status of the patient with the above parameters will guide further investigation.

Below are the most common tests ordered and potential indications for these tests. The tests and potential differential diagnosis are a guide rather than a definitive list.

Bedside tests
Electrocardiogram (ECG)

- Heart rate disturbance: bradycardia (HR <50 beats/min) or tachycardia (HR >100 beats/min)
- Arrhythmias/conduction defects: supraventricular or ventricular arrhythmias

Perioperative Medicine for the Junior Clinician, First Edition. Edited by Joel Symons, Paul Myles, Rishi Mehra and Christine Ball.
© 2015 John Wiley & Sons, Ltd. Published 2015 by John Wiley & Sons, Ltd.
Companion website: www.wiley.com/go/perioperativemed

- Hypotension (especially not responsive to treatment)
- Patients with a known history of CAD or HF
- Patients with postoperative cardiac symptoms – chest pain, dyspnoea or syncopal episode

Chest X-ray (CXR)

- Patients with increasing oxygen requirements
- Patients with decreased oxygen saturation ($<92\%$)
- Patients with dyspnoea
- Part of a postoperative septic screen
- To confirm the position of recently inserted central venous catheter, tracheal tube or thoracic drain tube (e.g. intercostal catheter)
- Surgical indications: thoracic surgery, cardiac surgery

Blood tests

Full blood examination (FBE)

- Patients with ongoing postoperative hypotension
- Large-volume bleeding via drain tubes
- Significant intraoperative blood loss
- Patients with known cardiac disease and significant perioperative blood loss
- Part of a septic screen to investigate a cause of infection in the perioperative period
- Part of a delirium screen in a patient with confusion or cognitive dysfunction in the perioperative period
- Patients presenting for emergency surgery
- Preoperative anaemia

Urea, electrolytes and creatinine (U&E)

- Investigate postoperative arrhythmias (especially K^+ and Mg^{2+})
- Investigate postoperative renal failure (acute and acute on chronic)
- Na^+ level to investigate hydration status of the patient. Serum Na^+ is a part of laboratory work assessment for investigation of perioperative hyponatraemia which can have a significant impact on a patient's clinical status
- To assess nutritional state of patients – especially those with chronic disease or surgery requiring prolonged hospital stay (e.g. burns patients, elderly patients having colorectal surgery)
- Patients receiving enteral or parenteral nutrition

Coagulation studies

- Unexplained postoperative bleeding
- Postoperative anaemia
- Patients who have received a blood transfusion in the postoperative period
- Patients anticoagulation medication (especially those who have had bridging therapy)
- Patients having surgery which could have an impact on coagulation function (e.g. hepatic surgery)

Liver function tests (LFTs)

- Patients having major intra-abdominal surgery (e.g. colorectal surgery, hepatic or biliary surgery) to assess any deterioration in liver function
- Patients having cardiac surgery
- Patients with known preoperative liver disease
- Patients prescribed multiple medications (e.g. antibiotics)
- Assessment of a patient's albumin and bilirubin – provides a guide to the liver's synthetic function and patient's nutritional state
- To investigate any patients with postoperative confusion
- Patients receiving blood transfusions or who have had a transfusion reaction

Blood sugar level (BSL)

- Patients with known type 1 or 2 diabetes
- Patients having hepatic and/or pancreatic surgery
- Immunosuppressed patients, those with wound infections or poor healing
- Patients receiving enteral or parenteral nutrition

Troponin/cardiac enzymes

- Patients with cardiac symptoms (e.g. chest pain, dyspnoea) or those with postoperative cardiac failure
- To investigate those patients who have potentially suffered an acute coronary syndrome:
  - persistent hypotension
  - postoperative arrhythmia (e.g. atrial fibrillation)
  - persistent tachycardia
- Patients with intraoperative or postoperative ECG changes

Patients receiving dual antiplatelet therapy having high-risk surgery (e.g. vascular surgery) with any of the above risks should have serial troponin measurements.

Arterial blood gas (ABG)

An ABG is a quick and easy test in the postoperative period to assess a patient's respiratory status, electrolytes, haemoglobin and BSL. Indications for an ABG include the following.

- Patients with postoperative hypoxaemia
- Patients requiring a high amount of supplemental oxygen
- Rapid assessment for postoperative anaemia (in conjunction with a FBE)
- To diagnose acid–base disturbances
- To guide a diagnosis of severe dehydration, shock or severe infection

Transthoracic echocardiogram (TTE)

In the postoperative setting, a TTE is useful to evaluate new dyspnoea, aid in diagnosis of cardiac failure or look for structural heart disease in the setting of a new arrhythmia. Focused TTE is also commonly used in the perioperative period to assess the patient's intravascular volume state.

Computed tomography (CT scan)

In the rare event that a patient fails to wake from anaesthesia or has clinical signs which indicate a possible cerebrovascular event, a CT scan can help in determining the diagnosis.

Conclusion

In summary, there is no evidence to support routine postoperative investigations. Rather, a change in a patient's postoperative course, suggested by accurate history and examination, will guide the clinician to the appropriate postoperative investigations.

Further reading

Scottish Intercollegiate Guidelines Network. *Postoperative Management in Adults: A Practical Guide to Postoperative Care for Clinical Staff*. Edinburgh: Scottish Intercollegiate Guidelines Network. www.sign.ac.uk

23

Part IV
Specific medication management and prophylaxis

Thromboprophylaxis

Amanda Davis

The Alfred Hospital and Monash University, Australia

Refer also to Chapter 25 Anticoagulants and antiplatelet agents.

Background risk of venous thromboembolism perioperatively

> When considering perioperative thromboprophylaxis, ask:
> * What is the risk of DVT and/or PE?
> * What are the risks of thromboprophylaxis?

In Australia about 30,000 people are hospitalised each year with venous thromboembolism (VTE) and approximately 2000 die from VTE. The majority of VTE cases requiring hospitalisation are related to previous hospital admissions for surgery or acute illness [1]. In the United States approximately one-third of the 150,000–200,000 VTE-related deaths per year occur following surgery [2].

The American College of Chest Physicians guidelines, most recently updated in 2012, provide a comprehensive review on the evidence base for thromboprophylaxis. There is significant discussion in these guidelines on how to estimate risk of VTE [2]. One important issue is whether symptomatic VTE and fatal PE are used to assess efficacy of therapy or whether asymptomatic DVT is also important [3].

Estimating individual patient risk

Thromboembolic risk is described by Virchow's triad of vessel injury, hypercoagulability and abnormal blood flow.

Venous thromboembolism risk can be estimated using the Caprini Score (Table 24.1). Using this scoring system, specific recommendations for thromboprophylaxis in patients undergoing general, gastrointestinal, urological, gynaecological and bariatric surgery are outlined in Table 24.2 [2].

Perioperative Medicine for the Junior Clinician, First Edition. Edited by Joel Symons, Paul Myles, Rishi Mehra and Christine Ball.
© 2015 John Wiley & Sons, Ltd. Published 2015 by John Wiley & Sons, Ltd.
Companion website: www.wiley.com/go/perioperativemed

Major orthopaedic surgery carries a significant risk of VTE with an estimated cumulative 35-day postoperative, untreated risk of symptomatic VTE of 4.3%, compared with a rate of 1.8% for those receiving low molecular weight heparin (LMWH) thromboprophylaxis.

For total hip and knee arthroplasty, a minimum of 10–14 days of thromboprophylaxis with any of LMWH, fondaparinux, apixaban, rivaroxaban, dabigatran, low-dose unfractionated heparin (UFH), adjusted dose vitamin K antagonist (VKA) (e.g. warfarin), aspirin or an intermittent pneumatic compression device (IPCD) is recommended. LMWH is the drug of choice in the guidelines, recommended for a period of 35 days, rather than only 10–14 days. The use of an IPCD in addition to chemical thromboprophylaxis is also encouraged during the hospital stay [4].

TABLE 24.1 Caprini risk assessment model

1 Point	2 Points	3 Points	5 Points
Age 41–60 y	Age 61–74 y	Age ≥75 y	Stroke (<1 mth)
Minor surgery	Arthroscopic surgery	History of VTE	Elective arthroplasty
BMI >25 kg/m²	Major open surgery (>45 min)	Family history of VTE	Hip, pelvis, or leg fracture
Swollen legs	Laparoscopic surgery (>45 min)	Factor V Leiden	Acute spinal cord injury (<1 mth)
Varicose veins	Malignancy	Prothrombin 20210A	
Pregnancy or postpartum	Confined to bed (>72 h)	Lupus anticoagulant	
History of unexplained or recurrent spontaneous abortion	Immobilising plaster cast	Anticardiolipin antibodies	
Oral contraceptives or hormone replacement	Central venous access	Elevated serum homocysteine	
Sepsis (<1 mth)		Heparin-induced thrombocytopenia	
Serious lung disease, including pneumonia (<1 mth)		Other congenital or acquired thrombophilia	
Abnormal pulmonary function			
Acute myocardial infarction			
Heart failure (<1 mth)			
History of inflammatory bowel disease			
Medical patient at bed rest			

Source: Gould et al. [2]. Reproduced with permission of American College of Chest Physicians.
BMI, Body Mass Index; VTE, venous thromboembolism.

	Risk and consequences of major bleeding complications	
Risk of symptomatic VTE	Average risk (~1%)	High risk (~2%) or severe consequences
Very low (<0.5%)	No specific prophylaxis	
Low (~1.5%)	Mechanical prophylaxis, preferably with IPC	
Moderate (~3.0%)	LDUH, LMWH, or mechanical prophylaxis, preferably with IPC	Mechanical prophylaxis, preferably with IPC
High (~6.0%)	LDUH or LMWH plus mechanical prophylaxis with ES or IPC	Mechanical prophylaxis, preferably with IPC, until risk of bleeding diminishes and pharmacologic prophylaxis can be added
High-risk cancer surgery	LDUH or LMWH plus mechanical prophylaxis with ES or IPC and extended-duration prophylaxis with LMWH postdischarge	Mechanical prophylaxis, preferably with IPC, until risk of bleeding diminishes and pharmacologic prophylaxis can be added
High risk, LDUH and LMWH contraindicated or not available	Fondaparinux or low-dose aspirin (160 mg); mechanical prophylaxis, preferably with IPC; or both	Mechanical prophylaxis, preferably with IPC, until risk of bleeding diminishes and pharmacologic prophylaxis can be added

Source: Gould et al. [2]. Reproduced with permission of American College of Chest Physicians.
ES, elastic stockings; IPC, intermittent pneumatic compression; LDUH, low-dose unfractionated heparin; LMWH, low molecular weight heparin; VTE, venous thromboprophylaxis.

The converse of the thrombotic risk is the bleeding risk. Estimating this is sometimes difficult and requires consideration of the operation type and patient risk factors. Direct consultation with the surgeon is recommended.

Thromboprophylaxis options

Chemical

A variety of anticoagulants are available for use as thromboprophylaxis [5,6]. The main therapies are UFH, LMWH, fondaparinux, VKAs, dabigatran, rivaroxaban and apixaban. A review of the clinical trial data for these last three novel oral anticoagulants is available [7]. Dosing is difficult in the obese patient [8].

When starting thromboprophylaxis after surgery, assessment of the bleeding risk should first be made. This should include reviewing the amount, type and progress of drainage on dressings or in surgical drains.

> The highest risk of bleeding occurs if thromboprophylaxis is given 4–8 hours compared with the intermediate interval of 12–24 hours postoperatively, and lowest when given at least 24 hours after surgery.

Mechanical

The use of mechanical devices to prevent VTE has limited data but theoretical benefit in terms of improving venous flow. Early mobilisation is likely to be helpful. Options include elastic stockings (Figure 24.1) and IPCDs (Figure 24.2). In the right setting, used correctly, there seems to be little risk to the patient from use of these devices. A large randomised trial using mechanical and chemical thromboprophylaxis compared with chemical thromboprophylaxis alone is required. Elastic stockings carry a potential risk of falls and pressure sores in the elderly population. Some limitations for use of mechanical devices include the need for an external power source unless battery powered, compliance and cost [2,4,9] (Video 24.1).

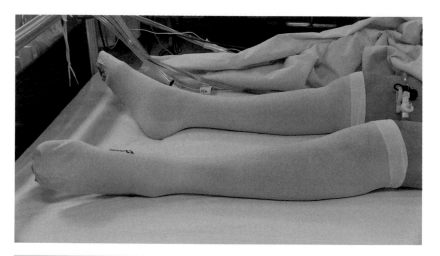

FIGURE 24.1 **Elastic stockings.**

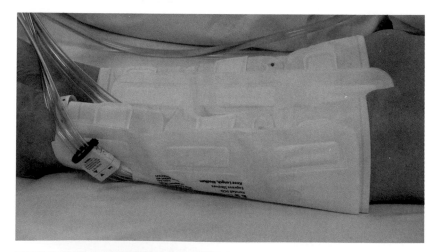

FIGURE 24.2 **Intermittent pneumatic compression device.**

www.wiley.com/go/perioperativemed

VIDEO 24.1 **Options to provide thromboprophylaxis include mechanical means such as elastic stockings and pneumatic compression devices and chemical means such as low molecular weight heparin.**

Current guidelines recommend against inferior vena cava (IVC) filter insertion for primary prevention in orthopaedic and non-orthopaedic surgery.

24

Options when bleeding risk outweighs benefit of thromboprophylaxis

When thromboprophylaxis is recommended but the bleeding risk is too high, options include delaying surgery, using mechanical devices or an IVC filter. Where possible, delaying surgery is the preferred option [2,4].

Surgery in the setting of acute VTE

A patient who has had a VTE in the last three months is at high risk of recurrence; if possible, delay surgery.

Should surgery proceed, thromboprophylaxis should be used postoperatively and when the bleeding risk is controlled, full-dose anticoagulation should be reintroduced. In the setting of acute VTE with DVT, an IVC filter may be useful. Consultation with a haematologist is recommended.

Thromboprophylaxis for those on long-term anticoagulation – role of 'bridging therapy'

Bridging anticoagulation refers to the use of a short-acting anticoagulant, either UFH or LMWH, during interruption of VKA therapy when the INR is not in the therapeutic range. Each patient's clinical situation must be carefully considered (Table 24.3) [10,11].

In general, vitamin K antagonists should be stopped approximately five days before surgery but may be continued for low-risk procedures such as minor dental procedures, minor dermatological procedures and cataract surgery.

TABLE 24.3 Suggested risk stratification for perioperative thromboembolism

Indication for VKA Therapy

Risk Stratum	Mechanical Heart Valve	Atrial Fibrillation	VTE
High[a]	• Any mitral valve prosthesis • Any caged-ball or tilting disc aortic valve prosthesis • Recent (within 6 mths) stroke or transient ischaemic attack	• CHADS$_2$ score of 5 or 6 • Recent (within 3 mths) stroke or transient ischaemic attack • Rheumatic valvular heart disease	• Recent (within 3 mths) VTE • Severe thrombophilia (e.g. deficiency of protein C, protein S, or antithrombin; antiphospholipid antibodies; multiple abnormalities)
Moderate	• Bileaflet aortic valve prosthesis and one or more of the following risk factors: atrial fibrillation prior stroke or transient ischaemic attack, hypertension, diabetes, congestive heart failure, age > 75 y	• CHADS$_2$ score of 3 or 4	• VTE within the past 3–12 mths • Nonsevere thrombophilia (e.g. heterozygous factor V Leiden or prothrombin gene mutation) • Recurrent VTE • Active cancer (treated within 6 mths or palliative)
Low	• Bileaflet aortic valve prosthesis without atrial fibrillation and no other risk factors for stroke	• CHADS$_2$ score of 0 to 2 (assuming no prior stroke or transient ischemic attack)	• VTE > 12 mths previous and no other risk factors

CHADS$_2$ = congestive heart failure, hypertension, age ≥ 75 years, diabetes mellitus, and stroke or transient ischemic attack; VKA = vitamin K antagonist.
[a] High risk patients may also include those with a prior stroke or transient ischaemic attack occuring >3 mths before the planned surgery and a CHADS$_2$ score <5, those with prior thromboembolism during temporary interruption of VKAs, or those undergoing certain types of surgery associated with an increased risk for stroke or other thromboembolism (e.g. cardiac valve replacement, carotid endarterectomy, major vascular surgery).
Source: Douketis et al. [10]. Reproduced with permission of American College of Chest Physicians.

> Bridging therapy with unfractionated heparin should be stopped 4–6 hours preoperatively and therapeutic dose LMWH should be stopped 24 hours preoperatively.

In patients who are receiving bridging anticoagulation for non-high bleeding risk surgery, therapeutic-dose LMWH may be resumed about 24 hours after surgery.

Usually vitamin K antagonists can be resumed 12–24 hours postoperatively after adequate haemostasis is achieved.

Surgeries/procedures considered to have an increased risk of bleeding during perioperative antithrombotic drug administration include urological surgery, pacemaker or implantable defibrillator implantation, colonic polyp resection > 1–2 cm, vascular organs such as kidney, liver, spleen, bowel resection, major surgery, e.g. cancer surgery, joint arthroplasty, reconstructive plastic surgery and cardiac, intracranial or spinal surgery. In these cases, therapeutic-dose LMWH should be resumed after 48–72 hours postoperatively.

Management of patients on novel oral anticoagulants

Novel oral anticoagulants include the direct thrombin inhibitor, dabigatran and the factor Xa inhibitors, rivaroxaban and apixaban. In most cases, it is reasonable to stop such therapies one to two days before elective surgery [12]. In those with renal impairment, three to five days may be necessary. In the case of dabigatran, a thrombin clotting time (TCT) can be performed and if normal, this would reflect the absence of any significant ongoing drug effect. Drug levels can be done in some laboratories.

References

1. National Health and Medical Research Council. *Clinical Practice Guideline for the Prevention of Venous Thromboembolism (Deep Vein Thrombosis and Pulmonary Embolism) in Patients Admitted to Australian Hospitals.* Melbourne, Australia: National Health and Medical Research Council, 2009.

2. Gould MK, Garcia DA, Wren SM, et al. Prevention of VTE in nonorthopedic surgical patients: Antithrombotic Therapy and Prevention of Thrombosis, 9th ed: American College of Chest Physicians Evidence-Based Clinical Practice Guidelines. *Chest*, 2012;**141**(2 Suppl): e227S–277S. doi:10.1378/chest.11-2297

3. Guyatt GH, Eikelboom JW, Gould MK, et al. Approach to outcome measurement in the prevention of thrombosis in surgical and medical patients: Antithrombotic Therapy and Prevention of Thrombosis, 9th ed: American College of Chest Physicians Evidence-Based Clinical Practice Guidelines. *Chest*, 2012;**141**(2 Suppl):e185S–194S. doi:10.1378/ chest.11-2298

4. Falck-Ytter Y, Francis CW, Johanson NA, et al. Prevention of VTE in orthopedic surgery patients: Antithrombotic Therapy and Prevention of Thrombosis, 9th ed: American College of Chest Physicians Evidence-Based Clinical Practice Guidelines. *Chest*, 2012;**141**(2 Suppl): e278S–2325S. doi:10.1378/chest.11-2404

5. Garcia DA, Baglin TP, Weitz JI, Samama MM. Parenteral anticoagulants: Antithrombotic Therapy and Prevention of Thrombosis, 9th ed: American College of Chest Physicians Evidence-Based Clinical Practice Guidelines. *Chest*, 2012;**141**(2 Suppl):e24S–43S. doi:10.1378/chest.11-2291

6. Ageno W, Gallus AS, Wittkowsky A, Crowther M, Hylek EM, Palareti G. Oral anticoagulant therapy: Antithrombotic Therapy and Prevention of Thrombosis, 9th ed: American College of Chest Physicians Evidence-Based Clinical Practice Guidelines. *Chest*, 2012;**141**(2 Suppl): e44S–88S. doi:10.1378/chest.11-2292

7. Garcia D, Libby E, Crowther MA. The new oral anticoagulants. *Blood*, 2010;**115**(1):15–20. doi:10.1182/blood-2009-09-241851

8. Patel JP, Roberts LN, Arya R. Anticoagulating obese patients in the modern era. *British Journal of Haematology*, 2011;**155**(2):137–149. doi:10.1111/j.1365-2141.2011.08826.x

9. Kakkos SK, Caprini JA, Geroulakos G, Nicolaides AN, Stansby GP, Reddy DJ. Combined intermittent pneumatic leg compression and pharmacological prophylaxis for prevention of venous thromboembolism in high-risk patients. *Cochrane Database of Systematic Reviews*, 2008;**4**:CD005258. doi:10.1002/14651858.CD005258.pub2

10. Douketis JD, Spyropoulos AC, Spencer FA, et al. Perioperative management of antithrombotic therapy: Antithrombotic Therapy and Prevention of Thrombosis, 9th ed: American College of Chest Physicians Evidence-Based Clinical Practice Guidelines. *Chest*, 2012;**141** (2 Suppl):e326S–350S. doi:10.1378/chest.11-2298

11. Ortel TL. Perioperative management of patients on chronic antithrombotic therapy. *Hematology: American Society of Hematology American Society of Hematology Education Program*, 2012;**2012**:529–535. doi:10.1182/asheducation-2012.1.529

12. Spyropoulos AC, Douketis JD. How I treat anticoagulated patients undergoing an elective procedure or surgery. *Blood*, 2012;**120**(15):2954–2962. doi:10.1182/Blood-2012-06-415943

Anticoagulants and antiplatelet agents

David Daly

The Alfred Hospital and Monash University, Australia

Many patients receive long-term anticoagulation therapy to prevent thromboembolism. The most common indications are atrial fibrillation (AF), the presence of a mechanical heart valve and venous thromboembolism. Oral anticoagulants include the coumarins (i.e. warfarin), direct thrombin inhibitors (i.e. dabigatran) and anti-Xa inhibitors (i.e. rivaroxaban and apixaban). Many patients receive antiplatelet agents to reduce the incidence and severity of myocardial infarction and stroke. Aspirin is commonly prescribed for primary and secondary prevention of cardiac events. Dual antiplatelet therapy is common after percutaneous coronary interventions.

The perioperative management of these patients involves balancing the risks of perioperative bleeding if anticoagulant and/or antiplatelet agents are continued against the risk of thromboembolism or myocardial infarction (MI) if these agents are interrupted.

Coagulation involves platelets and clotting factors. These are common targets of agents used to minimise venous thromboembolism in the perioperative period (Video 25.1).

Patients on warfarin

There is minimal increased risk of bleeding during surgery if the INR ≤1.5. Warfarin may not need to be interrupted for minor procedures where bleeding risk is low (i.e. cataract, dermatological or dental procedures) but when necessary, withhold warfarin for the preceding five days or give intravenous vitamin K the night before surgery. The use of prothrombin concentrates should be restricted to emergency surgical settings (Table 25.1) [1].

Managing anticoagulant therapy perioperatively requires an assessment of the risk of thrombosis due to temporary cessation of warfarin, versus the risk of bleeding if it is continued or modified. The risk of thromboembolism in patients with non-valvular AF (AF in the absence of rheumatic mitral stenosis, a mechanical or bioprosthetic heart

Perioperative Medicine for the Junior Clinician, First Edition. Edited by Joel Symons, Paul Myles, Rishi Mehra and Christine Ball.
© 2015 John Wiley & Sons, Ltd. Published 2015 by John Wiley & Sons, Ltd.
Companion website: www.wiley.com/go/perioperativemed

www.wiley.com/go/perioperativemed

VIDEO 25.1 Coagulation involves platelets and clotting factors. These are common targets of agents used to minimise venous thromboembolism in the perioperative period.

TABLE 25.1 Suggested dose of Prothrombinex-VF to reverse the anticoagulant effect of warfarin according to initial and targeted INR

Target INR	Initial INR			
	1.5–2.5	2.6–3.5	3.6–10.0	>10.0
0.9–1.3	30 IU/kg	35 IU/kg	50 IU/kg	50 IU/kg
1.4–2.0	15 IU/kg	25 IU/kg	30 IU/kg	40 IU/kg

Source: Tran et al. (1). Reproduced with permission from John Wiley & Sons Ltd.
INR, international normalised ratio; IU, international units.

valve or mitral valve repair) can be predicted by using the $CHADS_2$ score or with the CHA_2DS_2-VASc (Table 25.2). The American Heart Association has recently recommended the CHA_2DS_2-VASc score for assessment of stroke risk in patients with non-valvular AF [2].

Bridging therapy for patients on warfarin

Bridging therapy with UFH or LMWH aims to minimise the risks of both thromboembolism and surgical bleeding. Bridging therapy is associated with added risk of surgical bleeding, the risk of which should be considered in the context of disability resulting from stroke [3]. Refer to Table 25.3 for a current consensus approach to bridging therapy based on risk stratification.

Since management decisions are difficult without an adequate evidence base, guidelines are required. Table 25.4 summarises recommendations on the management of patients on warfarin undergoing invasive procedures, based on 2013 consensus guidelines [4].

Definition and scores for CHADS$_2$ and CHA$_2$DS$_2$-VASc		Stroke risk stratification with the CHADS$_2$ and CHA$_2$DS$_2$-VASc scores	
	Score		Adjusted stroke rate (% per year)
CHADS$_2$		**CHADS$_2$**	
Congestive heart failure	1	0	1.9%
Hypertension	1	1	2.8%
Age ≥ 75 y	1	2	4.0%
Diabetes mellitus	1	3	5.9%
Stroke/transient ischaemic attack/thromboembolism	2	4	8.5%
Maximum score	6	5	12.5%
		6	18.2%
CHA$_2$DS$_2$-VASc		**CHA$_2$DS$_2$-VASc**	
Congestive heart failure	1	0	0%
Hypertension	1	1	1.3%
Age ≥ 75	2	2	2.2%
Diabetes mellitus	1	3	3.2%
Stroke/transient ischaemic attack/thromboembolism	2	4	4.0%
Vascular disease (prior MI, PAD or aortic plaque)	1	5	6.7%
Age 65–74 years	1	6	9.8%
Sex category (e.g. female)	1	7	9.6%
Maximum score	9	8	6.7%
		9	15.2%

Source: Lip et al. [8]. Reproduced with permission from Elsevier Ltd.
MI, myocardial infarction; PAD, peripheral artery disease.

Patients on direct-acting oral anticoagulants

Bridging for patients on a direct-acting oral anticoagulant (DOAC) is not appropriate. For management of preoperative interruption of DOACs, refer to Table 25.5. It is essential to know the level of renal function/creatinine clearance (CrCl). (Normal or mild renal impairment CrCl ≥ 50 mL/min, moderate renal impairment CrCl 30–49 mL/min.)

For postoperative resumption of DOACs, resume 24 hours after low bleeding risk surgery and 48–72 hours after high bleeding risk surgery. A suggested management plan for patients receiving DOACs requiring urgent surgery is summarised in Figure 25.1.

TABLE 25.3 Does my patient need bridging therapy?

Risk of thromboembolism	Non-valvular AF	VTE	Mechanical heart valves
High Bridging therapy seems justified on current evidence	CHADS$_2$ score 5–6 Prior ischaemic stroke/ TIA, embolic events, intracardiac thrombus Rheumatic valvular heart disease	Recent VTE (<3 months) High risk thrombophilia#	Any mechanical mitral valve, two or more mechanical valves, non-bileaflet aortic valve replacement, or aortic-valve replacement with additional risk factors*
Low No bridging therapy required on current evidence	CHADS$_2$ score 0–2	VTE >3 months previously and no additional risk factors (e.g. active cancer)	Aortic valve replacement, bileaflet prosthesis, and no other additional risk factors*
Moderate Individualised by clinician	CHADS$_2$ score 3–4		Bileaflet aortic valve replacement with additional risk factor*

#*Deficiency of antithrombin, protein C or S, antiphospholipid syndrome, or homozygous or double-heterozygous factor V Leiden and prothrombin variant.*
**Additional risk factors include prior stroke, TIA, intracardiac thrombus or cardioembolic event.*
TIA, transient ischaemic attack; VTE, venous thromboembolism.

Managing epidural catheters in the setting of postoperative thrombosis prophylaxis

Management strategies for epidural catheters have been developed based on the pharmacokinetics of the various agents available for thrombosis prophylaxis [5]. The recommendations are based on drug half-life and time to reach maximum plasma concentration or maximum antithrombotic activity (T_{max}) (Table 25.6).

The removal of a neuraxial catheter should be delayed at least two half-lives plus the T_{max} for the specific anticoagulant involved. After two half-lives only 25% of the maximum antithrombotic activity remains.

Note that the elimination half-life of LMWH increases by approximately 40% in patients with a creatinine clearance of less than 30 mL/min.

It takes approximately eight hours for a platelet plug to stabilise and become resistant to antithrombotic agents. Therefore, one should wait at least eight hours less the T_{max} before restarting thrombosis prophylaxis.

Antiplatelet therapy

There are good data suggesting that antiplatelet therapy (APT) reduces morbid cardiac and neurological events when used for secondary prevention indications. The data supporting the use of APT for primary prevention are less clear, with concerns

Patient risk (thrombosis)	Preoperative (elective surgery)	Preoperative (emergency surgery)	Postoperative
Low	Stop warfarin 5 days before surgery Check INR day before surgery. If INR 2–3 give 3 mg vitamin K IV Day of surgery: if INR <1.5, proceed; if INR >1.5, defer surgery	Day of surgery: if INR <1.5, proceed; if INR >1.5, administer PCC; if PCC not available, FFP 10–15 mL/kg	Restart warfarin evening of surgery Usual thromboprophylaxis
High	Stop warfarin 5 days before surgery. When INR <2, start LMWH, i.e. enoxaparin 1 mg/kg twice daily (last dose at least 24 hours prior to surgery) or UFH intravenous infusion at treatment dose (stop infusion 6 hours before surgery) If patient INR is consistently 2–3 then another approach is: Day before surgery: give 3 mg vitamin K IV Day of surgery: if INR <1.5, proceed; if INR >1.5 defer surgery	Check INR before surgery. Administer PCC (see Table 25.1). If PCC not available, FFP 10–15 mL/kg	Restart warfarin the evening of surgery Start parenteral anticoagulation 12–24 hours postoperatively Continue parenteral anticoagulation for a minimum of 5 days and cease 48 hours after target INR is achieved If using LMWH, begin with prophylactic dose. Change to therapeutic dose LMWH 48–72 hours postoperatively If using UFH, avoid bolus and aim for APPT 1.5 times control If patient bleeding risk is high (e.g. intracranial or spinal surgery), consider using prophylactic dose LMWH or UFH only and cease 48 hours after target INR is reached

Source: Modified from Tran et al. [4].
APPT, activated partial prothrombin time; FFP, fresh frozen plasma; INR, international normalised ratio; IV, intravenous; LMWH, low molecular weight heparin; PCC, prothrombin complex concentrate; UFH, unfractionated heparin.

that side effects such as gastrointestinal haemorrhage may offset the benefits of these agents. The benefit of APT is increased when there is a higher incidence of cardiovascular disease, or risk factors for cardiovascular disease, in the population.

Should aspirin be used in the perioperative period?

The POISE-2 trial [6] randomly assigned 10,000 patients who were undergoing non-cardiac surgery and were at risk for vascular complications to receive either aspirin or placebo in the perioperative period. The eligibility criteria can be found in the POISE-2 Supplementary Appendix at nejm.org.

The primary outcome was a composite of death or MI at 30 days. The authors concluded that the administration of aspirin before surgery and throughout the early

Drug (dose)^	Renal function	Low bleeding risk surgery (2 or 3 drug half-lives between last dose and surgery)*	High bleeding risk surgery# (4 or 5 drug half-lives between last dose and surgery)
Dabigatran (150 mg twice daily)			
T½, 12–17 hr	Normal or mild↓	Last dose: 24 hr before surgery	Last dose: 48–72 hr before surgery
T½, 13–23 hr	Moderate↓	Last dose: 48–72 hr before surgery	Last dose: 96 hr before surgery
Rivaroxaban (20 mg once daily)			
T½, 5–9 hr	Normal or mild↓	Last dose: 24 hr before surgery	Last dose: 48–72 hr before surgery
T½, 9–13 hr	Moderate↓	Last dose: 48 hr before surgery	Last dose: 72 hr before surgery
Apixaban (5 mg twice daily)			
T½, 7–8 hr	Normal or mild↓	Last dose: 24 hr before surgery	Last dose: 48–72 hr before surgery
T½, 17–18 hr	Moderate↓	Last dose: 48 hr before surgery	Last dose: 72 hr before surgery

^Estimated half-life (T½) based on calculated renal clearance.
*Aiming for a moderate residual anticoagulation effect at surgery (<12–25%).
Aiming for no or minimal residual anticoagulant effect at surgery (<3–6%).
Source: Tran et al. [9]. Reproduced with permission from John Wiley & Sons Ltd.

postsurgical period had no significant effect on the rate of a composite of death or non-fatal MI but increased the risk of major bleeding.

Patients with a drug-eluting coronary stent (DES) less than one year before surgery and patients with a bare metal coronary stent (BMS) less than six weeks before surgery were excluded from the POISE-2 trial.

Antiplatelet therapy in patients with coronary stents undergoing non-cardiac surgery [7]

Coronary stent thrombosis (ST) usually results in significant MI or death and occurs due to non-endothelialisation of the stent struts. To avoid this devastating complication, wherever possible, continuation of APT is recommended in patients with prior coronary stenting undergoing non-cardiac surgery (refer to Chapter 31 Coronary artery disease and coronary stents).

- *Bare metal stents*: death, MI, stent thrombosis and the need for urgent revascularisation are increased if non-cardiac surgery is performed within six weeks of BMS placement. Elective surgery should therefore be deferred for at least six weeks and ideally three months following percutaneous coronary intervention (PCI) with BMS.
- *Drug-eluting stents*: if dual antiplatelet therapy is ceased and non-cardiac surgery performed within 12 months of DES placement, at least 5% of patients will experience MI, stent thrombosis and/or perioperative death. Accordingly, elective surgery should be deferred for 12 months following DES to minimise these complications.

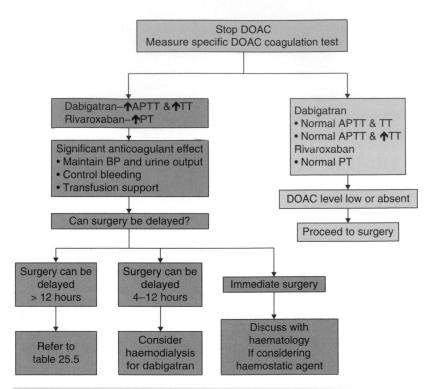

FIGURE 25.1 A suggested management plan for patients receiving direct-acting oral anticoagulant (DOAC) requiring urgent surgery. APTT, activated partial thromboplastin time; BP, blood pressure; PT, prothrombin time; TT, thrombin time.

TABLE 25.6 Pharmacokinetics of anticoagulants in patients with normal creatinine clearance

Medication	Half-life; hr	T_{max}; hr
UFH IV	1–2	Immediately
UFH SC	8–12	2–2.5
LMWH SC	4–6	3–4
Fondaparinux SC	17–21	1–2
Dabigatran oral	14–17	2–4
Rivaroxaban oral	5–9	2.5–4
Apixaban oral	8–15	3

Source: Adapted from Rosencher et al. [5]. Reproduced with permission from John Wiley & Sons Ltd. IV, intravenous; LMWH, low molecular weight heparin; SC, subcutaneous; UFH, unfractionated heparin.

References

1. Tran H, Collecutt M, Whitehead S, Salem HH. Prothrombin complex concentrates used alone in urgent reversal of warfarin anticoagulation. *Internal Medicine Journal*, 2011;**41**(4):337–343. doi:10.1111/j.1445-5994.2010.02237.x

2. January CT, Wann LS, Alpert JS, et al. 2014 AHA/ACC/HRS Guideline for the Management of Patients With Atrial Fibrillation: A Report of the American College of Cardiology/American Heart Association Task Force on Practice Guidelines and the Heart Rhythm Society. *Journal of the American College of Cardiology*, 2014;**64**(21):2246–2280. doi:10.1161/CIR.0000000000000040

3. Baron TH, Kamath PS, McBane RD. Management of antithrombotic therapy in patients undergoing invasive procedures. *New England Journal of Medicine*, 2013;**368**(22):2113–2124. doi:10.1056/NEJMra1206531

4. Tran HA, Chunilal SD, Harper PL, et al. An update of consensus guidelines for warfarin reversal. *Medical Journal of Australia*, 2013;**198**(4):198–199. doi:10.5694/mja12.10614

5. Rosencher N, Bonnet MP, Sessler DI. Selected new antithrombotic agents and neuraxial anaesthesia for major orthopaedic surgery: management strategies. *Anaesthesia*, 2007;**62**(11):1154–1160. doi:10.1111/j.1365-2044.2007.05195.x

6. Devereaux PJ, Mrkobrada M, Sessler DI, et al. Aspirin in patients undergoing noncardiac surgery. *New England Journal of Medicine*, 2014;**370**(16):1494–1503. doi:10.1056/NEJMoa1401105

7. Cardiac Society of Australia and New Zealand. Guidelines for the management of antiplatelet therapy in patients with coronary stents undergoing non-cardiac surgery. *Heart Lung Circulation*, 2010;**19**(1):2–10. doi:10.1016/j.hlc.2009.10.008

8. Lip GY, Tse HF, Lane DA. Atrial fibrillation. *Lancet*, 2012;**379**(9816):648–661. doi:10.1016/S0140-6736(11)61514-6

9. Tran H, Joseph J, Young L, et al. New oral anticoagulants: a practical guide on prescription, laboratory testing and peri-procedural/bleeding management. *Internal Medicine Journal*, 2014;**44**(6):525–536. doi:10.1111/imj.12448

26 Diabetes medication

Shane Hamblin

The Alfred Hospital, Western Health, Monash University
and The University of Melbourne, Australia

The traditional 'insulin sliding scale' is no longer recommended for the perioperative management of diabetes and hyperglycaemia. Perioperative diabetes management can be complicated; a generic recipe does not exist.

Key considerations for perioperative management

- Type of diabetes
- Type of medication
- Type of surgery
- HbA$_1$c result
- Presence or absence of diabetes complications

People with diabetes have a higher rate of asymptomatic heart disease [1]. Peripheral neuropathy is also important because of the risk of pressure injury to the heels.

Type of diabetes

This is a critical step. It should not be assumed that an older person taking insulin has type 2 diabetes. Diabetic ketoacidosis (DKA) will occur perioperatively in type 1 diabetes if insulin is withheld for days. Small doses of quick-acting insulin usually will not prevent this.

Important information includes:

- age at diagnosis
- did insulin therapy commence within a year of diagnosis?
- history of DKA or acid in the blood with high glucose readings?
- a diagnosis of type 1 diabetes.

Perioperative Medicine for the Junior Clinician, First Edition. Edited by Joel Symons, Paul Myles, Rishi Mehra and Christine Ball.
© 2015 John Wiley & Sons, Ltd. Published 2015 by John Wiley & Sons, Ltd.
Companion website: www.wiley.com/go/perioperativemed

Uncertainty may remain because type 1 diabetes can occur in older patients and in patients previously on oral agents (latent autoimmune diabetes of adults). Although rare, DKA can occur in type 2 diabetes. In uncertain cases, it is safer to manage a patient as if they have type 1 diabetes.

Patients with HbA_1c levels above 10% or a blood glucose over 15 mmol/L should be postponed if possible.

Type of medication

Treatment for type 2 diabetes is changing rapidly, with many classes of oral hypoglycaemics now available (Table 26.1) plus a variety of injectables (Table 26.2).

Type 1 diabetes is most commonly treated with 'basal-bolus' insulin (subcutaneous long-acting basal insulin once or twice daily with boluses of prandial quick-acting insulin). Continuous subcutaneous quick-acting insulin infusion (CSII) pumps are becoming more common. A diminishing number use premixed insulin regimens.

Type of surgery

Same-day ('minor') surgery requires clear and complete communication; preadmission clinic assessment or advice from the patient's usual diabetes team is critical. A written plan should be provided to the patient and documented in the medical record.

TABLE 26.1 **Oral hypoglycaemic agents**

Drug	Main mode of action
Metformin	Suppresses hepatic glucose output
Sulphonylureas Gliclazide Glimepiride Glipizide Glibenclamide (Glibenclamide also available in tablet with metformin)	Stimulate insulin release from pancreatic beta cells
Acarbose	Delays carbohydrate absorption by alpha-glucosidase inhibition in small intestine
Thiazolidinediones Pioglitazone (Actos) Rosiglitazone (Avandia) (Rosiglitazone available in tablet with metformin)	Improve insulin sensitivity through PPAR-gamma receptor
DPP4 inhibitors Sitagliptin (Januvia) Linagliptin (Trajenta) Saxagliptin (Onglyza) Vildagliptin (Galvus) Alogliptin (Nesina) (Most available in tablet with metformin)	Prolong endogenous incretin action (mainly GLP-1)
SGLT2 inhibitors Dapagliflozin (Forxiga) Empagliflozin (Jardiance)	Promote glycosuria by inhibition of renal sodium-glucose co-transporter-2

TABLE 26.2 Pharmacokinetics of subcutaneous injectables used for diabetes

Injectable	Onset	Peak	Offset
Quick-acting insulin analogues Apidra Humalog NovoRapid	10–20 minutes	1–3 hours	3–5 hours
Soluble human insulin Actrapid Humulin R	20–30 minutes	1–3 hours	6–8 hours
Intermediate-acting insulin Humulin NPH Protaphane	1.5–2 hours	4–12 hours	Up to 24 hours
Long-acting insulin Lantus (Glargine) Levemir (Detemir)	2–4 hours 2–4 hours	6–8 hours 6–8 hours	24 hours 12–24 hours
Premixed insulin Mixtard 30/70; 50/50 NovoMix30 Humulin 30/70 HumalogMix25 HumalogMix50	10–20 minutes	1–4 hours	Up to 24 hours
GLP-1 analogues Byetta (exenatide) twice daily Bydureon (extended-release exenatide) weekly	10–20 minutes 10–20 minutes 10–20 minutes	2 hours Peak 1–2 hours Peak 2–6 weeks	10 hours 8–10 weeks (single injection). Weekly injections steady state at 8 weeks
Victoza (liraglutide) daily		8–12 hours	24 hours

Multi-day admission ('major') surgery generally implies a greater risk of instability and complications.

Medication management

Note: This information does not replace local hospital guidelines. Refer to Figure 26.1 for a summary of perioperative diabetes management.

> **The goal of therapy in people with diabetes postoperatively is to maintain blood glucose levels between 5 and 10 mmol/L.**
>
> **It is never appropriate to write up insulin orders for days in advance without reviewing the effectiveness of those orders every day (preferably in person).**
>
> **Insulin infusion is often the best treatment postoperatively (with 5% dextrose infusion) but only if a well-supervised area is available.**

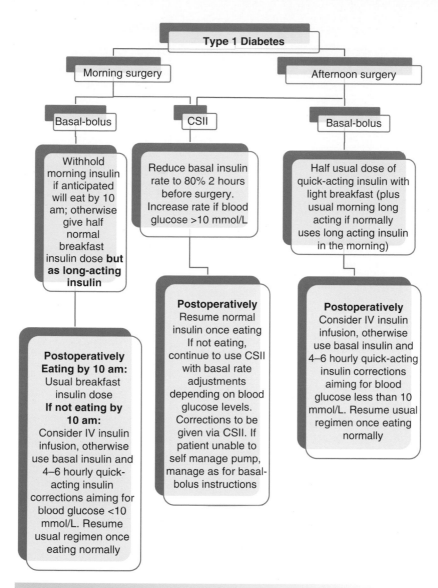

FIGURE 26.1 Perioperative diabetes management for type 1 and type 2 diabetes.
For patients treated with insulin as well as OHAs and/or GLP-1 analogues, follow both sides of the chart. Where there is doubt regarding type of diabetes, treat the patient as if they have type 1 diabetes. *Note*: In type 1 patients treated with premixed insulin or insulin combinations in a syringe, for morning surgery give half normal morning dose as long-acting insulin on admission to the hospital; for afternoon surgery give half usual dose at home with light breakfast. Basal-bolus, long-acting subcutaneous insulin with prandial quick-acting insulin; CSII, continuous subcutaneous insulin infusion ('insulin pump'); OHA, oral hypoglycaemic agents.

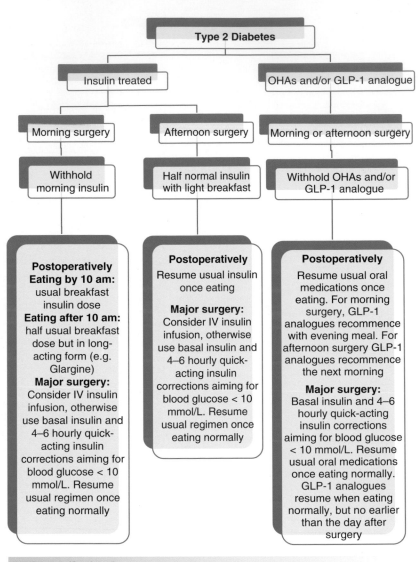

```
                         ┌──────────────────┐
                         │  Type 2 Diabetes │
                         └──────────────────┘
             ┌──────────────────┐      ┌──────────────────────────┐
             │  Insulin treated │      │  OHAs and/or GLP-1 analogue │
             └──────────────────┘      └──────────────────────────┘
```

Type 2 Diabetes

- **Insulin treated**
  - **Morning surgery**
    - **Withhold morning insulin**
  - **Afternoon surgery**
    - **Half normal insulin with light breakfast**
- **OHAs and/or GLP-1 analogue**
  - **Morning or afternoon surgery**
    - **Withhold OHAs and/or GLP-1 analogue**

Postoperatively
Eating by 10 am: usual breakfast insulin dose
Eating after 10 am: half usual breakfast dose but in long-acting form (e.g. Glargine)
Major surgery: Consider IV insulin infusion, otherwise use basal insulin and 4–6 hourly quick-acting insulin corrections aiming for blood glucose < 10 mmol/L. Resume usual regimen once eating normally

Postoperatively Resume usual insulin once eating
Major surgery: Consider IV insulin infusion, otherwise use basal insulin and 4–6 hourly quick-acting insulin corrections aiming for blood glucose < 10 mmol/L. Resume usual regimen once eating normally

Postoperatively Resume usual oral medications once eating. For morning surgery, GLP-1 analogues recommence with evening meal. For afternoon surgery GLP-1 analogues recommence the next morning
Major surgery: Basal insulin and 4–6 hourly quick-acting insulin corrections aiming for blood glucose < 10 mmol/L. Resume usual oral medications once eating normally. GLP-1 analogues resume when eating normally, but no earlier than the day after surgery

FIGURE 26.1 (Continued)

Type 2 diabetes

Minor surgery

Morning procedure

- Withhold diabetic medication (including insulin) on the morning of surgery.
- *Oral agents and/or GLP-1 analogues:* if surgery has occurred early and the patient is recovered and eating by 10 am, give normal morning medications with that meal except for GLP-1 analogues (these can cause delayed gastric emptying and

PONV). Otherwise, withhold morning medication, administer subcutaneous quick-acting insulin, just before the patient has something to eat, provided the blood glucose is above 6 mmol/L, (e.g. 4–6 units). Give usual medications in the evening if the patient is eating normally.

- *Insulin:* give normal morning dose of insulin postoperatively if the patient is eating by 10 am. Otherwise, give half the normal morning dose as long-acting insulin; supplement with quick-acting insulin if required.

Afternoon procedure
- No oral agents or GLP-1 analogues preoperatively.
- *Insulin:* give half the normal insulin dose with a light breakfast.
- Continue with the patient's usual treatment once they are eating, apart from GLP-1 analogues which should be withheld until the next day.

Major surgery

Preoperative management is the same as above.

Postoperatively, intravenous insulin infusion is recommended in settings where there are experienced staff and the capacity to regularly monitor blood glucose.

Otherwise:

- if the patient is taking insulin, give the usual dose of long-acting insulin subcutaneously. If the patient is using premixed insulin, administer the long-acting proportion as glargine
- if the patient is not treated with insulin, start with 10 units glargine
- administer four to six hourly quick-acting insulin supplements as required
- resume usual diabetes treatment once the patient is eating normally
- delay administration of GLP-1 analogues until the next day
- restart metformin when the patient is haemodynamically stable and renal function returns to baseline.

Type 1 diabetes

> **Principle:** To avoid ketoacidosis, there must always be insulin action present.

Morning procedure (patients taking basal-bolus insulin)

- Give the normal evening dose of long-acting insulin the night before surgery (10% less if there is a tendency for low fasting glucose).
- If the patient will eat by 10 am, delay the usual morning insulin until then.
- Otherwise, give half the normal breakfast quick-acting dose *as long-acting insulin.*
- Blood glucose two hourly preoperatively to observe blood glucose trend (if the BSL > 10 mmol/L, administer small doses of subcutaneous quick-acting insulin four to six hourly).
- Alternatively, if experienced staff are available, a variable rate IV insulin infusion (with concomitant 5% dextrose IV) may be used.
- If prolonged fasting is experienced preoperatively (e.g. more than four hours after missed breakfast), intravenous 5% dextrose infusion should be commenced.

Afternoon procedure

Half the usual quick-acting insulin is given with a light breakfast along with usual long-acting insulin (if long-acting morning insulin normally taken). Check blood glucose two hourly prior to surgery. If it is above 10 mmol/L, small corrective doses of subcutaneous quick-acting insulin may be given every four to six hours.

Postoperative care

- If an IV insulin infusion is not feasible, subcutaneous long-acting (usual basal dose) insulin with supplements of quick-acting insulin (proportionate to the patient's usual prandial doses) should be given every four to six hours.
- While the patient is nil orally, provide a continuous dextrose infusion, preferably via a dedicated line.
- When the patient is eating normally, resume usual basal-bolus insulin regimen, with supplemental quick-acting insulin given along with the usual prandial quick-acting insulin.
- Whether eating normally or not, at least *daily review* of the adequacy of insulin treatment is essential. Adjust the regimen appropriately, increasing or reducing the usual dose based on how much supplemental insulin was required the previous day.
- Check blood ketone levels (or if unavailable, urine ketones) at least daily while not eating.

Insulin pumps (CSII) (Video 26.1)

These should only be used if the patient can self-manage them pre- and postoperatively. Staff need to be shown how to stop the pump in case severe hypoglycaemia occurs. These pumps should be reduced to 80% basal rate two hours before surgery and two-hourly blood glucose checked. If blood glucose >10 mmol/L, correct it with the pump. Ensure the anaesthetist is aware that a CSII is being used. Site the CSII cannula away from the surgical site.

www.wiley.com/go/perioperativemed

VIDEO 26.1 Insulin pumps come in a variety of forms and allow continuous insulin absorption and improved blood glucose control. They may need to be reprogrammed in the perioperative period.

Dexamethasone

Although widely used for PONV prophylaxis (refer to Chapter 79 Postoperative nausea and vomiting), dexamethasone should be avoided in type 1 diabetes. The anaesthetic record should be checked carefully if the patient experiences marked postoperative hyperglycaemia despite appropriate insulin management.

Reference

1. Koistinen MJ. Prevalence of asymptomatic myocardial ischaemia in diabetic subjects. *BMJ*, 1990;**301**(6743):92–95. doi:10.1136/bmj.301.6743.92

Further reading

American Association of Clinical Endocrinologists and American Diabetes Association. Consensus statement on inpatient glycemic control. *Diabetes Care*, 2009;**32**(6):1119–1131.

Australian Diabetes Society. *Peri-operative Diabetes Management Guidelines*. www.diabetessociety. com.au/position-statements.asp

Dhatariya K, Flanagan D, Hilton L, et al. *Management of Adults with Diabetes Undergoing Surgery and Elective Procedures: Improving Standards.* www.diabetes.org.uk/Documents/ Professionals/Reports%20and%20statistics/Management%20of%20adults%20with%20 diabetes%20undergoing%20surgery%20and%20elective%20procedures%20-%20 improving%20standards.pdf

26

Steroid medication

Shane Hamblin

The Alfred Hospital, Western Health, Monash University
and The University of Melbourne, Australia

Careful management of perioperative steroid medication prevents significant adverse outcomes. Many patients require chronic glucocorticoid therapy ('steroid medication') for a variety of medical conditions. A proportion of these develop iatrogenic secondary hypoadrenalism due to chronic suppression of the hypothalamic-pituitary-adrenal axis (refer to Chapter 102 Case Study 7 Addisonian crisis). Secondary adrenal insufficiency may also occur due to pituitary failure (e.g. pituitary tumour or haemorrhage, pituitary irradiation, trauma). A small group of patients have primary adrenal failure (e.g. Addison's disease).

Normal stress response

Rises in cortisol (along with the other 'counter-regulatory' hormones: adrenaline, glucagon and growth hormone) occur when a person is subject to stress. Common causes of physical stress include injury and illness. Psychological stresses which usually generate a cortisol rise include fear and pain. There is marked variability in the cortisol increase depending on the type and duration of the stress as well as individual factors.

Perioperative cortisol responses

Hospitalised patients have multiple influences promoting cortisol release: pain, surgery, sepsis, emotional distress. Interestingly, the major rise in cortisol occurs on tracheal extubation and in the hours after surgery, rather than during surgery itself [1].

Adults usually have cortisol responses proportionate to the type and duration of surgery. They have less cortisol rise with minor procedures requiring only sedation, compared with major surgery and full general anaesthesia. The cortisol stress response to sedation and anaesthesia in the paediatric age group is not as well characterised. Cortisol rises in children appear to be similar, irrespective of the type of sedation or whether the procedure is for imaging, endoscopy or minor surgery [2]. Some studies report little change in cortisol in healthy children undergoing surgery with general anaesthesia [3].

The mean adult daily unstressed cortisol output from the adrenal glands is approximately 15 mg [4]. The most commonly used steroids in clinical practice are prednisolone and dexamethasone. In terms of glucocorticoid activity, 15 mg

Perioperative Medicine for the Junior Clinician, First Edition. Edited by Joel Symons, Paul Myles, Rishi Mehra and Christine Ball.
© 2015 John Wiley & Sons, Ltd. Published 2015 by John Wiley & Sons, Ltd.
Companion website: www.wiley.com/go/perioperativemed

hydrocortisone is roughly equivalent to 4 mg prednisolone or 0.6 mg dexamethasone. It seems likely that previous guidelines for steroid replacement were overgenerous and that lower replacement doses may be sufficient.

Management of steroid medication

Addison's disease

Routine medical management of Addison's disease includes ensuring the patient knows the importance of increasing steroid cover at times of illness. Patients are encouraged to wear a bracelet or 'dog tag' to identify that they have this condition. However, many patients do not like wearing them. In such cases, a card stating the diagnosis placed next to their licence or other identification will alert medical staff, should they present with an altered conscious state and be incapable of giving a medical history.

High-dose hydrocortisone has sufficient mineralocorticoid action to make fludrocortisone dose increases unnecessary. Dexamethasone, however, is a pure glucocorticoid with minimal mineralocorticoid action, so increased doses of mineralocorticoid are required if dexamethasone is the only glucocorticoid being used at the time of increased stress.

Minor procedures
Assuming well-controlled stable Addison's disease, minor procedures only require doubling of the dose of oral glucocorticoid on the day of the procedure. For colonoscopy, an increase (doubling) in glucocorticoid dose from the day before (during the bowel preparation phase) as well as the day of the procedure is advisable. Altered absorption of the oral medication is not usually a problem with the bowel preparation. It is not necessary to increase the mineralocorticoid dose (fludrocortisone). It is advisable to also give hydrocortisone (50–100 mg IV) at the time of the procedure.

Same-day surgery
For adult patients undergoing same-day surgical procedures requiring anaesthesia, IV hydrocortisone (50–100 mg) is usually given by the anaesthetist at the start of the procedure. These patients do not usually require additional parenteral steroid replacement after surgery. Postoperatively, the patient's usual oral glucocorticoid dose is doubled for one to two days, depending on their clinical status.

If there is vomiting postoperatively, IV hydrocortisone (e.g. 50 mg) should be given eight hourly until the patient is tolerating oral intake. There should be a low threshold to keep such patients in hospital overnight.

Multi-day admissions
The same initial treatment applies regarding IV hydrocortisone given at the start of surgery. Postoperatively, IV hydrocortisone 50 mg eight hourly is usually recommended. The dose is progressively reduced over the next couple of days, depending on the extent and type of surgery and the patient's clinical state.

If surgery prevents oral intake for a prolonged period (e.g. bowel resection), IV hydrocortisone should continue until oral intake is re-established. The dose of IV glucocorticoid is progressively reduced over several days postoperatively.

If clinical setbacks occur (e.g. infection, pulmonary embolism), the dose of glucocorticoid should be temporarily increased to cover additional stress requirements (e.g. revert to 50 mg eight hourly IV), then progressively reduced as the clinical situation stabilises.

Patients treated with long-term steroids

A patient is at risk of clinically relevant adrenal suppression if a daily dose of prednisolone 10 mg or more (dexamethasone dose 1.5 mg) has been used for more than three weeks.

When surgical procedures are required, it is wise to manage such patients as being adrenally insufficient using the guidelines above. If time permits, adrenal reserve may be assessed preoperatively with an adrenocorticotrophic hormone (ACTH) stimulation test.

Hypopituitarism

A patient with known secondary hypoadrenalism from pituitary disease is managed the same way as for Addison's disease.

Perioperative management of a patient undergoing selective pituitary adenoma removal has been a matter of debate over the past decade. Traditional blanket coverage with hydrocortisone postoperatively has been challenged (unless the patient has pituitary-dependent Cushing's disease). Most patients do not require glucocorticoid in this setting, if they were eupituitary preoperatively, as hypopituitarism is unusual with modern neurosurgical techniques. If routine glucocorticoid cover is not given, daily postoperative morning cortisol measurements are recommended to ensure the levels are satisfactory [5].

Glucocorticoid management for various procedures is summarised in Table 27.1.

Safe perioperative management of patients requiring steroid medication is achievable, provided appropriate dose adjustments are made according to the extent of surgery and the patient is carefully reviewed.

TABLE 27.1 **Glucocorticoid management for various procedures**

Gastroscopy; interventional radiology procedures	Colonoscopy	Same-day surgery	Multi-day admission surgery
Double oral dose on day of procedure	Double oral dose day before and on day of procedure	IV hydrocortisone 50–100 mg at time of procedure	IV hydrocortisone 50–100 mg at time of procedure
IV hydrocortisone 50 mg at time of procedure	IV hydrocortisone 50 mg at time of procedure	Double oral dose for 1–2 days postoperatively	IV hydrocortisone 50 mg 8 hourly after surgery. Progressive reduction over 2–4 days
			Oral therapy (2–3 times normal dose initially) when able to eat. Reduce to normal dose over a few days

References

1. Udelsman R, Norton JA, Jelenich SE, et al. Responses of the hypothalamic-pituitary-adrenal and renin-angiotensin axes and the sympathetic system during controlled surgical and anesthetic stress. *Journal of Clinical Endocrinology and Metabolism*, 1987;**64**(5):986–994. doi:10.1210/jcem-64-5-986

2. Hsu AA, von Elten K, Chan D, et al. Characterization of the cortisol stress response to sedation and anesthesia in children. *Journal of Clinical Endocrinology and Metabolism*, 2012;**97**(10):E1830–1835. doi:10.1210/jc.2012-1499

3. Taylor LK, Auchus RJ, Baskin LS, Miller WL. Cortisol response to operative stress with anesthesia in healthy children. *Journal of Clinical Endocrinology and Metabolism*, 2013;**98**(9):3687–3693. doi:10.1210/jc.2013-2148

4. Esteban NV, Loughlin T, Yergey AL, et al. Daily cortisol production rate in man determined by stable isotope dilution/mass spectrometry. *Journal of Clinical Endocrinology and Metabolism*, 1991;**72**(1):39–45. doi:10.1210/jcem-72-1-39

5. Inder WJ, Hunt PJ. Glucocorticoid replacement in pituitary surgery: guidelines for perioperative assessment and management. *Journal of Clinical Endocrinology and Metabolism*, 2002;**87**(6):2745–2750. doi: 10.1210/jcem.87.6.8547

28 Opioids and opioid addiction

Meena Mittal[1], Nicholas Christelis[2] and David Lindholm[1]

[1] The Alfred Hospital, Australia
[2] The Alfred Hospital and Epworth Hospitals and Monash University, Australia

Opioids are the mainstay of analgesic therapy after moderate to major surgery. They are widely and effectively used for the management of acute pain, malignant pain and, in carefully selected patients, chronic non-malignant pain.

Opioid-dependent patients include those using prescription opioids for chronic pain, substitution opioids for addiction to illicit substances and illicit opioids, both prescription and non-prescription.

Refer to Box 28.1 for a description of terms used in this chapter.

Access to appropriate and effective pain control should be considered a human right, even in opioid-tolerant patients, but these patients can be challenging in the perioperative setting (Box 28.2).

Preoperative assessment

In addition to a routine history, a specific pain-related history should be taken.

- What surgery is planned? Expected analgesic requirement post surgery?
- Previous experience of acute pain (what worked)
- Experience of chronic pain – pain diagnosis, usual pain scores, usual function
- Patient's expectation of analgesia after surgery
- Prescribed and non-prescribed opioids (illicit, alcohol, nicotine) and doses and duration of use
- Contact details of prescriber and dispensing pharmacy
- Non-opioid medications
- History of misuse and addiction, withdrawal, social network
- Allergies

Perioperative Medicine for the Junior Clinician, First Edition. Edited by Joel Symons, Paul Myles, Rishi Mehra and Christine Ball.
© 2015 John Wiley & Sons, Ltd. Published 2015 by John Wiley & Sons, Ltd.
Companion website: www.wiley.com/go/perioperativemed

BOX 28.1 Glossary

Opiate	Refers *only* to natural alkaloid drugs derived from the opium poppy plant (*Papaver somniferum*), e.g. morphine, codeine
Opioid	Refers to all endogenous (neuropeptides) or exogenous substances with morphine-like properties that are blocked by antagonists such as naloxone, e.g. oxycodone, fentanyl, methadone
Opioid-induced tolerance	Exposure to the same amount of drug results in a diminished effect or there is need for markedly increased amounts of the drug to achieve the same desired effect
Opioid-induced hyperalgesia	A paradoxical response to opioid agonists, which results in heightened pain sensitivity rather than analgesia
Opioid withdrawal	Refers to the wide range of syndromes that occur after sudden reduction or cessation of opioids after heavy and/or prolonged use. Physical symptoms include restlessness, insomnia, headaches, abdominal cramps, vomiting, diarrhoea, perspiration, muscle and joint pain, tremors, rhinitis, tachycardia, yawning. Psychological symptoms include anxiety, depression, cravings, poor concentration, irritability, agitation, mood swings and suicidal ideation.
Addiction/substance dependence	Addiction (termed substance dependence by the American Psychiatric Association) is a maladaptive pattern of substance use, leading to clinically significant impairment or distress, as manifested by three or more of the following occurring in a 12-month period (DSM 4 criteria) [7]

a) Tolerance
b) Withdrawal (physiological dependence)
c) The substance is taken in larger amounts or over a longer period than intended
d) There is persistent desire or unsuccessful efforts to cut down or control substance use
e) A great deal of time is spent in activities necessary to obtain the substance
f) Important social, occupational or recreational activities are given up or reduced because of substance use
g) The substance use is continued despite knowledge of harm caused by it

28

BOX 28.2 Perioperative issues related to opioid-tolerant and opioid-addicted patients

Adequate management of postoperative acute pain	Poor acute pain control leads to slower postsurgical recovery, increased pulmonary complications (infection, atelectasis), slower mobilisation, delayed discharge and increased incidence of persistent postsurgical chronic pain Chronic opioid use leads to higher pain scores, increased opioid consumption postoperatively and challenging acute pain management
Opioid tolerance	Tolerance may develop due to prolonged use of high-dose opioids; treat with liberal doses of appropriate analgesics including opioids [8] *Note*: Patients may display incomplete cross-tolerance (ICT) and are not necessarily tolerant to another opioid. The advantage of ICT is that if someone becomes tolerant to opioids, e.g. cancer pain, a *new* opioid can have beneficial effects and analgesia but also cause new side effects including sedation and respiratory depression
Opioid withdrawal	Risk of withdrawal secondary to abrupt cessation of opioids is high, particularly with long-term high-dose opioids (refer to Chapter 99 Case Study 4 Opioid withdrawal).
Opioid-induced adverse effects	The side effect profile (e.g. sedation, respiratory depression, nausea and constipation) can limit opioid use in high doses. Close monitoring for opioid toxicity is required
Pain assessment	Pain scores may not be accurate in patients with chronic pain; baseline 5/10 (NRS) may be normal for a chronic pain patient
Confounding factors	It is important to exclude a surgical or medical cause leading to exacerbation of pain postoperatively before attributing it to opioid tolerance or patient behaviour. Depression, anxiety, psychosis, personality disorders co-exist in patients with chronic pain and can worsen pain perception and pain experience in the postoperative period
Patient behaviour	Patients may be demanding or mistrustful due to the effect of illicit substances, poor social circumstances, personality or previous negative experiences involving judgemental attitude of health professionals
Physician attitude	A patient history of illicit substance use may lead to more cautious use of opioids by physicians and undertreatment of pain

Perioperative management of opioid analgesics

> The key to managing these patients is consistency of care. Develop an individualised management strategy with the acute pain service (APS), anaesthetist, surgical team and other physicians caring for the patient.

Clear communication and documentation are vital. Adopt a non-judgemental, caring approach and gain patient trust; respect privacy whilst setting clear boundaries and realistic expectations for the patient. To manage demanding behaviour, a contract may be formed with the patient highlighting the proposed treatment plan [1–3].

Preoperatively

Identify opioid dependence (have a high index of suspicion and consider all patients on oral or IV opioids to be opioid tolerant to some degree). Verify the opioid type and baseline dose and document these clearly. Continue the baseline opioid dose even when the patient is fasting. Continue usual opioids (oral, patch, epidural, intrathecal) on the morning of surgery. Involve the APS early and formulate a management plan. Finally, educate the patient about the potential for increased postoperative pain and alternatives to opioids, including regional analgesia. Address patient fears of inadequate pain control with reassurance.

Intraoperatively

Maintain baseline opioids, including transdermal or intrathecal ones. Anticipate higher requirements of short-acting opioids. Avoid direct heat to fentanyl patches (this increases uptake). Be aware of drugs interacting with opioids and avoid them if possible.

Postoperatively

Inform the APS early. Involve drug and alcohol and psychiatric services if relevant. Continue the usual dose of opioid (or a modest increase of 20–30% for major surgery) as background to prevent opioid withdrawal. If the patient is nil orally, the oral dose will require appropriate equivalent conversion to appropriate IV opioid. Continue transdermal opioid if it was used preoperatively. Give additional short-acting opioid for analgesia for breakthrough pain, anticipating higher requirements. Commence patient-controlled analgesia (PCA) in the recovery room and titrate opioids aggressively to achieve adequate pain control. Requirements may be two to four times the dose needed in the opioid-naïve patient but no data suggest the exact predictability [4].

Maintain appropriate monitoring of vitals and the sedation score to monitor for overmedication and withdrawal. Consider admission to the HDU especially if a background opioid infusion is used. Monitor functional activity score (FAS) for objective pain assessment as pain scores on the 11-point numerical rating scale (NRS) (0–10) are subjective and may be unreliable.

Formulate a plan for weaning to reach preoperative doses two to four weeks post discharge. Consider conversion to methadone to reduce excessive doses of opioid, reduce tolerance, prevent opioid rotation and control behavioural issues of dependence. Monitor for opioid-induced hyperalgesia (this requires a dose reduction in opioids, not an increase).

Perioperative management of non-opioid analgesics

There is strong evidence supporting the use of multimodal analgesia to manage pain effectively postsurgically and also to minimise opioid use.

Preoperatively

Continue use of usual non-opioid analgesics unless contraindicated by surgery, e.g. COX-2 inhibitors or gabapentinoids. Consider regional anaesthesia/analgesia, e.g. neuraxial catheter, local tissue infiltration, nerve and plexus blockade unless there is a patient or surgical contraindication. Consider a preoperative loading dose of non-opioid such as pregabalin. Preliminary evidence suggests this is beneficial in reducing opioid consumption in the first 24 hours postoperatively [5].

Intraoperatively

Use regional anaesthesia/analgesia or wound infiltration wherever possible. Consider the use of adjuvants like ketamine infusion, IV COX-2 inhibitors (e.g. parecoxib) and/or IV tramadol.

Postoperatively

Use multimodal analgesia (refer to Chapter 93 Acute pain). These include a combination of the following.

- *Simple analgesics*
  - Paracetamol, NSAIDS, tramadol.
- *Complex analgesics*
  - Gabapentinoids (pregabalin/ gabapentin) – there is evidence to suggest that gabapentinoids are opioid sparing in the acute setting and may reduce progression to persistent postsurgical pain [6].
  - Antidepressants (amitriptyline, nortriptyline, duloxetine) for neuropathic pain or hyperalgesic states.
  - Ketamine infusion as an opioid sparing, antineuropathic agent with a role in reduction of opioid tolerance and opioid-induced hyperalgesia.
  - Lignocaine infusion as an antineuropathic agent. Limited evidence suggests an opioid-sparing benefit but it may be used when the patient is opioid unresponsive.
  - Clonidine for management of withdrawal, tolerance and small analgesic benefit.
- *Regional analgesia*
  - Continue nerve blockade and/or neuraxial analgesia. Always have a low threshold for using local anaesthetic techniques in opioid-tolerant patients as these can provide effective analgesia and greatly reduce the amount of systemic analgesic required. *Discuss this early with the anaesthetist, pain service or perioperative physician.*
- Management should include *non-pharmacotherapy*
  - Information provision (education), stress/tension reduction (relaxation and hypnotic strategies) and cognitive-behavioural interventions.

The patient on buprenorphine

The pharmacodynamic properties of high-dose buprenorphine, e.g. 4–32 mg/day, are unique. It is a partial opioid agonist with a high affinity for the opioid receptor and a long half-life. This means that it binds to the opioid receptor firmly but does not cause any meaningful analgesia and does not dissociate from other opioids like morphine. This makes supplemental analgesia with other opioids very difficult, i.e. *opioids generally do not work in this group.*

These patients should be managed by experts (pain specialists, anaesthetists, addiction specialists).

Note: Doses of methadone or buprenorphine should not be altered without support from pain or addiction specialists. These drugs, particularly methadone, have unpredictable pharmacodynamics, can have multiple interactions with other drugs and the complications can include unpredictable and even delayed respiratory depression.

Discharge planning

Aim to discharge the patient on their preoperative oral opioid dose if they have chronic pain. Consider methadone/buprenorphine if there is illicit substance use or behavioural issues of dependence (even in chronic pain patients). This transition can be challenging so liaise with APS and drug and alcohol services for guidance. Organise follow-up with a chronic pain clinic or drug and alcohol clinic.

> It is vital to communicate with the general practitioner and provide details of the management issues in the hospital and the plan for weaning from medications.

28

References

1. Ballantyne JC, LaForge KS. Opioid dependence and addiction during opioid treatment of chronic pain. *Pain*, 2007;**129**(3):235–255. doi:10.1016/j.pain.2007.03.028

2. May JA, White HC, Leonard-White A, Warltier DC, Pagel PS. The patient recovering from alcohol or drug addiction: special issues for the anesthesiologist. *Anesthesia and Analgesia*, 2001;**92**(6):1601–1608.

3. Rosenblatt AB, Mekhail NA. Management of pain in addicted/illicit and legal substance abusing patients. *Pain Practice*, 2005;**5**(1):2–10. doi:10.1111/j.1533-2500.2005.05102.x

4. Carroll IR, Angst MS, Clark JD. Management of perioperative pain in patients chronically consuming opioids. *Regional Anesthesia and Pain Medicine*, 2004;**29**(6):576–591. doi:10.1016/j.rapm.2004.06.009

5. Zhang J, Ho KY, Wang Y. Efficacy of pregabalin in acute postoperative pain: a meta-analysis. *British Journal of Anaesthesia*, 2011;**106**(4):454–462. doi:10.1093/bja/aer027

6. Clarke H, Bonin RP, Orser BA, Englesakis M, Wijeysundera DN, Katz J. The prevention of chronic postsurgical pain using gabapentin and pregabalin: a combined systematic review and meta-analysis. *Anesthesia and Analgesia*, 2012;**115**(2):428–442. doi:10.1213/Ane.0b013e318249d36e

7. Bailey JA, Hurley RW, Gold MS. Crossroads of pain and addiction. *Pain Medicine*, 2010;**11**(12):1803–1818. doi:10.1111/j.1526-4637.2010.00982.x

8. Basbaum AI. Insights into the development of opioid tolerance. *Pain*, 1995;**61**(3):349–352. doi:10.1016/0304-3959(95)00009-H

Antibiotic prophylaxis

Allen Cheng

The Alfred Hospital and Monash University, Australia

Antibiotic prophylaxis is one of many measures that prevent surgical site infection (including good surgical technique, aseptic practices intraoperatively and effective skin disinfection). The use of prophylactic antibiotics should be distinguished from their therapeutic use for established infection.

- Antibiotic prophylaxis, when given at the appropriate time and dose, reduces the risk of surgical site infection.
- The choice of antibiotic should be determined at a hospital or regional level to cover the most likely infecting organisms for the procedure, while minimising adverse effects on the patient or antibiotic resistance.
- Systems should be implemented to ensure antibiotic prophylaxis is administered, with attention to the choice, dose, duration and timing prior to surgery.

Evidence supporting efficacy of prophylaxis

Short-course antibiotic prophylaxis reduces surgical site infections (and other common hospital-acquired infections) by around 50–60% compared with patients who do not receive prophylaxis. The relative benefit appears to be consistent across different types of surgery. However, there is a diminishing benefit for surgical procedures that are associated with a low risk of infection, such as elective inguinal hernia repair.

Studies suggest that lower infection rates are seen when antibiotics are administered preoperatively (within one to two hours of the surgical incision) compared to when given during the procedure or postoperatively. However, prolonged antibiotic prophylaxis does not confer any added benefit in reducing infection compared to antibiotic prophylaxis for up to 24 hours.

Antibiotic choice

In general, prophylactic antibiotics should have a spectrum of activity that covers the most common infecting organisms, and to be effective need to be present at adequate concentrations from the time that the initial incision is made until

Perioperative Medicine for the Junior Clinician, First Edition. Edited by Joel Symons, Paul Myles, Rishi Mehra and Christine Ball.
© 2015 John Wiley & Sons, Ltd. Published 2015 by John Wiley & Sons, Ltd.
Companion website: www.wiley.com/go/perioperativemed

TABLE 29.1 **Examples of recommended antibiotics for use in selected surgical procedures**

Procedure	Antimicrobial, dose	Comments
Obstetrics – caesarean section	Cephazolin 2 g IV	
Gynaecology – hysterectomy	Cephazolin 2 g IV AND metronidazole 500 mg IV	Repeat dosing if operation time >3 hours, and two postoperative doses
Orthopaedic	Cephazolin 2 g IV	Repeat dosing if operation time >3 hours, and two postoperative doses
Cardiothoracic	Cephazolin 2 g IV	Repeat dosing if operation time >3 hours, and give two postoperative doses
Colorectal	Cephazolin 2 g IV AND metronidazole 500 mg IV	Repeat dosing if operation time >3 hours, and two postoperative doses
Urological – prostatectomy	Gentamicin 2 mg/kg IV	

Source: Adapted from Expert Group [2].

completion of surgery. Ideally, prophylactic antibiotics should have minimal adverse effects in the surgical patient, and minimal effects on the ecology of antibiotic resistance. Some examples of recommended antibiotics for common procedures are listed in Table 29.1. More comprehensive national guidelines are also available [1–3].

The use of modified regimens, particularly vancomycin to cover methicillin-resistant *Staphylococcus aureus* (MRSA), should be limited where possible to groups of patients at higher risk of MRSA infection. If the risk is sufficiently high, screening and/or decolonisation may be considered.

Timing and repeat dosing

For antibiotics with a short half-life, dosing should be repeated at an interval equal to one to two times the half-life. In practice, this is the case for prolonged cardiac, orthopaedic and neurosurgical procedures, for antibiotics that are rapidly eliminated. An exception is gentamicin, in which a higher dose is given if prolonged prophylaxis is required. Some characteristics of commonly used antibiotics are listed in Table 29.2.

Special situations

Vancomycin poses particular problems when used perioperatively, because of the requirement for slow infusion. Rapid infusion (> 10 mg/min) is associated with 'red man syndrome' characterised by histamine release, flushing and hypotension. Some evidence suggests that it is not necessary to have completed the infusion at the time of incision, but the lowest infection rate was seen when the infusion was commenced between 15 and 60 minutes prior to surgery [4]. An alternative agent is teicoplanin, which can be administered as a slow push, but this is more expensive and its use is less well supported by evidence.

Lower uterine segment caesarean sections are associated with a high rate of infection, and prophylactic antibiotics have been shown to reduce infection [5].

TABLE 29.2 **Characteristics of antibiotics commonly used for surgical prophylaxis**

Antibiotic	Dose	Predominant mode of elimination	Half-life (hours)
Cephazolin	2 g	Renal	2
Cefuroxime	750 mg	Renal	1.5
Cefoxitin	2 g	Renal	1
Clindamycin	600 mg	Hepatic	2–3
Metronidazole	500 mg	Hepatic	6–14
Vancomycin	15–25 mg/kg	Renal	4–6
Gentamicin	2–5 mg/kg	Renal	2–3
Aztreonam	1 g	Renal	2

However, despite being associated with lower infection rates, the safety of administering antibiotics prior to surgical incision (compared to after clamping of the cord) has been questioned, as there is a potential for antibiotics to cross the placenta (and mask sepsis in the neonate) and for maternal anaphylaxis compromising neonatal outcomes. Nevertheless, most guidelines recommend preincision antibiotics as the risk of infection is felt to outweigh the small risks involved [5].

Where infections with resistant organisms are common, for example where MRSA is endemic or during an MRSA outbreak, it may be necessary to change or add to prophylactic antibiotic regimens. In general, this should be part of a wider investigation and response to elevated infection rates.

Systems to ensure appropriate use

Surveillance systems are required to define infection rates for high-risk procedures and for antibiotic resistance to determine the optimal antibiotic choices. Because of the need to regularly review these data, a system should ideally exist to formulate and review a hospital-wide policy to determine guidelines for the use of antibiotic prophylaxis, incorporating surgeons, anaesthetists, infectious diseases physicians, pharmacists, microbiologists and infection control practitioners. Recommendations should cover all common procedures, subgroups at risk of different organisms (e.g. diabetics, hospitalised patients) and alternative choices in patients who have allergies to beta-lactam antibiotics. Where such policies do not exist, regional or national policies may serve as a default guideline.

Systems should be implemented to ensure that antibiotic prophylaxis is administered, at the correct dose and timing, where it is indicated. This may include the use of preoperative checklists ('time out'), deciding on antibiotic choice at preadmission clinics and having policies that allow anaesthetists to administer antibiotic prophylaxis without direction from a surgeon.

In high-risk surgery (such as joint replacement surgery and cardiac surgery), and where a cluster of infection has been identified, a process of auditing should occur. This should collate data on the appropriateness of antibiotic choice, dose and timing relative to surgical incision, with feedback to the treating surgical unit, anaesthetists and clinical governance units.

Areas of uncertainty

The timing of vancomycin dosing remains controversial with data based only on an observational study in cardiac surgical patients [4]. The use of tourniquets in knee joint replacement may interfere with the circulation of antibiotics to the site of surgery.

Many of the studies that established the efficacy of antibiotic prophylaxis were conducted in an era where obesity was less prevalent, and many studies suggest that body weight is a risk factor for infection. This epidemiological evidence, as well as pharmacokinetic principles, suggests that dosing should be based on body weight. However, this has yet to be tested in a controlled clinical trial, and the pharmacodynamics of antibiotics when used as prophylaxis is only incompletely understood.

References

1. Bratzler DW, Dellinger EP, Olsen KM, et al. Clinical practice guidelines for antimicrobial prophylaxis in surgery. *American Journal of Health-System Pharmacy*, 2013;**70**(3):195–283. doi:10.2146/ajhp120568

2. Antibiotic Writing Group. *Therapeutic Guidelines: Antibiotic*, 15th edn. Melbourne, Australia: Therapeutic Guidelines Ltd, 2014. www.tg.org.au/

3. Scottish Intercollegiate Guidelines Network. *Antibiotic Prophylaxis in Surgery.* www.sign.ac.uk/guidelines/

4. Garey KW, Dao T, Chen H, et al. Timing of vancomycin prophylaxis for cardiac surgery patients and the risk of surgical site infections. *Journal of Antimicrobial Chemotherapy*, 2006;**58**(3):645–650. doi:10.1093/jac/dkl279

5. Costantine MM, Rahman M, Ghulmiyah L, et al. Timing of perioperative antibiotics for cesarean delivery: a metaanalysis. *American Journal of Obstetrics and Gynecology*, 2008;**199**(3):301, e1–6. doi:10.1016/j.ajog.2008.06.077

30 Antibiotic prophylaxis for endocarditis

Denis Spelman

The Alfred Hospital and Monash University, Australia

Recommendations for prevention of endocarditis have been promulgated by specialist groups for over 50 years. These include the American Heart Association (AHA) [1], the British Society of Antimicrobial Chemotherapy (BSAC) [2] and European guidelines [3]. In Australia there are the regularly updated *Therapeutic Guidelines: Antibiotics* [4].

In the most recent versions, there has been a decrease in the number of patient categories for which prophylaxis is now recommended. The current over-riding strategy targets antibiotic endocarditis prophylaxis for those patients at increased risk of adverse outcomes from endocarditis.

There are differences between these recommendations. For example, in the AHA guidelines four cardiac conditions are listed as requiring antibiotic prophylaxis, but the Australian guidelines also include indigenous Australians with rheumatic heart disease.

There is no Level 1 evidence (including no randomised controlled trials) to support these recommendations, which are generally based on expert committee consensus. The impact of antibiotic prophylaxis use on evolving antibiotic resistance is uncertain.

Pathogenesis

Organisms gain access to the bloodstream either from the operative wound or from invasive devices, including intravascular cannulae or indwelling urinary catheters. The risk of bacteraemia may differ from the risk of endocarditis, which may change with the bacterial inoculum and duration of the bacteraemia. Blood-borne organisms can adhere to the cardiac endothelium, with specific organisms (e.g. *Staphylococcus aureus*) having increased ability to adhere to heart valves.

Some, but not all, cardiac conditions are especially at risk. Similarly some, but not all, operative procedures are considered high risk of producing bacteraemia and endocarditis.

Perioperative Medicine for the Junior Clinician, First Edition. Edited by Joel Symons, Paul Myles, Rishi Mehra and Christine Ball.
© 2015 John Wiley & Sons, Ltd. Published 2015 by John Wiley & Sons, Ltd.
Companion website: www.wiley.com/go/perioperativemed

Strategies for the prevention of perioperative endocarditis

- Optimal gum and dental care with regular ongoing evaluation: dental sepsis should be treated prior to any operative procedure.
- Aseptic insertion and early removal of intravascular and indwelling urinary catheters postoperatively.
- Any concurrent infection should be adequately treated, ideally preoperatively.
- Antibiotic prophylaxis as below.

Antibiotic prophylaxis

> Perioperative endocarditis antibiotic prophylaxis is *only* recommended for patients:
> - with specific cardiac conditions which are associated with the highest risk of adverse outcome from endocarditis (Box 30.1)
> - who are undergoing specified dental and operative procedures associated with a high incidence of bacteraemia (Box 30.2).

Antibiotic prophylaxis is *not* recommended for cardiac conditions not included in Box 30.1 (e.g. mitral valve prolapse) nor for any patient undergoing dental or surgical procedures not included in Box 30.2.

For dental procedures, there is variation and lack of clarity between guidelines as to the definition of high-risk dental procedures. The BSAC defines this as 'all dental procedures involving dento-gingival manipulation' [2]. The AHA refers to 'All dental procedures that involve manipulation of gingival tissue or the periapical region of teeth or perforation of the oral mucosa' [1]. The Australian *Therapeutic Guidelines* divide multiple dental procedures into three categories for which prophylaxis is always required, required in some circumstances or not required [4]. Box 30.2 includes a summary of dental conditions in which prophylaxis is 'always required' [4].

BOX 30.1 Cardiac conditions for which antibiotic prophylaxis is recommended for patients undergoing a high-risk procedure (see Box 30.2)

Mechanical or biological cardiac valve surgery or prosthetic material used for valve repair
Previous endocarditis
Specific congenital heart disease*
Valvopathy in the setting of cardiac transplantation
Rheumatic heart disease in indigenous Australians

*For details see Antibiotic Writing Group [4].

An infectious diseases physician may recommend prophylaxis in circumstances not covered by these guidelines, for example a patient who is undergoing prolonged or multiple procedures.

Antibiotic choice (refer to Table 30.1) is determined by:

• patient allergy, e.g. penicillin or other antibiotic. Vancomycin is an alternative to penicillins in the presence of allergy to beta-lactam antibiotics

TABLE 30.1 Examples of recommended regimens for patients with a cardiac condition (Box 30.1) undergoing a high-risk procedure (see Box 30.2)

Procedure	Antibiotic	Dose	Route	Timing
Dental procedure	Amoxicillin	2 g (child 50 mg/kg up to 2 kg)	Oral	1 hour before procedure
Dental procedure + beta-lactam allergy	Clindamycin	600 mg (child 15 mg/kg up to 600 mg)	Oral	1 hour before procedure
Respiratory tract procedure	Amoxicillin	2 g (child 50 mg/kg up to 2 kg)	IV	Just before the procedure
Respiratory tract procedure + beta-lactam allergy	Clindamycin	600 mg (child 15 mg/kg up to 600 mg)	IV	Over 20 minutes just before procedure
Genitourinary and gastrointestinal procedures	Amoxicillin	2 g (child 50 mg/kg up to 2 kg)	IV	Just before the procedure
Genitourinary and gastrointestinal procedures + beta-lactam allergy	Vancomycin	25 mg/kg up to 1.5 g (child less than 12 years 30 mg/kg up to 1.5 g)	IV slow infusion	With infusion ending before procedure

- surgery type: with intra-abdominal surgery gram-negative bacilli are most likely, in contrast to oral surgery when antibiotic choice targets oropharyngeal streptococci
- knowledge that the patient has had colonisation or infection with a specific bacterium, e.g. MRSA.

Antibiotic regimen scenarios

Generally, there is no need for a second dose of antibiotic intraoperatively or postoperatively, except for a prolonged procedure. If a person is already receiving long-term antibiotics, e.g. penicillin for the prevention of rheumatic fever, he/she may have oral streptococci relatively resistant to penicillin. Such a patient should therefore receive a dose of an antibiotic from a different class, such as clindamycin, for invasive procedures involving the oral cavity or upper respiratory tract. If a patient is already receiving IV antibiotic therapy at the time of a planned operative procedure (see Box 30.2), the timing of antibiotic dosing should be optimised such that a dose is given 30–60 minutes preoperatively.

In many cases the usual surgical antibiotic prophylaxis will suffice for endocarditis prophylaxis. However, on occasion, such as with intra-abdominal surgery, there may be a need for the addition of endocarditis prophylaxis with an agent (e.g. amoxicillin) active against Enterococcus.

References

1. Wilson W, Taubert KA, Gewitz M, et al. Prevention of infective endocarditis: guidelines from the American Heart Association: a guideline from the American Heart Association Rheumatic Fever, Endocarditis, and Kawasaki Disease Committee, Council on Cardiovascular Disease in the Young, and the Council on Clinical Cardiology, Council on Cardiovascular Surgery and Anesthesia, and the Quality of Care and Outcomes Research Interdisciplinary Working Group. *Circulation*, 2007;**116**(15):1736–1754. doi:10.1161/CIRCULATIONAHA.106.183095

2. Gould FK, Elliott TS, Foweraker J, et al. Guidelines for the prevention of endocarditis: report of the Working Party of the British Society for Antimicrobial Chemotherapy. *Journal of Antimicrobial Chemotherapy*, 2006;**57**(6):1035–1042. doi:10.1093/jac/dkl121

3. Habib G, Hoen B, Tornos P, et al. Guidelines on the prevention, diagnosis, and treatment of infective endocarditis (new version 2009): the Task Force on the Prevention, Diagnosis, and Treatment of Infective Endocarditis of the European Society of Cardiology (ESC). Endorsed by the European Society of Clinical Microbiology and Infectious Diseases (ESCMID) and the International Society of Chemotherapy (ISC) for Infection and Cancer. *European Heart Journal*, 2009;**30**(19):2369–2413. doi:10.1093/eurheartj/ehp285

4. Antibiotic Writing Group. *Therapeutic Guidelines: Antibiotic*, 15th edn. Melbourne, Australia: Therapeutic Guidelines Ltd, 2014. www.tg.org.au/

30

Part V
Perioperative management of organ dysfunction and specific population groups

Coronary artery disease and coronary stents

Sesto Cairo

The Alfred Hospital and Monash University, Australia

Perioperative myocardial ischaemia/infarction

Myocardial ischaemia and infarction are major causes of perioperative morbidity and mortality, particularly in high-risk patients. The incidence of major perioperative cardiovascular complications ranges from 0.8% in patients without known coronary artery disease (CAD), to 4% with known CAD and up to 6.7% in high-risk patients [1].

A major contributing factor is the perioperative stress response, with increased catecholamines leading to an increase in HR and BP (and hence myocardial oxygen demand) while at the same time promoting a relative hypercoagulable state.

Key features of perioperative myocardial ischaemia/infarction [2,3]

Ischaemia peaks during the early postoperative period. Intraoperative ischaemia is less common and infrequently associated with perioperative myocardial ischaemia/infarction (PMI). PMI is mostly (50%) silent, meaning without typical clinical features such as angina chest pain. The early ECG changes of tachycardia and ST depression generally resolve so the PMI may not be diagnosed unless serum troponins are routinely measured. The relatively silent nature of PMI may be attributed to distracting postoperative pain, postoperative analgesia and misinterpreting the symptoms as being related to the surgery or anaesthesia.

Perioperative myocardial ischaemia/infarction is far more likely to be non-ST elevation MI (NSTEMI) rather than ST elevation MI (STEMI). Most PMIs are not caused by plaque rupture but coronary plaque disruption occurs in more than half of fatal PMIs. The majority of PMIs occur within the first 24–48 hours after surgery with a mortality rate of about 10–15%. Postoperative MI, as identified

Perioperative Medicine for the Junior Clinician, First Edition. Edited by Joel Symons, Paul Myles, Rishi Mehra and Christine Ball.
© 2015 John Wiley & Sons, Ltd. Published 2015 by John Wiley & Sons, Ltd.
Companion website: www.wiley.com/go/perioperativemed

by silent troponin elevation, is common in high-risk cardiac patients undergoing non-cardiac surgery and is often preceded by prolonged postoperative ischaemia. This is associated with both early (six months) and long-term (five years) morbidity and mortality even if a PMI is not formally diagnosed. Such patients should have their risk factors aggressively managed (refer to Chapter 11 The cardiac patient for non-cardiac surgery and Chapter 88 Myocardial injury after non-cardiac surgery).

Diagnosis and management of perioperative myocardial infarction

The WHO criteria for MI in non-surgical patients require that at least two of the following three conditions be met [4].

1. History of ischaemic-type chest pain
2. Serial ECG changes
3. Elevated serum cardiac markers

Since these are sometimes difficult to determine in the surgical patient, the following diagnostic criteria for patients undergoing non-cardiac surgery have been proposed [2].

1. A typical rise in the troponin level or a typical fall in an elevated troponin level detected at its peak after surgery in a patient without a documented alternative explanation for an elevated troponin (e.g. PE, HF or sepsis). This criterion requires that at least one of the following criteria must also be present:
   • ischaemic signs or symptoms (e.g. chest pain, shortness of breath [SOB], acute pulmonary oedema [APO])
   • development of pathological Q waves on an ECG
   • ECG changes indicative of ischaemia
   • coronary artery intervention
   • new or presumed new cardiac wall motion abnormality on echo, or new or presumed new fixed defect on radionuclide scanning.
2. Pathological findings of an acute or healing MI.
3. Development of new pathological Q waves on an ECG if troponin levels were not obtained or obtained at times that could have missed the clinical event.

Traditional cardiac biomarkers (e.g. creatine kinase MB fraction [CKMB]) have low specificity in surgical patients and have been largely replaced by troponin I and T. An increased cardiac troponin (> 99th percentile, laboratory specific) may remain elevated for 10–14 days.

Initial treatment of NSTEMI includes medical stabilisation followed by risk stratification. The treatment of unstable NSTEMI or STEMI is either PCI or fibrinolysis, with PCI obviously preferable in the perioperative setting [3,5].

Prevention of perioperative myocardial ischaemia/infarction

Strategies to potentially modify the stress response and reduce perioperative cardiovascular complications in patients with (or at risk of) CAD include the following.

Beta-blockers

Beta-blockers should be continued in patients perioperatively [6]. However, initiation of beta-blocker therapy on the day of surgery may reduce the risk of myocardial infarction/ischaemia but increase all-cause mortality, predominantly due to stroke [1].

Patients with proven or at high risk of CAD should receive beta-blockade for long-term outcome benefits, irrespective of any impending surgery. These should be started well before rather than at the time of surgery. If CAD is only recognised at the time of admission for elective surgery, it is inappropriate to start (aggressive) beta-blockade. Perioperative beta-blockers should be titrated carefully to avoid severe bradycardia and hypotension.

Statins

These drugs reduce serum cholesterol and reduce reinfarction in patients with CAD. Patients on statins should continue them perioperatively as this is likely to reduce cardiac risk [6].

Alpha-2 agonists

Alpha-2 agonists produce sedation, anxiolysis and analgesia. However, the recently published POISE-2 trial does not support the use of clonidine to decrease perioperative cardiac complications as the risks of hypotension appear to outweigh the benefits [7].

Anaemia and hypothermia

Anaemia is associated with increased postoperative MI. Whether more aggressive transfusion lowers this risk is unclear. Paradoxically, both anaemia and transfusion are independently associated with organ injury and increased morbidity. Hypothermia is also associated with postoperative MI.

Preoperative coronary revascularisation

The indications for coronary artery bypass graft (CABG) and PCI are identical to those in the non-operative setting; performing coronary revascularisation to 'get the patient through surgery' is not indicated and may increase perioperative morbidity and mortality.

Management of patients with coronary stents requiring non-cardiac surgery (Videos 31.1 and 31.2)

The increasing number of patients with coronary artery stents now presenting for non-cardiac surgery creates unique perioperative problems, particularly as the majority are DES. It is recommended that patients with a DES remain on dual antiplatelet therapy (aspirin and clopidogrel, or equivalent) for 12 months to prevent late 'in-stent' thrombosis [8]. Bare metal stents require at least six weeks of dual antiplatelet therapy (refer to Chapter 25 Anticoagulants and antiplatelet agents). Since perioperative stent thrombosis carries significant morbidity and mortality, any elective non-cardiac surgery should be performed after the recommended duration of antiplatelet therapy has been completed.

www.wiley.com/go/perioperativemed

VIDEO 31.1 **Coronary stents in the management of coronary artery disease.**

www.wiley.com/go/perioperativemed

VIDEO 31.2 **This video discusses an approach to the management of patients who need surgery within the recommended period of dual antiplatelet therapy.**

References

1. POISE Study Group, Devereaux PJ, Yang H, Yusuf S, et al. Effects of extended-release metoprolol succinate in patients undergoing non-cardiac surgery (POISE trial): a randomised controlled trial. *Lancet*, 2008;**371**(9627):1839–1847. doi:10.1016/S0140-6736(08)60601-7

2. Devereaux PJ, Goldman L, Cook DJ, Gilbert K, Leslie K, Guyatt GH. Perioperative cardiac events in patients undergoing noncardiac surgery: a review of the magnitude of the problem, the pathophysiology of the events and methods to estimate and communicate risk. *Canadian Medical Association Journal*, 2005;**173**(6):627–634. doi:10.1503/cmaj.050011

3. Adesanya AO, de Lemos JA, Greilich NB, Whitten CW. Management of perioperative myocardial infarction in noncardiac surgical patients. *Chest*, 2006;**130**(2):584–596. doi:10.1378/chest.130.2.584

4. Alpert JS, Thygesen K, Jaffe A, White HD. The universal definition of myocardial infarction: a consensus document: ischaemic heart disease. *Heart*, 2008;**94**(10):1335–1341. doi:10.1136/hrt.2008.151233

5. Berger PB, Bellot V, Bell MR, et al. An immediate invasive strategy for the treatment of acute myocardial infarction early after noncardiac surgery. *American Journal of Cardiology*, 2001;**87**(9):1100–1102, A6, A9. doi:10.1016/s0002-9149(01)01469-2

6. Fleisher LA, Fleischmann KE, Auerbach AD, et al. 2014 ACC/AHA Guideline on Perioperative Cardiovascular Evaluation and Management of Patients Undergoing Noncardiac Surgery: A Report of the American College of Cardiology/American Heart Association Task Force on Practice Guidelines. *Journal of the American College of Cardiology*, 2014;**64**(22):e77–e137. doi:10.1016/j.jacc.2014.07.944

7. Devereaux PJ, Sessler DI, Leslie K, et al. Clonidine in patients undergoing noncardiac surgery. *New England Journal of Medicine*, 2014;**370**:1504–1513. doi:10.1056/NEJMoa1401106

8. Bornemann H, Pruller F, Metzler H. The patient with coronary stents and antiplatelet agents: what to do and how to deal? *European Journal of Anaesthesiology*, 2010;**27**(5):406–410. doi:10.1097/EJA.0b013e328335b284

31

Hypertension

Steven Fowler[1] and Terry Loughnan[2]

[1] The Alfred Hospital, Australia
[2] Peninsula Health, Australia

Hypertensive patients are more haemodynamically unstable perioperatively and are at greater risk of myocardial ischaemia [1].

Definition and pathophysiology

Blood pressure (BP) is dependent on the pumping action of the heart, filling (which is dependent on volume and venous tone) and resistance (compliance) of the arterial tree.

Hypertension is defined as a BP greater than 140/90 mmHg [2]. Reduced compliance of the arterial tree with ageing leads to an increase in systolic BP, pulse pressure and BP lability.

Epidemiology

Perioperative hypertension is a very common condition. It is associated with pre-existing hypertension, advanced age, obesity, type 2 diabetes and vascular disease. It is more commonly seen in patients undergoing cardiothoracic, vascular, head and neck surgery, renal transplantation and neurosurgical procedures. There is a strong link between hypertension and increased cardiovascular risk (CAD, stroke and renal failure) in the general population, but in the perioperative setting the situation is not as clear-cut.

Aetiology

This is summarised in Box 32.1.

Complications of perioperative hypertension

Perioperative hypertension is an independent predictor of inpatient morbidity and mortality as well as unplanned ICU admission [3]. It may lead to:

- myocardial ischaemia/infarction
- systolic heart failure
- left ventricular hypertrophy and diastolic dysfunction → pulmonary oedema
- arrhythmias

Perioperative Medicine for the Junior Clinician, First Edition. Edited by Joel Symons, Paul Myles, Rishi Mehra and Christine Ball.
© 2015 John Wiley & Sons, Ltd. Published 2015 by John Wiley & Sons, Ltd.
Companion website: www.wiley.com/go/perioperativemed

- surgical bleeding and haematoma
- cerebral haemorrhage/hyperperfusion syndrome
- aortic dissection/vascular graft disruption
- renal failure
- unplanned ICU admission.

Management

Preoperative phase

Patients should have their BP checked, and hypertension treated before surgery.

In general, antihypertensive medications should be given on the day of surgery. For those undergoing major surgery in which fluid shifts occur, it is advisable to withhold ACE inhibitors and ARBs on the day of surgery [4]. Acute drug withdrawal (e.g. beta-blocker, clonidine) can precipitate a hypertensive crisis or myocardial ischaemia.

Isolated preoperative hypertension does not seem to significantly alter anaesthetic risk [1,5] and so deferment or cancellation is unnecessary. Surgery should be postponed in those patients with evidence of unstable angina or new-onset kidney injury.

The extent and urgency of surgery and presence of other co-morbidities need to be considered. For very poorly controlled hypertension (e.g. diastolic BP >110 mmHg), consider invasive arterial pressure monitoring and postoperative high-dependency monitoring.

Preoperative BP reduction by no more than 20% should be the aim and can be achieved with IV antihypertensive therapy in combination with a benzodiazepine for anxiolysis. IV beta-blocker or clonidine are suitable agents (Table 32.1).

TABLE 32.1 **Suggested options to treat perioperative hypertension**

Drug	Class	Dose	Route	Side effects	Pros	Cons
Labetalol	Selective alpha-1 and non-selective beta-adrenergic blocker	20 mg boluses up to 100 mg	IV	Bradycardia, hypotension, bronchospasm (rare)	Stable HR and smooth effect; useful in pregnancy; maintains cerebral, renal and coronary blood flow	Contraindicated in patients with severe sinus bradycardia, heart failure, heart block (higher grades), caution in asthma/COPD
Clonidine	Alpha-2 agonist	50 mcg boluses up to 150 mcg	IV, oral	Sedation, transient hypertension, dry mouth	Analgesia, usually lowers heart rate	Sedation (may or may not be useful); contraindicated in heart block (higher grades)
Metoprolol	Beta-1 selective adrenergic blocker	1–2 mg boluses up to 5 mg	IV, oral	Bradycardia, hypotension, bronchospasm (rare)	Reduces myocardial ischaemia; heart rate	Contraindicated as per labetalol; exaggerated effect with Ca²⁺ blockers
Hydralazine	Direct arteriolar vasodilator	2.5–5 mg boluses up to 20 mg	IV, oral	Hypotension, headache, flushing	Useful in pregnancy	Long half-life, tachycardia, myocardial ischaemia, cerebral vasodilation
Glyceryl trinitrate (GTN)	Venodilator	25, 50 mg patch or 10–100 mcg/min infusion	Sublingual or patch or IV infusion	Hypotension, headache, dizziness	Useful in pulmonary oedema	Reflex tachycardia, cerebral vasodilation, tolerance, toxicity

COPD, chronic obstructive pulmonary disease; HR, heart rate; IV, intravenous.

Intraoperative phase

Particular attention should be paid to adequate anaesthesia, analgesia and volume status.

Hypertension related to surgical tourniquet discomfort is difficult to control but usually resolves on deflation of the cuff. Judicious intraoperative treatment with IV beta-blocker or clonidine may be indicated.

Note also that intraoperative *hypo*tension is more common in patients receiving antihypertensive medications. This may make the intraoperative management of BP quite challenging.

Postoperative phase

Acute postoperative hypertension is defined as a relative change >20% above preoperative baseline or a systolic BP > 190 mmHg and/or diastolic BP >100 mmHg on two consecutive readings [6].

Postoperative hypertension is common and often requires therapeutic intervention. It usually begins within 20–30 minutes of emergence and lasts up to eight hours. It is believed to be caused by neurohumoral activation along with reversal of the vasodilatory effects of anaesthesia. There may also be altered baroreceptor function/responsiveness (e.g. carotid surgery). It is likely that acute postoperative hypertension is a greater risk to the patient than preoperative hypertension.

Patient assessment

First, measure BP and exclude artefact. Check the size of the NIBP cuff, or for an inaccurate transducer (height, zero, resonance). Exclude iatrogenic drug errors.

Take a history, noting specifically the presence of headache or chest pain, the level of preoperative (baseline) BP, co-morbidities, and medications taken on the day of surgery.

Examine the patient, looking for pain or agitation. Check HR and RR. Is there cardiac failure? Is there a distended bladder?

Consider the following investigations: ABG (check PaO_2 and $PaCO_2$ and $Na^+/K^+/Hb$), 12-lead resting ECG, screening transthoracic echocardiography and troponin.

Postoperative treatment

A target BP within 10% of the preoperative level should ideally be achieved but a systolic BP up to 160 mmHg can usually be accepted for several hours as an expected response to surgical stress.

Consider a treatment threshold on an individual patient basis. In cardiac and aortic surgical patients, systolic BP should be maintained < 130 mmHg, and < 110 mmHg, respectively.

Initially focus on addressing the possible causes.

- IV analgesia, e.g. alfentanil bolus (or lignocaine via spinal, epidural or perineural catheter).
- Drain the bladder.
- Oxygenation and ventilation (i.e. type I or type II respiratory failure).

- Warming.
- Manage volume overload and pulmonary oedema.
- Correct hypovolaemia.
- Anxiolysis.
- Consider secondary causes (refer to aetiology above).
- High acuity placement with an arterial line or non-invasive ventilation (e.g. continous positive airway pressure [CPAP], bilevel positive airway pressure [BiPAP]) may be considered.

Drug treatment may be required to decrease the likelihood of myocardial ischaemia or an intracerebral event.

Administer missed antihypertensive doses (oral or IV equivalent).

The agent of choice will often depend on the clinical situation (including absolute and relative contraindications).

- IV clonidine 50 mcg can be given every 15 minutes up to 150 mcg or
- IV metoprolol 1 mg every 10 minutes up to 5 mg or
- IV labetalol 20 mg every 5 minutes up to 100 mg.

If higher doses or multiple agents are required, seek assistance from a senior colleague. Excessive antihypertensive therapy may cause cerebral ischaemia. If combination therapy fails, it is appropriate to consider secondary causes of hypertension.

References

1. Howell SJ, Sear JW, Foex P. Hypertension, hypertensive heart disease and perioperative cardiac risk. *British Journal of Anaesthesia*, 2004;**92**(4):570–583. doi:10.1093/Bja/Aeh091

2. James PA, Oparil S, Carter BL, et al. 2014 evidence-based guideline for the management of high blood pressure in adults: report from the panel members appointed to the Eighth Joint National Committee (JNC 8). *JAMA*, 2014;**311**(5):507–520. doi:10.1001/jama.2013.284427

3. Rose DK, Cohen MM, DeBoer DP. Cardiovascular events in the postanesthesia care unit: contribution of risk factors. *Anesthesiology*, 1996;**84**(4):772–781. doi:10.1097/00000542-1996 04000-00003

4. Drenger B, Fontes ML, Miao YH, et al. Patterns of use of perioperative angiotensin-converting enzyme inhibitors in coronary artery bypass graft surgery with cardiopulmonary bypass effects on in-hospital morbidity and mortality. *Circulation*, 2012;**126**(3):261–269. doi:10.1161/ Circulationaha.111.059527

5. Spahn DR, Priebe HJ. Editorial II: Preoperative hypertension: remain wary? 'Yes' – cancel surgery? 'No'. *British Journal of Anaesthesia*, 2004;**92**(4):461–464. doi:10.1093/bja/aeh085

6. Varon J, Marik PE. Perioperative hypertension management. *Vascular Health and Risk Management*, 2008;**4**(3):615–627. www.ncbi.nlm.nih.gov/pubmed/18827911

Arrhythmias

Andrew Robinson

The Mercy Hospital for Women, Australia

Arrhythmias are not uncommon in the perioperative period. Pre-existing arrhythmias need appropriate investigation and optimisation before surgery, and postoperative arrhythmias can lead to significant morbidity and mortality, as well as delaying the postoperative course.

Preoperative assessment

Assessment of an arrhythmia in the preoperative patient should include standard history, examination and investigations. A measure of functional exercise capacity is often useful (refer to Chapter 11 The cardiac patient for non-cardiac surgery); this is often expressed in terms of metabolic equivalents (METs) [1] (Box 33.1). Exercise tolerance of less than 4 METs is associated with an increase in postoperative cardiopulmonary complications [2,3].

As a general rule, antiarrhythmic medications should be continued in the preoperative period. Most patients with arrhythmias should be considered for anaesthetic review prior to elective surgery.

Specific arrhythmias
Sinus tachycardia

Sinus tachycardia is defined as a sinus rhythm greater than 100 beats per minute. It is not an uncommon perioperative rhythm. Frequently this is ascribed to anxiety or pain, but more serious aetiologies must be considered, as a number of them can progress to life-threatening conditions (Box 33.2).

Sinus bradycardia

Sinus bradycardia is diagnosed when the ECG demonstrates a normal P wave, narrow complex QRS complex and a rate of less than 60 beats per minute. It is rarely significant until the rate drops to less than 50 beats per minute. Athletes and trained individuals may have 'normal' rates in the 40 beats per minute range.

If required, it can be treated with atropine 0.6–1.2 mg IV. If the rate is very slow, response to agents will be slow, and cardiopulmonary resuscitation (CPR) may be required to move peripherally administered drugs to the heart before an effect is seen.

Perioperative Medicine for the Junior Clinician, First Edition. Edited by Joel Symons, Paul Myles, Rishi Mehra and Christine Ball.
© 2015 John Wiley & Sons, Ltd. Published 2015 by John Wiley & Sons, Ltd.
Companion website: www.wiley.com/go/perioperativemed

Atrial fibrillation

Atrial fibrillation (AF) is the most common postoperative arrhythmia with significant consequences for patient health. It complicates up to 8% of non-cardiac surgery, up to 30% of non-cardiac thoracic surgery and up to 45% of cardiac surgery. It is associated with longer hospital stays and increased morbidity and mortality [4].

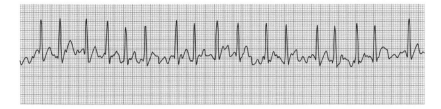

FIGURE 33.1 Atrial fibrillation with rapid ventricular response.

Atrial fibrillation is often associated with other cardiac disease including coronary artery disease, valvular disease and heart failure. Additional investigations may be appropriate in the preoperative period (refer to Chapter 13 Preoperative cardiac testing and Chapter 31 Coronary artery disease and coronary stents).

Many patients with AF will be on anticoagulant medications that may require cessation or conversion to other forms of anticoagulant. The CHADS$_2$ score is useful in stratifying perioperative risk (refer to Chapter 25 Anticoagulants and antiplatelet agents).

Atrial fibrillation is sometimes first noted in the work-up for surgery. This would usually require further investigation with at least a 12-lead ECG, TTE (to exclude structural heart disease) and blood tests to assess thyroid, renal and hepatic function [5]. Other tests such as exercise ECG, Holter monitor and transoesophageal echocardiography (TOE) (to exclude left atrial thrombus) may also be indicated.

Acute AF can be managed via rate control or by reversion to sinus rhythm. Reversion can be achieved with drugs or synchronised direct cardioversion (DC) shock. Most patients (around 60%) with acute postoperative AF will spontaneously revert within 24 hours [6].

The patient with AF and a rapid ventricular response (Figure 33.1) can be haemodynamically unstable and may require urgent treatment. Usually, this should be managed prior to anything other than life-saving surgery.

The decision to either rate control or restore sinus rhythm is mostly based around the risk of left atrial thrombus, which is low in the first 24–48 hours after initiation of AF, and higher thereafter [6]. Drugs that can be used to control rate include beta-blockers or non-dihydropyridine calcium channel antagonists (verapamil, diltiazem). Where there is co-existent heart failure, digoxin or amiodarone may be better choices.

If there is significant haemodynamic compromise, associated myocardial ischaemia or rapid AF in a patient with Wolff–Parkinson–White syndrome (WPW), DC reversion with a synchronised shock (100–200 J biphasic) is indicated; this has a small but significant (1–7%) risk of thromboembolism [6].

Heart block

First-degree heart block (PR interval >0.20 seconds = 5 small squares) is rarely of clinical significance (Figure 33.2).

Second-degree block is of slightly more concern. Mobitz type I (Wenckebach) is normally benign and occurs mostly in the context of increased vagal tone (Figure 33.3). Occasionally this will require a vagolytic drug such as atropine (600 mcg IV) when the heart rate is significantly compromised.

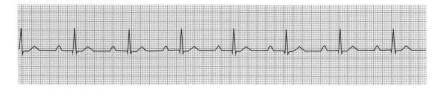

FIGURE 33.2 **First-degree heart block.**

The PR intervals become longer (solid arrows) until a dropped beat occurs (open arrow)

Dropped beat. P wave with no QRS complex

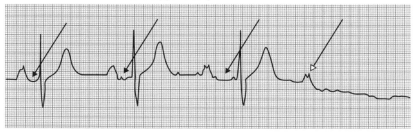

FIGURE 33.3 Second-degree heart block – Mobitz type I.

The PR intervals remain the same length (solid arrows) until a dropped beat occurs (open arrow)

Dropped beat (open arrow). P wave with no QRS complex.

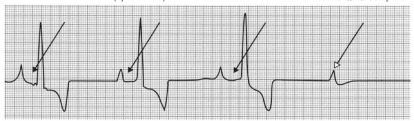

FIGURE 33.4 Second-degree heart block – Mobitz type II.

Mobitz type II (Figure 33.4) is a more significant finding and is associated with conducting system disease distal to the atrioventricular node. Where there is also a widened QRS complex, suggesting a bundle branch block, it is not uncommon to find symptoms of near-syncopal or syncopal attacks. If these are present, evaluation by a cardiologist for consideration of a permanent pacemaker prior to surgery is very reasonable [7]. If the surgery is felt to be too urgent to consider this, facilities for transcutaneous pacing should be available, in case the block progresses to complete heart block intraoperatively [7].

Third-degree or complete heart block (Figure 33.5) should have a pacemaker inserted prior to surgery in all but the most urgent of circumstances.

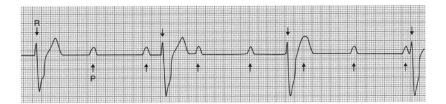

FIGURE 33.5 **Complete heart block.** The arrows at the top of the diagram indicate the ventricular rate (R wave) of about 40 beats per minute whilst the lower arrows (P wave) indicate the atrial rate (about 100 beats per minute).

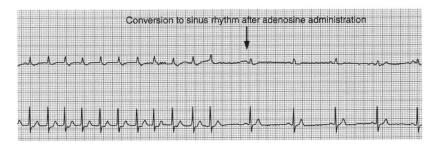

FIGURE 33.6 **Supraventricular tachycardia.**

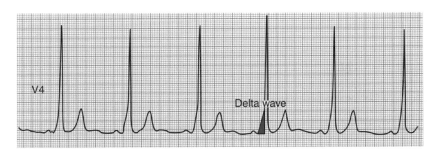

FIGURE 33.7 **Wolff–Parkinson–White (WPW) syndrome.** Note how the delta wave broadens the QRS complex and shortens the PR interval.

Paroxysmal supraventricular tachycardias (SVT) including WPW syndrome

Patients at risk of SVT (Figure 33.6) in the perioperative period include those with atrioventricular node re-entrant tachycardia (60% of paroxysmal SVT) and WPW syndrome (Figure 33.7) (30% of paroxysmal SVT). Most of these patients will be on some form of antiarrhythmic medication – often beta-blockers. This should be continued in the perioperative period.

Should such a patient develop an SVT, termination of the tachycardia is achieved by transiently blocking the atrioventricular node. A first step would usually be to apply a vagal manoeuvre such as carotid sinus massage or the valsalva manoeuvre. If this is unsuccessful, adenosine (6–12 mg IV) will usually terminate the arrhythmia.

If the arrhythmia is not terminated or recurs quickly, pretreatment with a beta-blocker or calcium channel blocker followed by more adenosine can be used.

If there is significant haemodynamic compromise, synchronised cardioversion could be used. Whenever adenosine is used, facilities for defibrillation should be present.

In the setting of known WPW syndrome, the treatment of tachyarrhythmias is more complex, with the additional risk of ventricular fibrillation occurring as a result of adenosine therapy. Further consultation should be sought from a cardiologist before treatment. Haemodynamically unstable patients should be defibrillated rather than attempting medical therapy.

Long QT syndrome

Long QT syndromes are either congenital or acquired. Most are acquired and are secondary to drugs. Patients with a prolonged QT interval are at risk of lethal ventricular arrhythmias; this risk is increased by an extensive number of drugs. A full listing can be found at http://www.QTdrugs.org

A patient with known long QT interval who presents for elective surgery should not cease beta-blocker therapy. For those who are not beta-blocked already, perioperative beta-blockade should be considered in consultation with a cardiologist.

If a patient with previously unknown long QT is picked up at routine preoperative ECG, elective surgery should be postponed until cardiology review. If surgery must proceed, avoid drugs that can worsen QT prolongation, consider perioperative beta-blockade and have a defibrillator immediately available. Droperidol is relatively contraindicated.

Ventricular rhythms

Ventricular rhythms are usually life-threatening and require basic then advanced life support. Ventricular tachycardia (VT) (Figure 33.8) can be associated with a cardiac output, but ventricular fibrillation (VF) (Figure 33.9) is not.

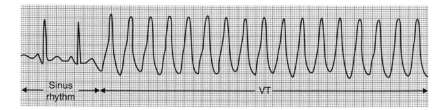

FIGURE 33.8 **Ventricular tachycardia.**

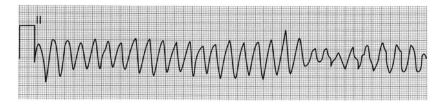

FIGURE 33.9 **Ventricular fibrillation.**

The local medical emergency protocol ('Code Blue') should be activated and appropriate CPR commenced. Time to defibrillation and effective CPR are critical determinants of outcome. Refer to Appendix B for basic and advanced cardiac life support algorithms.

References

1. Ainsworth BE, Haskell WL, Herrmann SD, et al. 2011 Compendium of physical activities: a second update of codes and MET values. *Medicine and Science in Sports and Exercise*, 2011;**43**(8):1575–1581. doi:10.1249/MSS.0b013e31821ece12

2. Girish M, Trayner E Jr, Dammann O, Pinto-Plata V, Celli B. Symptom-limited stair climbing as a predictor of postoperative cardiopulmonary complications after high-risk surgery. *Chest*, 2001;**120**(4):1147–1151. doi:10.1378/chest.120.4.1147

3. Reilly DF, McNeely MJ, Doerner D, et al. Self-reported exercise tolerance and the risk of serious perioperative complications. *Archives of Internal Medicine*, 1999;**159**(18):2185–2192. doi:10.1001/archinte.159.18.2185

4. Mayson SE, Greenspon AJ, Adams S, et al. The changing face of postoperative atrial fibrillation prevention: a review of current medical therapy. *Cardiology in Review*, 2007;**15**(5):231–241. doi:10.1097/CRD.0b013e31813e62bb

5. January CT, Wann LS, Alpert JS, et al. 2014 AHA/ACC/HRS Guideline for the Management of Patients With Atrial Fibrillation: A Report of the American College of Cardiology/American Heart Association Task Force on Practice Guidelines and the Heart Rhythm Society. *Journal of the American College of Cardiology*, 2014;**64**(21):2246–2280. doi:10.1161/CIR.0000000000000040

6. Fuster V, Ryden LE, Cannom DS, et al. ACC/AHA/ESC 2006 Guidelines for the Management of Patients with Atrial Fibrillation: a report of the American College of Cardiology/American Heart Association Task Force on Practice Guidelines and the European Society of Cardiology Committee for Practice Guidelines (Writing Committee to Revise the 2001 Guidelines for the Management of Patients With Atrial Fibrillation): developed in collaboration with the European Heart Rhythm Association and the Heart Rhythm Society. *Circulation*, 2006;**114**(7):e257–354. doi:10.1161/circulationaha.106.177292

7. Epstein AE, DiMarco JP, Ellenbogen KA, et al. ACC/AHA/HRS 2008 Guidelines for Device-Based Therapy of Cardiac Rhythm Abnormalities: a report of the American College of Cardiology/American Heart Association Task Force on Practice Guidelines (Writing Committee to Revise the ACC/AHA/NASPE 2002 Guideline Update for Implantation of Cardiac Pacemakers and Antiarrhythmia Devices) developed in collaboration with the American Association for Thoracic Surgery and Society of Thoracic Surgeons. *Journal of the American College of Cardiology*, 2008;**51**(21):e1–62. doi:10.1016/j.jacc.2008.02.032

34 Pacemakers and implanted defibrillators

Andrew Robinson

The Mercy Hospital for Women, Australia

Improvements in technology, such as battery life and miniaturisation, have led to an expanding list of indications for both pacemakers and implanted cardioverter-defibrillators such that the prevalence of these devices is increasing. In the US, more than 115,000 cardiac rhythm management devices are implanted per year.

The perioperative management of these devices continues to be problematic, with a lack of evidence on best practice and conflicting advice from experts. In addition, some institutions have ready access to pacemaker technicians, while others do not. This creates difficulties in transposing guidelines from one institution to another. It is useful to identify local contacts and procedures with respect to management of these devices.

The recommendations below are taken from the HRS/ASA consensus statement on the perioperative management of patients with implantable defibrillators and pacemakers [1]. This document is available online (www.hrsonline.org/content/download/1432/20125/file/2011-HRS_ASA%20Perioperative%20Management.pdf) and also contains specific advice for particular procedures.

Management of pacemakers

The overall purpose is to maintain pacemaker function, where required, and avoid damage to the pacemaker itself or the lead system (Video 34.1).

The preoperative assessment of a patient with a pacemaker should determine:

- presence of device
- the type of device
- the level of pacemaker dependency
- that the pacemaker is functioning as expected
- the likelihood of electromagnetic interference (EMI) during the procedure.

The presence and type of device do not usually pose any difficulties. Most patients carry details of the device they have inserted. If there is any doubt, and other

Perioperative Medicine for the Junior Clinician, First Edition. Edited by Joel Symons, Paul Myles, Rishi Mehra and Christine Ball.
© 2015 John Wiley & Sons, Ltd. Published 2015 by John Wiley & Sons, Ltd.
Companion website: www.wiley.com/go/perioperativemed

www.wiley.com/go/perioperativemed

medical documentation is unavailable, devices can be identified by chest X-ray or by pacemaker interrogators that any pacemaker clinic would have available.

The crucial issue is whether the patient is pacemaker dependent.

If the patient is dependent, then it is recommended that the pacemaker be reprogrammed to an asynchronous mode (AOO, DOO or VOO; Table 34.1) without rate responsiveness if EMI is likely to occur during the procedure. This is best achieved by a cardiac technician and pacemaker programmer but can also *usually* be achieved by placing a pacemaker magnet over the pacemaker. For most but not all pacemakers, this will activate an asynchronous mode at a predetermined rate without rate responsiveness. The rate may be affected by programming and battery level.

Consultation with a pacemaker cardiologist or pacemaker company representative can give more specific information regarding the behaviour of a particular device.

Where possible, intraoperative EMI should be minimised with the following manoeuvres (Video 34.2).

- Minimise the use of diathermy – short, irregular bursts at the lowest energy level.
- Consider the use of bipolar diathermy or harmonic scalpel.
- Avoid the diathermy current path crossing the pacemaker system.

The main danger of EMI is inappropriate suppression of pacemaker function, leading to inadequate cardiac output (Figure 34.1). Other rarer complications include damage to the device or lead–tissue interface.

If pacing is suppressed by diathermy or other EMI, it will nearly always return on cessation of the interference. If it does not return, and the patient is pacemaker dependent, CPR will be required as will equipment for emergency pacing. A magnet may put the pacemaker into an effective pacing mode.

TABLE 34.1 Generic pacemaker and implanted cardioverter-defibrillator (ICD) codes

NASPE/BPEG pacemaker codes (2002)

Pacing chamber	Sensing chamber	Response to sense	Programmability	Multisite pacing
O = none	O = none	O = none	O = none	O = none
A = atrium	A = atrium	I = inhibited	R = rate modulation	A = atrium
V = ventricle	V = ventricle	T = triggered		V = ventricle
D = dual	D = dual	D = dual (T+I)		D = dual

Position V, Multisite Pacing, is new in the 2002 revision. It implies that a second chamber is paced. An example would be DDDRV for a rate-responsive biventricular pacemaker.

NASPE/BPEG defibrillator codes (1993)

Shock chamber	Antitachycardia pacing chamber	Tachycardia detection	Antibradycardia pacing chamber
O = none	O = none	E = electrogram	O = none
A = atrium	A = atrium	H = haemodynamic	A = atrium
V = ventricle	V = ventricle		V = ventricle
D = dual	D = dual		D = dual

Source: Bernstein et al. [3,4]. Reproduced with permission from John Wiley & Sons, Ltd.

www.wiley.com/go/perioperativemed

VIDEO 34.2 **Operative considerations for pacemakers.**

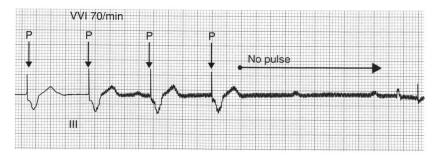

FIGURE 34.1 **Suppression of pacemaker function by diathermy.**

The effect of EMI on device function is an important consideration in the perioperative period.

> If a patient with a pacemaker requires defibrillation, this can be performed. Avoid defibrillation directly over pacemakers.

If programming is altered, it should be returned to previous settings as soon as practicable postoperatively. If dysfunction has occurred, formal pacemaker testing should take place.

Implanted cardioverter-defibrillators

Implanted cardioverter-defibrillators (ICDs, sometimes 'automatic' = AICDs) are used in patients who have survived cardiac arrest, but also in a growing number of conditions as a primary preventive strategy. Such conditions include cardiomyopathies, long QT syndrome and other electrophysiological disorders.

They work by sensing arrhythmias and managing them according to individualised programming by either defibrillation/cardioversion or, in some cases, overdrive pacing. They are generally also capable of pacing, although this function is frequently not required.

Implanted cardioverter-defibrillators are also vulnerable to EMI, but instead of suppression of normal pacing, this may lead to inappropriate defibrillation. Because of this, most cardiologists would recommend reprogramming prior to surgery to disable shock therapy. This is particularly important if the patient is also dependent on the device for pacing, as a magnet will not cause an asynchronous pacing mode.

The application of a magnet to an ICD will generally temporarily disable tachyarrhythmia therapy. However, for some devices, the programming will be permanently disabled, and tachyarrhythmia therapy will not return on removal of the magnet. In addition, there is generally no way of knowing if a magnet is correctly applied to an ICD to be sure that therapies are disabled.

Where a patient with an ICD cannot have their device reprogrammed prior to surgery, the same measures to decrease EMI as for pacemakers should be used. In addition, the patient's cardiologist or pacemaker company representative should be contacted to urgently reprogram the device or at least advise as to the effect of a magnet.

Obviously, when the device has been turned off, equipment for external defibrillation should be immediately available.

Emergency management of an unknown device

If information regarding a pacemaker cannot be found from the patient, the medical record, the pacemaker company representative or the relevant cardiologist, and an urgent procedure must be performed, significant information can be obtained via a chest X-ray and 12-lead ECG [2] (Figure 34.2).

The first step is to identify the type of device, pacemaker or ICD. To this end, implanted defibrillators generally have a thicker distal region of the right ventricular

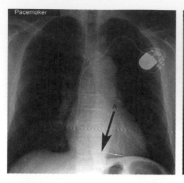
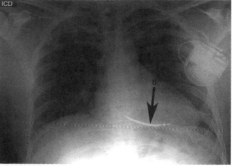

FIGURE 34.2 X-ray appearance of pacemaker and ICD. Arrow A shows the right ventricular lead of a pacemaker (dual chamber). Arrow B demonstrates the thicker radiodense coil of an ICD. Source: Crossley et al. [1]. Reproduced with permission from Elsevier Ltd.

TABLE 34.2 Management of a patient with an unknown type of pacemaker or ICD

	Pacemaker (*not* ICD)	Implanted defibrillator
Pacemaker dependent	• Use short diathermy bursts • Place magnet over pacemaker for extensive electrosurgery or procedures above umbilicus • Have magnet available for procedures below umbilicus • Place transcutaneous pacing pads (anterior-posterior) • Monitor ECG *and pulse* via plethysmography or arterial line	• Place magnet over device to suspend tachyarrhythmia detection • Use short diathermy bursts • Place transcutaneous pacing pads (anterior-posterior) • Monitor ECG *and pulse* via plethysmography or arterial line
Not dependent	• Have magnet immediately available • Monitor ECG *and pulse* via plethysmography or arterial line • Place transcutaneous pacing pads (anterior-posterior)	• Place magnet over device to suspend tachyarrhythmia detection • Use short diathermy bursts • Place transcutaneous pacing pads (anterior-posterior) • Monitor ECG *and pulse* via plethysmography or arterial line

ECG, electrocardiogram.

lead – the defibrillator coil. Occasionally, an additional atrial lead will also have this appearance in dual coil defibrillators.

The number and position of leads will also inform as to the kind of pacemaker – single or dual chamber, ventricular or biventricular.

A 12-lead ECG will assist in defining whether the patient is dependent on the pacemaker or not; if there are pacemaker spikes in front of most/all of the P waves or QRS complexes, assume the patient is pacemaker dependent.

Management can then be commenced according to Table 34.2.

Further advice should be sought from a cardiologist as soon as feasible and in all cases the device should be interrogated and assessed before the patient leaves a cardiac monitored environment [1].

References

1. Crossley GH, Poole JE, Rozner MA, et al. The Heart Rhythm Society (HRS)/American Society of Anesthesiologists (ASA) Expert Consensus Statement on the perioperative management of patients with implantable defibrillators, pacemakers and arrhythmia monitors: facilities and patient management this document was developed as a joint project with the American Society of Anesthesiologists (ASA), and in collaboration with the American Heart Association (AHA), and the Society of Thoracic Surgeons (STS). *Heart Rhythm*, 2011;**8**(7):1114–1154. doi:10.1016/j.hrthm.2010.12.023

2. Jacob S, Shahzad MA, Maheshwari R, Panaich SS, Aravindhakshan R. Cardiac rhythm device identification algorithm using X-Rays: CaRDIA-X. *Heart Rhythm*, 2011;**8**(6):915–922. doi:10.1016/j.hrthm.2011.01.012

3. Bernstein AD, Daubert JC, Fletcher RD, et al. The revised NASPE/BPEG generic code for antibradycardia, adaptive-rate, and multisite pacing. North American Society of Pacing and Electrophysiology/British Pacing and Electrophysiology Group. *Pacing and Clinical Electrophysiology*, 2002;**25**(2):260–264. doi:10.1046/j.1460-9592.2002.00260.x

4. Bernstein AD, Camm AJ, Fisher JD, et al. North American Society of Pacing and Electrophysiology policy statement. The NASPE/BPEG defibrillator code. *Pacing and Clinical Electrophysiology*, 1993;**16**(9):1776–1780. www.ncbi.nlm.nih.gov/pubmed/7692407

34

35 Heart failure

Vanessa van Empel and Dion Stub

The Alfred Hospital, Australia

Definition and diagnosis

Heart failure (HF) is a complex clinical syndrome that can result from any structural or functional cardiac disorder leading to the heart failing to meet the oxygen demand of tissues. HF is a syndrome in which patients have symptoms (breathlessness, ankle swelling, fatigue) and signs (elevated jugular venous pressure, pulmonary crackles).

Recently the classification of HF has been divided into HF-REF (heart failure with reduced ejection fraction) and HF-PEF (heart failure with preserved ejection fraction).

The proposed criteria for the diagnosis of both include [1]:

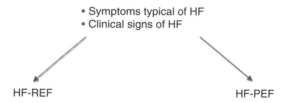

• Symptoms typical of HF
• Clinical signs of HF

HF-REF

• Reduced left ventricular ejection fraction (LVEF <50%)

HF-PEF

• Preserved LVEF >50%
• Evidence of abnormal LV diastolic function on imaging +/– supported by elevated BNP

Epidemiology and aetiology

Refer to Table 35.1.

Approximately 1.5–2% of the Australian population has HF [2]. Prevalence rises with advancing age, increasing up to 10% among persons of 70 years and older. Approximately 50% of all HF patients have a normal or only slightly reduced LVEF, e.g. HF-PEF. HF-PEF patients are, as a group, older, more often female and more

Perioperative Medicine for the Junior Clinician, First Edition. Edited by Joel Symons, Paul Myles, Rishi Mehra and Christine Ball.
© 2015 John Wiley & Sons, Ltd. Published 2015 by John Wiley & Sons, Ltd.
Companion website: www.wiley.com/go/perioperativemed

TABLE 35.1 Epidemiology and aetiology of heart failure

Common	Less common
Coronary artery disease	Viral myocarditis
Hypertension	Alcohol-related cardiomyopathy
Diabetes	Idiopathic dilated cardiomyopathy
Valvular heart disease	Infiltrative disorders, e.g. amyloid, sarcoid

TABLE 35.2 Clinical evaluation of heart failure

Symptoms	Signs
Highly suggestive	*Left heart failure*
Orthopnoea	Displayed apical impulse
Paroxysmal nocturnal dyspnoea	Third heart sound
Common – less discriminating	Pulmonary congestion
Breathlessness	*Right heart failure*
Exertional dyspnoea	Elevated jugular venous pressure
Fatigue	Ascites/hepatomegaly
Ankle swelling	Peripheral oedema
Anorexia/abdominal fullness	

frequently have systolic hypertension and atrial fibrillation [3]. Patients with HF-PEF still have a better prognosis compared to patients with HF-REF.

Clinical evaluation

Refer to Table 35.2.

Investigations to consider in the preoperative evaluation of suspected heart failure

Refer to Table 35.3.

Risk assessment

Several risk indices have been developed relating the clinical characteristics to perioperative cardiac mortality and morbidity. Whilst beyond the scope of this chapter, most of these models recognise decompensated HF as a major clinical risk, which requires intensive management and may result in delay or cancellation of non-urgent surgery.

Treatment and perioperative care of heart failure patients

There is limited evidence on the optimal management of HF in the perioperative period. We therefore recommend a similar approach to that used for the general management of HF.

TABLE 35.3 Preoperative investigations in patients with suspected heart failure

Investigation	Remarks
Electrocardiogram (ECG)	Although a completely normal ECG makes a diagnosis of HF due to LV systolic dysfunction less likely, it does not exclude other causes of HF. The ECG provides information which can help with the aetiology of HF but can also be important for decisions about treatment (e.g. rate control)
Transthoracic echocardiography (TTE)	Whilst TTE is not necessary for clinically asymptomatic patients, all patients with suspected HF require a TTE. It provides immediate information on chamber volumes, ventricular systolic and diastolic function, wall thickness and valve function
Biochemistry	Standard biochemical (sodium, potassium, creatinine) and haematological (haemoglobin, haematocrit, ferritin, leucocytes and platelets) analysis, as well as thyroid function, liver enzymes and blood glucose, should be done routinely in every patient with suspected HF. Measurement of BNP (or NT-proBNP) is of additional value. BNP is increased when the heart is diseased or the load of one of the heart chambers is increased. This can be due to AF or pulmonary embolism but also non-cardiovascular conditions such as renal failure
Assessment of ischaemia and viability	If myocardial ischaemia is suspected, additional assessment is required. Detection of myocardial ischaemia and viability can include stress test (stress ECG, stress echo or stress nuclear study) or coronary angiography
Assessment of functional capacity	A pivotal feature of preoperative evaluation is the assessment of functional capacity. Functional capacity is measured in metabolic equivalents (METs). Exercise testing provides an objective measurement of functional capacity. Without exercise testing, functional capacity can be estimated based on the ability to perform everyday activities, such as watching television (1 MET) or climbing two flights of stairs (4 METs). Poor functional capacity is considered the inability to perform activity equal to 4 METs, and is associated with increased incidence of postoperative cardiac events [9]. When functional capacity is high, the prognosis is excellent, even in the presence of stable CAD or risk factors [10]

AF, atrial fibrillation; BNP, brain natriuretic peptide; CAD, coronary artery disease; HF, heart failure; LV, left ventricle; NT-proBNP, N-terminal prohormone of brain natriuretic peptide.

Angiotensin Converting Enzyme (ACE) inhibition [4]

ACE inhibitors form the foundation of all medical management and are considered first-line therapy for nearly all HF patients, including those with LV systolic dysfunction without symptoms.

Although the perioperative use of ACE inhibitors carries a risk of hypotension under anaesthesia, in particular following induction and concomitant beta-blocker use, it is recommended that ACE inhibitors are continued during non-cardiac surgery in stable patients with LV systolic dysfunction and only in patients with hypotension should transient discontinuation be considered.

Beta-blockade

Long-term HF outcomes are improved with beta-blocker therapy [5–7]. Patients who are already receiving and tolerating beta-blockers should generally continue such therapy perioperatively. Routine initiation of perioperative beta-blocker therapy is of unproven benefit and associated with potential harm [8]. There is some evidence supporting benefit in patients who are at high cardiac risk, and in the presence of coronary artery disease. In such patients, beta-blocker therapy should be initiated and titrated to heart rate and blood pressure in the weeks before surgery.

Diuretics

Diuretic therapy is frequently used in HF patients to treat and prevent fluid retention. The possibility of electrolyte disturbances should be considered, and correction is necessary before surgery. The volume status in patients with HF should be carefully monitored in the perioperative period and loop diuretics (e.g. furosemide) may be given intravenously to control volume overload. Diuretics should be continued in HF patients up to the day of surgery, continued IV if nil orally, and continued orally when possible.

References

1. McMurray JJ, Adamopoulos S, Anker SD, et al. ESC guidelines for the diagnosis and treatment of acute and chronic heart failure 2012: The Task Force for the Diagnosis and Treatment of Acute and Chronic Heart Failure 2012 of the European Society of Cardiology. Developed in collaboration with the Heart Failure Association (HFA) of the ESC. *European Heart Journal*, 2012;**33**(14):1787–1847. doi:10.1093/eurheartj/ehs104

2. National Heart Foundation of Australia and the Cardiac Society of Australia and New Zealand. Chronic Heart Failure Guidelines Expert Writing Panel. *Guidelines for the Prevention, Detection and Management of Chronic Heart Failure in Australia*. 2011. www.heartfoundation.org.au/SiteCollectionDocuments/Chronic_Heart_Failure_Guidelines_2011.pdf

3. Phan TT, Shivu GN, Abozguia K, Sanderson JE, Frenneaux M. The pathophysiology of heart failure with preserved ejection fraction: from molecular mechanisms to exercise haemodynamics. *International Journal of Cardiology*, 2012;**158**(3):337–343. doi:10.1016/j.ijcard.2011.06.113

4. Groban L, Butterworth J. Perioperative management of chronic heart failure. *Anesthesia and Analgesia*, 2006;**103**(3):557–575. doi:10.1213/01.ane.0000226099.60493.d9

5. [No authors listed] Effect of metoprolol CR/XL in chronic heart failure: Metoprolol CR/XL Randomised Intervention Trial in Congestive Heart Failure (MERIT-HF). *Lancet*, 1999;**353**(9169):2001–2007. doi:10.1016/s0140-6736(99)04440-2

6. Mori TA, Croft KD, Puddey IB, Beilin LJ. An improved method for the measurement of urinary and plasma F2-isoprostanes using gas chromatography-mass spectrometry. *Analytical Biochemistry*, 1999;**268**(1):117–125. doi:10.1006/abio.1998.3037

7. Packer M, Fowler MB, Roecker EB, et al. Effect of carvedilol on the morbidity of patients with severe chronic heart failure: results of the carvedilol prospective randomized cumulative survival (COPERNICUS) study. *Circulation*, 2002;**106**(17):2194–2199. doi:10.1161/01.cir.0000035653.72855.bf

35

8. Devereaux PJ, Yang H, Yusuf S, et al. Effects of extended-release metoprolol succinate in patients undergoing non-cardiac surgery (POISE trial): a randomised controlled trial. *Lancet*, 2008;**371**(9627):1839–1847. doi:10.1016/S0140-6736(08)60601-7

9. Biccard BM. Relationship between the inability to climb two flights of stairs and outcome after major non-cardiac surgery: implications for the pre-operative assessment of functional capacity. *Anaesthesia*, 2005;**60**(6):588–593. doi:10.1111/J.1365-2044.2005.04181.x

10. Morris CK, Ueshima K, Kawaguchi T, Hideg A, Froelicher VF. The prognostic value of exercise capacity: a review of the literature. *American Heart Journal*, 1991;**122**(5):1423–1431. doi:10.1016/0002-8703(91)90586-7

36 Aortic stenosis

Rishi Mehra

The Alfred Hospital and Monash University, Australia

Aortic stenosis (AS) is a condition in which the aortic valve is narrowed (stenosed). It is the most common cardiac valvular condition in the developed world [1].

Severe AS carries a high risk of mortality and morbidity for non-cardiac surgery. The American Heart Association/American College of Cardiology (AHA/ACC) guidelines estimate severe AS has a 30-day mortality of >5% (refer to Chapter 11 The cardiac patient for non-cardiac surgery).

Pathophysiology of AS

The aortic valve is a trileaflet cardiac valve, situated at the base of the aortic root. All stroke volume ejected from the left ventricle (LV) passes through the aortic valve (AV). A normal AV offers only minimal impedance to ejection but as stenosis occurs, ejection requires more ventricular work. Over time, the LV compensates by hypertrophy.

Aortic stenosis represents a spectrum of disease severity, ranging from a normal aortic valve to mild leaflet thickening without flow impairment (aortic sclerosis) to severe stenosis.

Measures of severity

Aortic valve area

While the AV is a three-dimensional structure, the narrowest point exists within a plane, so one measurement of AS severity is the AV area (AVA). A normal AVA is 2.8–4.2 cm^2. Severe AS is an AVA <0.7 cm^2.

Pressure gradient

As the AVA reduces, the pressure required to overcome impedance to ejection from the LV increases. This additional pressure requirement is called a pressure gradient [2].

When the AVA is <1.0 cm^2, even minor decreases in valve area lead to rapid increases in pressure gradients. The result is greater cardiac work to overcome the impedance of the narrowed AV. Eventually, the demand on the LV outstrips the work that can be delivered, resulting in LV failure and increased risk of death.

Once the patient with AS is symptomatic, survival is limited. Median survival for a patient with angina and untreated severe AS is less than one year.

Perioperative Medicine for the Junior Clinician, First Edition. Edited by Joel Symons, Paul Myles, Rishi Mehra and Christine Ball.
© 2015 John Wiley & Sons, Ltd. Published 2015 by John Wiley & Sons, Ltd.
Companion website: www.wiley.com/go/perioperativemed

Symptoms and signs of aortic stenosis (Box 36.1)

The onset of symptoms of AS heralds a poor prognosis. The mean time intervals from symptom onset to death are:

- heart failure – two years
- syncope – three years
- angina – five years.

Once severe aortic stenosis exists, if the patient develops symptoms, their life expectancy is dramatically reduced. This is the time when the patient requires aortic valve replacement.

Aetiology of aortic stenosis

Aortic stenosis in the developed world is commonly caused by the following (Video 36.1):

- bicuspid aortic valve disease
- calcific aortic valve disease
- rheumatic heart disease.

Bicuspid aortic valve disease (5.4%)

Bicuspid aortic valve disease is the most common congenital form of cardiac disease; 1–2% of the general population have a bicuspid AV. This typically leads to a

www.wiley.com/go/perioperativemed

VIDEO 36.1 **Aetiology of aortic stenosis.**

'fish mouth' appearance of the AV, where two leaflets are present instead of three. The result is premature calcification of the AV, with severe stenosis typically arising in 50–60-year-old adults.

Calcific aortic valve disease (81.9%)

This has similar pathophysiology to atherosclerosis, with lipid and cholesterol deposition within the AV leaflets and reduction in AVA. The SEAS trial found no evidence for the use of statins or other lipid/triglyceride lowering methods to slow progression of AS or prevent treatment of calcific AV disease [3].

Rheumatic heart disease (11.2%)

This arises from infection with group A beta-haemolytic streptococcal infection. Following streptococcal throat infection, antibodies are generated for M protein, which shares a similar antigenic structure to proteins found on cardiac valve leaflets. The result is destruction of cardiac valves and premature calcification. Most commonly, the mitral valve is involved (70% of patients); the AV is additionally involved in 20–25% of patients. Tragically, rheumatic heart disease can be prevented by a single intramuscular injection of penicillin once streptococcal throat infection occurs [4].

The burden of rheumatic heart disease falls on poorer socioeconomic areas of the world. These include Asia, the Indian subcontinent, Eastern Europe, Africa and parts of the Pacific Islands and the indigenous populations of Australia and New Zealand.

Rare causes (0.6%)

- Homozygous type II hyperlipoproteinaemia
- Irradiation
- Metabolic, e.g. Fabry's disease
- Systemic lupus erythematosus
- Alkaptonuria

TABLE 36.1 Severity of aortic stenosis

Degree of aortic stenosis	Mean gradient (mmHg)	Peak velocity (metres/second)	Aortic valve area (cm²)
Normal aortic valve	<5	<2.5	2.8–4.0
Mild aortic stenosis	<25	2.5–3.0	>1.5–2.8
Moderate aortic stenosis	25–40	3.0–4.0	1.0–1.5
Severe aortic stenosis	>40	>4	<1.0

Classification of disease severity

Aortic stenosis severity is described by echocardiographic parameters: AVA, mean and peak pressure gradients and the jet velocity of blood passing through the stenosed valve. As AVA reduces, jet velocity increases (Table 36.1).

Other methods of measuring severity include angiographic catheter measurements (LV pullback and aortic root pressures) and less common non-invasive imaging modalities (e.g. cardiac CT, cardiac MRI).

Treatment of aortic stenosis

Four treatment options exist.

- Conservative management with serial reviews and evaluation.
- *Balloon valvuloplasty*. A catheter and balloon force open the AV with short-term improvement, but recurrence of AS is almost complete by 12 months.
- *Surgical aortic valve replacement (AVR)*. This is the gold standard for treatment. Thirty-day mortality for surgical AVR is 2–5%. AVR is only undertaken when the risk of death from AS is greater than the risk of AVR. Surgical valve implantation is of two types: a metal prosthetic valve or a bioprosthetic valve. A bioprosthetic valve is a porcine valve tissue that is treated to remove antigens and woven onto a metal skeleton. It requires anticoagulation for only three months, unlike the prosthetic valves which require lifelong anticoagulation.
- *Transcatheter aortic valve implantation (TAVI)*. This is a newer technique, usually as an alternative in those deemed to be at high surgical risk.

Implications of aortic stenosis for the perioperative patient

Intrathoracic, intra-abdominal and some vascular surgical procedures can lead to a large amount of tissue trauma, resulting in an increase in cardiac output for 24–72 hours postoperatively. The increased demand on the LV in the face of surgery and a raised afterload result in LV failure and death.

Perioperative management of the patient with aortic stenosis

Management consists of early recognition of increased risk and planning for surgery. Diagnosis and referral to cardiology should occur with a view to grading severity and exploring treatments.

Patients who present with a prosthetic valve replacement *in situ* will also need an appropriate anticoagulation plan. This should involve a haematologist and the patient may need appropriate bridging therapy (refer to Chapter 25 Anticoagulants and antiplatelet agents). Appropriate antibiotic prophylaxis may be required (refer to Chapter 30 Antibiotic prophylaxis for endocarditis).

> Severe aortic stenosis carries one of the highest risks for non-cardiac surgical morbidity and mortality in the perioperative period. Diagnosis and management of this condition are essential for optimal perioperative patient outcomes.

References

1. Manning WJ. Asymptomatic aortic stenosis in the elderly: a clinical review. *JAMA*, 2013;**310**(14):1490–1497. doi:10.1001/jama.2013.279194

2. Carabello BA. Clinical practice. *Aortic stenosis*. *New England Journal of Medicine*, 2002;**346**(9):677–682. doi:10.1056/NEJMcp010846

3. Rossebo AB, Pedersen TR, Boman K, et al. Intensive lipid lowering with simvastatin and ezetimibe in aortic stenosis. *New England Journal of Medicine*, 2008;**359**(13):1343–1356. doi:10.1056/NEJMoa0804602

4. Robertson KA, Volmink JA, Mayosi BM. Antibiotics for the primary prevention of acute rheumatic fever: a meta-analysis. *BMC Cardiovascular Disorders*, 2005;**5**(1):11. doi:10.1186/1471-2261-5-11

36

Pulmonary hypertension

Mark Buckland

The Alfred Hospital and Monash University, Australia

Definition and aetiology

Pulmonary hypertension (PH) is a haemodynamic and pathophysiological state found in a number of medical conditions. It is defined as a mean pulmonary artery pressure (mPAP) ≥25 mmHg at rest, measured by right heart catheter.

The clinical conditions associated with PH are divided into five categories.

1. Pulmonary arterial hypertension (PAH); includes idiopathic PH and that secondary to connective tissues diseases like scleroderma
2. PH secondary to left heart disease
3. PH due to chronic lung disease and/or hypoxia
4. Chronic thromboembolic PH (CTEPH)
5. PH due to unclear multifactorial mechanisms (Box 37.1)

The response to the increases in PAP, regardless of aetiology, is borne by the right side of the heart. It responds to this increased pulmonary vascular resistance (PVR) initially with hypertrophy and dilation of the right ventricle (RV). As this progresses, there is backpressure causing incompetence of the tricuspid valve (tricuspid regurgitation – TR) and increased right atrial pressure (RAP). Ultimately the RV will start to fail. The reduced ability of the RV to pump blood through the lungs to prime the left ventricle (LV) will lead to a rapidly declining spiral with decreased cardiac output and organ perfusion, including blood flow to the RV.

While this can occur in all the above groups, it is usually more severe in patients with PAH who often have PAP equal to or above systemic blood pressure. It is this and their relatively non-specific clinical picture that make the PAH group the most challenging to manage perioperatively. In fact, they can appear deceptively well.

Patients from the other groups will have the underlying illness as a clue to consider PH as a potential problem in their management; its occurrence in such patients is always a poor prognostic sign.

Diagnosis

Pulmonary arterial hypertension should be considered in those patients who have breathlessness or exertional dyspnoea, *after* exclusion of the other associated causes. If they also have symptoms and signs of right heart failure, such as

Perioperative Medicine for the Junior Clinician, First Edition. Edited by Joel Symons, Paul Myles, Rishi Mehra and Christine Ball.
© 2015 John Wiley & Sons, Ltd. Published 2015 by John Wiley & Sons, Ltd.
Companion website: www.wiley.com/go/perioperativemed

BOX 37.1 Classification of pulmonary hypertension

1. Pulmonary arterial hypertension
   - Idiopathic PAH
   - Heritable PAH
     - **BMPR2**
     - **Other genes such as SMAD9**
     - Unknown
   - Drug and toxin Induced
   - Associated with:
     - Connective tissue disease
     - HIV infection
     - Portal hypertension
     - Congenital heart diseases
     - Schistosomiasis
   - Pulmonary veno-occlusive disease and/or pulmonary capillary hemangiomatosis
   - **Persistent pulmonary hypertension of the newborn (PPHN)**
2. Pulmonary hypertension due to left heart disease
   - Left ventricular systolic dysfunction
   - Left ventricular diastolic dysfunction
   - Valvular disease
   - **Congenital/acquired left heart inflow/outflow tract obstruction and congenital cardiomyopathies**
3. Pulmonary hypertension due to lung diseases and/or hypoxia
   - Chronic obstructive pulmonary disease
   - Interstitial lung disease
   - Other pulmonary diseases with mixed restrictive and obstructive pattern
   - Sleep-disordered breathing
   - Alveolar hypoventilation disorders
   - Chronic exposure to high altitude
   - Developmental lung diseases
4. Chronic thromboembolic pulmonary hypertension (CTEPH)
5. Pulmonary hypertension with unclear multifactorial mechanisms
   - Hematologic disorders: chronic hemolytic anemia, myeloproliferative disorders, splenectomy
   - Systemic disorders: sarcoidosis, pulmonary histiocytosis, lymphangioleiomyomatosis
   - Metabolic disorders: glycogen storage disease, Gaucher disease, thyroid disorders
   - Others: tumoral obstruction, fibrosing mediastinitis, chronic renal failure, segmental PH

*5th WSPH Nice 2013. Main modifications to the previous Dana Point classification are in bold. BMPR = bone morphogenic protein receptor type II; HIV = human Immunodeficiency virus; PAH = pulmonary arterial hypertension.
Source: Simonneau et al. [1]. Reproduced with permission from Elsevier Ltd.

37

peripheral oedema, abdominal distension or discomfort, fatigue and findings of elevated JVP, palpable RV impulse, loud P2 and murmur consistent with TR, then the most useful investigation to consider is a TTE. This not only allows assessment of the left heart, but also indirect measurement of the RV systolic pressure, which reflects PAP, will give the RV size and function, and demonstrate presence of RV hypertrophy.

A perioperative patient with the above findings, who has not been fully worked up or diagnosed (unlikely), must be referred to a unit specialising in the management of PH; in most centres either respiratory physicians or cardiologists. The subsequent diagnostic pathway is geared toward excluding/confirming conditions from groups 2–5 above and ultimately a right heart catheter to accurately measure pulmonary vascular pressure and responsiveness to vasodilator therapy (Figure 37.1).

The importance of identifying those patients with significant PH (PAH or others) is the very high risk of perioperative morbidity and mortality (20–30% and 7–9% respectively) in patients undergoing all but the most minor of surgical procedures. These poor outcomes occur despite patients being managed in specialised units with expertise in caring for such patients and despite use of contemporary treatments and medications. In the majority of cases, the mechanism of death or morbidity is acute RV failure.

Pharmacological management

Those patients who are diagnosed with PAH will be on a range of therapies. General measures include supervised exercise training (limiting strenuous activity); oxygen supplementation – if SpO_2 is low; diuretic therapy for oedema and RV volume overload; digoxin and oral anticoagulants – all shown to improve survival.

If at the time of right heart catheter, they are found to be vasoactive responders, they will be on high-dose calcium channel blockers (CCB). Less than 20% of patients with PAH fall into this group. Unfortunately, in many the response is not sustained in the long term.

Non-responders are treated with specific therapies aimed at reducing the PVR and PAP. There are three broad groups.

1. Drugs acting on the endothelin pathway (shown to be activated in PAH patients) antagonising the endothelin receptors – effective in oral forms.
   • Bosentan
   • Ambrisentan
2. Drugs inhibiting phosphodiesterase-5 (PDEA-5 inhibitors) such as sildenafil that increase levels of cyclic guanine monophosphate (cGMP) and thus increase levels of vasodilatory nitric oxide (NO) – orally active.
3. Drugs acting via the prostacyclin pathway, itself a potent vasodilator – active intravenously or inhaled.
   • Epoprostenol (synthetic prostacyclin) administered by long-term infusion
   • Iloprost (prostacyclin analogue) administered by either intravenous or inhaled routes

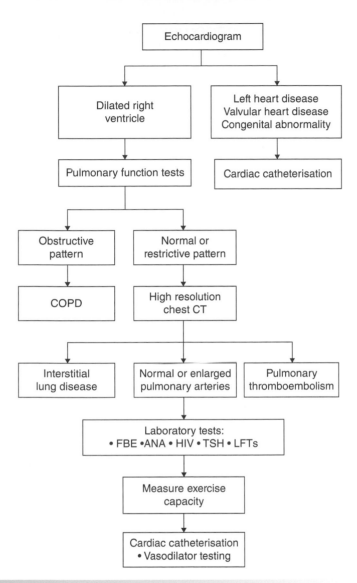

FIGURE 37.1 **Management algorithm for pulmonary hypertension. ANA, antinuclear antibody; FBE, full blood examination; COPD, chronic obstructive pulmonary disease; CT, computed tomography; HIV, human immunodeficiency virus; LFT, liver function test; TSH, thyroid-stimulating hormone.**

Patients often start on a drug from group 1 or 2 as tolerated along with the general medications mentioned above. As the disease progresses, they have another oral therapy added, but many eventually progress to a continuous infusion of a prostacyclin via a permanent intravascular catheter.

Perioperative management

The aims here are to match the patient's disease severity, with the right procedure in the appropriate facility. These patients should have all but minor, superficial procedures (e.g. skin lesion excision under local anaesthetic) carried out in an experienced unit.

On admission, once the diagnosis of PAH is obvious, the patient should be referred to the PH specialists within the hospital as well as notifying the departments of anaesthesia and probably critical care.

Their routine therapy should be continued and only modified in consultation with the PH specialists.

Investigations should include U&Es, FBE, coagulation, especially if on warfarin, and probably echocardiography (especially if it has not been done in the last three months or their condition has changed significantly). This will give an estimate of the actual PAP and show how the right heart is coping – vital information for perioperative management.

As the risk of a poor perioperative outcome in these patients is high, there should be a multidisciplinary discussion about the planned procedure, its appropriateness and whether a simpler alternative exists. The patient should have input to this decision.

Part of this process should include postoperative planning. The patient should be cared for in a closely monitored environment, ideally HDU or ICU. Analgesia planning is key; anaesthetists familiar with caring for such patients should oversee this. Patients should be returned to their regular therapy for PAH as rapidly as possible.

Reference

1. Simonneau G, Gatzoulis MA, Adatia I, et al. Updated clinical classification of pulmonary hypertension. *Journal of the American College of Cardiology*, 2013;**62**(25S). doi: 10.1016/j.jacc.2013.10.029

Further reading

Rich S. Pulmonary hypertension. In: Longo D, Fauci A, Kasper D, et al., editors. *Harrison's Principles of Internal Medicine*, 18th edn. New York: McGraw-Hill, 2011.

Teo YW, Greenhalgh DL. Update on anaesthetic approach to pulmonary hypertension. *European Journal of Anaesthesiology*, 2010;**27**(4):317–323. doi:10.1097/EJA.0b013e328335474e

38 Endocarditis, myocarditis and cardiomyopathy

Enjarn Lin

The Alfred Hospital and Monash University, Australia

Endocarditis

Infective endocarditis (IE) is an infection of the endocardial surface of the heart [1]. It usually affects the heart valves but may also occur on septal defects, patent ductus arteriosus, mural endocardium and intracardiac devices.

Epidemiology

In developing nations, IE usually affects young adults with rheumatic valve disease, usually due to Streptococcus species. In developed nations, older patients are seen, particularly with degenerative valves, valve prosthesis, injective drug use and medical procedures. These are commonly Staphylococcus species.

Pathophysiology

The characteristic lesion is a vegetation composed of micro-organisms, inflammatory cells, fibrin and platelets. These develop characteristically where blood accelerates towards a narrowing (i.e. cardiac valve), causing turbulence, a jet effect and inflammation, which may become secondarily infected during bacteraemia. Vegetations commonly occur on the atrial surface of mitral and tricuspid valves, on the ventricular surface of aortic and pulmonary valves or in other areas of traumatic endothelial damage seen with electrodes, catheters, degenerative changes and rheumatic inflammation.

Clinical presentation

Usual presentation is relapsing fever without an obvious focus of infection, with new or varying murmurs in 85% of patients. Features such as splinter haemorrhages are less common and usually seen with left-sided heart lesions (Box 38.1). Atypical presentation is more common in the elderly or those who are immunocompromised. There are a number of risk factors for adverse outcome (Box 38.2).

Perioperative Medicine for the Junior Clinician, First Edition. Edited by Joel Symons, Paul Myles, Rishi Mehra and Christine Ball.
© 2015 John Wiley & Sons, Ltd. Published 2015 by John Wiley & Sons, Ltd.
Companion website: www.wiley.com/go/perioperativemed

BOX 38.1 Signs and symptoms of infective endocarditis

Constitutional

Fever (90%)
Cardiac failure (40–50%)
Haematuria (60–70%)
Conduction disorder (10–20%)
Splenomegaly (30–40% if long-standing)
Cerebral and systemic emboli (7–15%)

Specific

Murmurs (85% new or changed murmur)
Vascular and immunological phenomena (30%)

* Petechial rash (40–50% transient)
* Petechial haemorrhages (20–30% mucous membranes/Roth's spots on fundi)
* Splinter haemorrhages (10%)
* Clubbing (10% if long-standing)
* Osler's nodes (5%)

BOX 38.2 Risk factors for adverse outcome in infective endocarditis (IE)

Patient characteristics

Older age
Prosthetic valve IE
Insulin-dependent diabetes mellitus
Other co-morbidity

Presence of complications

Heart failure
Renal failure
Stroke
Septic shock
Periannular complications (abscess or rupture)

Micro-organism

Staph. aureus
Fungi
Gram-negative bacteria

Echocardiographic features

Periannular complications
Severe left-sided valve regurgitation
Low left ventricular ejection fraction
Pulmonary hypertension
Large vegetations
Severe prosthetic valve dysfunction
Premature mitral valve closure and signs of elevated diastolic pressures

Diagnosis

The accurate diagnosis of IE is reliant upon history, examination, timely investigations (including blood cultures and echocardiography), and a high index of suspicion (Box 38.3; Video 38.1).

BOX 38.3 Modified Duke criteria for infective endocarditis (IE)

Major criteria	Blood cultures positive for IE:
	• typical micro-organisms consistent with IE from two separate blood cultures
	Evidence of endocardial involvement:
	• echocardiography positive for IE
	   ○ vegetation
	   ○ abscess
	   ○ dehiscence of prosthetic valve
	• new valvular regurgitation

Minor criteria	Predisposition (heart condition, injecting drug use) Fever (temperature >38°C) Vascular phenomena Immunological phenomena Microbiological evidence
Diagnosis of IE is *definite* in the presence of 2 major criteria, or 1 major and 3 minor criteria, or 5 minor criteria	Diagnosis of IE is *possible* in the presence of 1 major and 1 minor criteria, or 3 minor criteria

Source: Adapted from Habib et al. [1].

www.wiley.com/go/perioperativemed

VIDEO 38.1 **Endocarditis is a pathological condition in which the endocardial layers of the heart are infected. Most commonly, this involves the cardiac valves.**

Management

Patients with IE often require multidisciplinary treatment under the care of infectious disease specialists in tertiary referral centres. Referral to other medical specialties is required when specific organ involvement occurs. Treatment is centred around bactericidal antimicrobial regimes, generally two to six weeks for native valve disease and at least six weeks if prosthetic valve IE occurs [2]. Surgical intervention is high risk and the timing controversial but around 50% of patients will require surgical intervention for severe complications, principally the presence and/or prevention of heart failure, uncontrolled infection or thromboembolism. If possible, surgery should be postponed for one to two weeks after the initiation of appropriate antibiotic therapy.

Antibiotic prophylaxis

Antibiotic prophylaxis is now only recommended in very specific circumstances (refer to Chapter 30 Antibiotic prophylaxis for endocarditis).

Myocarditis and cardiomyopathy

Myocarditis and cardiomyopathy are relatively rare diseases of the myocardium which are challenging to diagnose and treat. They have significant morbidity and mortality and are both associated with heart failure and sudden death. Dilated cardiomyopathy is the leading indication for heart transplantation in children and adults.

Myocarditis

Myocarditis is an inflammatory disease of the myocardium caused by infectious, immune and toxic triggers [3]. It is a leading cause of sudden cardiac death in young adults and progresses to dilated cardiomyopathy in 20% of patients.

Aetiology

In developed nations, the most common causes of myocarditis are acute viral infections or postviral immune-mediated responses, usually associated with adenoviruses and enteroviruses (coxsackie B). In developing nations, causes include rheumatic myocarditis, Chagas' disease and advanced HIV (Table 38.1).

Pathophysiology

The pathophysiology of myocarditis can be divided into three phases: the acute phase (viral prodrome), the subacute phase (inflammation, immune system activation and myocardial dysfunction) followed by a chronic phase characterised by myocardial remodelling and the development of dilated cardiomyopathy. In the majority of patients, the virus is cleared by the immune system and ventricular function returns to normal.

Clinical presentation

Symptoms of myocarditis range from asymptomatic, with abnormalities only detected on echocardiography, to severe life-threatening heart failure. Patients may present with a viral prodrome or chest discomfort due to pericarditis, palpitations due to arrhythmias or sudden death.

TABLE 38.1 Causes of myocarditis

Infectious	Non-infectious
Viruses:	Autoimmune disorders:
• Coxsackie B	• giant cell arteritis
• HIV	• hypereosinophilic syndrome
• EBV	• Kawasaki's disease
• CMV	• coeliac disease
• HSV	• Crohn's disease
• Parvovirus B-19	• SLE
Bacteria:	• dermatomyositis
• Chlamydia	• rheumatoid arthritis
• *Corynebacterium diphtheriae*	• sarcoidosis
• Legionella	• scleroderma
• Mycoplasma	• ulcerative colitis
• *Mycobacterium tuberculosis*	Hypersensitivity reactions to drugs:
• Staphylococcus	• antibiotics (penicillin, ampicillin,
• Streptococcus	cephalosporins, tetracyclines,
Protozoa:	sulfonamides)
• *Trypanosoma cruzi* (Chagas' disease)	• methyldopa
	• clozapine
Spirochete:	• loop and thiazide diuretics
• *Borrelia burgdoferi*	Toxic reactions to drugs:
• Leptospira	• amphetamines and cocaine
• *Treponema pallidium*	• chemotherapeutic agents (anthracyclines,
	doxorubicin, 5-fluorouracil)
	• ethanol
	Others:
	• metals (lead, copper, iron)
	• arsenic
	• radiotherapy

CMV, cytomegalovirus; EBV, Epstein–Barr virus; HSV, herpes simplex virus; HIV, human immunodeficiency virus; SLE, systemic lupus erythematosus.

Diagnosis

- *Biomarkers and viral serology*: cardiac enzymes, acute phase reactants
- *ECG*: non-specific T wave and ST changes mimicking STEMI or acute pericarditis, LBBB. QT prolongation is an independent predictor of poor outcome in myocarditis
- *Cardiac imaging*: echocardiography (structure and function), cardiac MRI (identification of myocardial inflammation and oedema)
- *Endomyocardial biopsy*: gold standard for diagnosis. Myocarditis is defined by the presence of lymphocytic (or other cell) infiltrates in association with myocyte necrosis

Management

Specific treatment involves immunosuppression, antiviral therapy and heart transplantation. Supportive treatment involves heart failure therapy, insertion of permanent pacemaker (PPM)/ICD and circulatory support (refer to Chapter 34 Pacemakers and implanted defibrillators, and Chapter 35 Heart failure).

Cardiomyopathy

The cardiomyopathies represent a heterogeneous group of primary heart muscle disorders, defined by the presence of abnormal myocardial structure and/or function and the absence of significant coronary artery disease and conditions such as hypertension, valvular and congenital heart disease. Though these conditions may lead to myocardial dilation and poor function, they are not primary cardiomyopathies.

Classification

Historically, the cardiomyopathies were classified by their clinical features or phenotype but now genotype is included where possible [4,5]. Recently, arrhythmogenic right ventricular dysplasia/cardiomyopathy (ARVD/C) has been recognised and characterised as a separate cardiomyopathy. Some cardiomyopathies are yet to be classified.

Genetics of cardiomyopathy

Since the first point mutation causing hypertrophic cardiomyopathy (HCM) was found in 1990, more than 600 rare genetic variants associated with cardiomyopathy have been found. However, variable penetrance with incomplete gene expression is common, even in the autosomal dominant forms of cardiomyopathy. Environmental factors and other modifier genes further influence the overall clinical phenotype.

Clinical presentation

The clinical presentation of the cardiomyopathies is varied and dependent somewhat on the underlying diagnosis. Patients may be asymptomatic and investigated due to family history while others present *in extremis* with cardiogenic shock. Heart failure can be due to systolic dysfunction, diastolic dysfunction or a combination of both affecting one or both ventricles. Clinically, there is a great deal of overlap in terms of myocardial dysfunction amongst the cardiomyopathies. Diastolic dysfunction is a hallmark of restrictive cardiomyopathy but also a feature of dilated cardiomyopathy and HCM.

Diagnosis

Examination and baseline investigations may reveal features of specific cardio-myopathies, but the mainstay of diagnosis in cardiomyopathy is echocardiography [6] (Table 38.2; Figure 38.1; Video 38.2). Diagnosis is supported by genetic testing, other forms of cardiac imaging (including MRI and gated blood pool scan) and endomyocardial biopsy to exclude myocarditis.

Management

Similar to myocarditis, supportive treatment includes heart failure therapy, insertion of biventricular pacemakers for cardiac resynchronisation therapy, insertion of ICDs (refer to Chapter 34 Pacemakers and implanted defibrillators and Chapter 35 Heart failure), and anticoagulation for the primary or secondary prevention of arrhythmias and thromboembolic disease respectively; genetic counselling should be offered to patients and family members. Mechanical circulatory support such as extracorporeal membrane oxygenation or ventricular assist devices remain the realm of tertiary referral centres. Surgical interventions such as septal ablation for HCM may be offered to alleviate symptoms, but heart transplantation remains the only definitive treatment.

TABLE 38.2 **Features of specific cardiomyopathies**

	Echocardiographic features	Prevalence	Other features
Hypertrophic cardiomyopathy	Increased LV wall thickness/mass Absence of abnormal loading conditions (hypertension, valve disease) Maximal wall thickness ≥15 mm	Relatively common 1:500 general population	Most affected individuals are asymptomatic Differential diagnosis: • hypertensive heart disease • 'athlete's heart' Hypertrophy may be concentric or eccentric Affected individuals may have progressive heart failure due to diastolic dysfunction and systolic dysfunction due to obstruction Historically called hypertrophic obstructive cardiomyopathy (HOCM)
Dilated cardiomyopathy	LV dilation LV dysfunction Absence of abnormal loading conditions Absence of coronary artery disease	1:2500 general population	Global LV systolic impairment RV dilation may be present but not necessary for diagnosis Third most common cause of heart failure Most common cause of heart transplantation
Restrictive cardiomyopathy (RCM)	Normal ventricular wall thickness Normal or reduced diastolic volumes Presence of restrictive ventricular physiology (severe diastolic dysfunction)	Less common	Classic RCM is infiltrative in nature as typified by cardiac amyloidosis Infiltration causes ventricular stiffening, diastolic dysfunction, elevated filling pressures and heart failure Bi-atrial dilation and pulmonary hypertension is associated Systolic function said to be preserved but rare for systolic function to be truly normal
Arrhythmogenic right ventricular dysplasia/ cardiomyopathy	Right ventricular dilation with wall motion abnormalities LV involvement also seen	Exact prevalence unknown Estimated to affect 1 in 1000–5000	True incidence unknown due to clinically silent cases Familial cases account for majority of cases Patchy fatty infiltration of the RV results in areas of fibrosis and scarring Structural abnormalities of RV results in ventricular arrhythmias, sudden cardiac death, or progressive dysfunction

LV, left ventricle; RV, right ventricle.

38

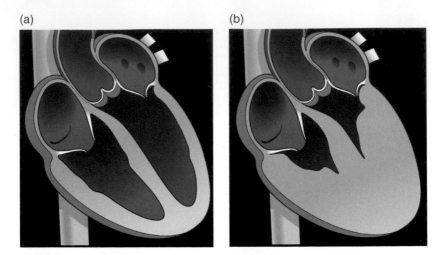

FIGURE 38.1 (A) A normal heart. (B) This heart demonstrates features typical of hypertrophic cardiomyopathy, with a hypertrophied septum and increase in ventricular mass. The septal hypertrophy often results in a degree of obstruction to the left ventricular outflow tract, impeding cardiac output.

www.wiley.com/go/perioperativemed

VIDEO 38.2 **Cardiomyopathies are a diverse group of diseases that affect the muscular tissue of the heart. The various types of cardiomyopathy are typically distinguished by echocardiographic features.**

References

1. Habib G, Hoen B, Tornos P, et al. Guidelines on the prevention, diagnosis, and treatment of infective endocarditis (new version 2009): the Task Force on the Prevention, Diagnosis, and Treatment of Infective Endocarditis of the European Society of Cardiology (ESC). Endorsed by the European Society of Clinical Microbiology and Infectious Diseases (ESCMID) and the International Society of Chemotherapy (ISC) for Infection and Cancer. *European Heart Journal*, 2009;**30**(19):2369–2413. doi:10.1093/eurheartj/ehp285

2. Antibiotic Writing Group. *Therapeutic Guidelines: Antibiotic*, 14th edn. Melbourne, Australia: Therapeutic Guidelines Ltd, 2010. www.tg.org.au/

3. Kindermann I, Barth C, Mahfoud F, et al. Update on myocarditis. *Journal of the American College of Cardiology*, 2012;**59**(9):779–792. doi:10.1016/j.jacc.2011.09.074

4. Elliott P, Andersson B, Arbustini E, et al. Classification of the cardiomyopathies: a position statement from the European Society Of Cardiology Working Group on Myocardial and Pericardial Diseases. *European Heart Journal*, 2008;**29**(2):270–276. doi:10.1093/eurheartj/ehm342

5. Maron BJ, Towbin JA, Thiene G, et al. Contemporary definitions and classification of the cardiomyopathies: an American Heart Association Scientific Statement from the Council on Clinical Cardiology, Heart Failure and Transplantation Committee; Quality of Care and Outcomes Research and Functional Genomics and Translational Biology Interdisciplinary Working Groups; and Council on Epidemiology and Prevention. *Circulation*, 2006;**113**(14):1807–1816. doi:10.1161/CIRCULATIONAHA.106.174287

6. Gersh BJ, Maron BJ, Bonow RO, et al. 2011 ACCF/AHA Guideline for the Diagnosis and Treatment of Hypertrophic Cardiomyopathy: a report of the American College of Cardiology Foundation/American Heart Association Task Force on Practice Guidelines. Developed in collaboration with the American Association for Thoracic Surgery, American Society of Echocardiography, American Society of Nuclear Cardiology, Heart Failure Society of America, Heart Rhythm Society, Society for Cardiovascular Angiography and Interventions, and Society of Thoracic Surgeons. *Journal of the American College of Cardiology*, 2011;**58**(25):e212–260. doi:10.1016/j.jacc.2011.06.011

39 Acute lung injury

Paul Nixon[1] and David Tuxen[2]

[1] The Alfred Hospital, Australia
[2] The Alfred Hospital and Monash University, Australia

Acute lung injury (ALI) describes an inflammatory process in the lungs in response to a variety of disease states. When ALI meets the criteria below, it is termed acute respiratory distress syndrome (ARDS) [1] (Table 39.1).

Pathophysiology

Acute lung injury is a diffuse inflammatory process with increased pulmonary vascular permeability, alveolar and interstitial oedema and increased lung weight. Widespread alveolar collapse occurs, predominantly in dependent regions, with an increased shunt fraction. A decrease in the total volume of aerated lung tissue develops with increased distention of ventilated lung segments and capillary endothelial damage, resulting in an increase in physiological dead space. The clinical features of severe ALI (ARDS) are hypoxaemia, bilateral radiographic opacities, increased minute ventilation requirements and decreased lung compliance.

Aetiology

Acute lung injury can be caused by disease processes directly affecting the lungs (intrinsic or direct ALI) or by systemic processes (extrinsic or indirect ALI); the pathophysiological process and outcomes are similar between the two groups [2] (Table 39.2).

Management

Management involves treating the underlying cause, supportive care and minimising ventilator-induced lung injury. Multiple agents have been investigated to modify the inflammatory process, but none has established benefits. Antibiotics are not routinely indicated, but are essential when pneumonia or sepsis is the cause.

Perioperative Medicine for the Junior Clinician, First Edition. Edited by Joel Symons, Paul Myles, Rishi Mehra and Christine Ball.
© 2015 John Wiley & Sons, Ltd. Published 2015 by John Wiley & Sons, Ltd.
Companion website: www.wiley.com/go/perioperativemed

TABLE 39.1 **ARDS diagnostic criteria and mortality prediction**

ARDS diagnostic criteria

An acute process (less than 1 week)

Bilateral opacities on chest X-ray

Origin of oedema not fully explained by cardiac failure or fluid overload

Level of severity

	Mild	Moderate	Severe
Oxygenation: PF ratio	>200 to ≤300 mmHg	>100 to ≤200 mmHg	≤100 mmHg
PEEP setting (intubated)	≥5 cmH₂O (if on NIV: CPAP ≥5 cmH₂O)	≥5 cmH₂O	≥5 cmH₂O
Predicted mortality	27%	32%	45%

CPAP, continuous positive airway pressure; NIV, non-invasive ventilation; PEEP, positive end expiratory pressure; PF ratio, PaO₂/FiO₂.

TABLE 39.2 **Common causes of acute lung injury**

Intrinsic process	Extrinsic process
Pneumonia	Sepsis
Aspiration	Major trauma
Pulmonary contusion	Severe burns
Near drowning	Multiple blood product transfusions
Smoke inhalation	Pancreatitis
Amniotic fluid embolism	Drug reaction
Fat embolism	

Ventilator-induced lung injury

> Mechanical ventilation is required in all but the mildest forms of ALI, but can also contribute to lung injury.

This process is known as ventilator-induced lung injury (VILI) and attempts should be made to prevent it in all ventilated patients, but especially those with an established lung insult. The lung is not simply a passive receiver of this injury, but can generate injurious cytokines that contribute to multiple organ failure, the most common cause of death in ARDS. Much of the current management of ALI is now based on ventilator strategies that reduce this secondary lung insult with resultant survival improvements.

Although the lungs may appear uniformly injured on plain chest X-ray, CT scanning has revealed three functionally distinct zones [3]. These zones develop as oedematous lung regions collapse, a result of their increased weight.

Zone 3 (most dependent lung regions):

- remains collapsed throughout tidal ventilation
- as much as 50–60% of lung volume
- most prone to lung cyst formation, the precursor of pneumothoraces, thought to be initiated by microabscess formation.

Zone 1 (least dependent lung regions):

- remains inflated throughout tidal ventilation
- receives 80–90% of tidal volume
- at risk of overdistension of alveoli (volutrauma, resulting in capillary permeability changes and alveoli cell apoptosis).

Zone 2 (intermediate zone):

- inflates during inspiration and collapses during expiration
- cyclical opening and closing of small airways and alveoli (atelectrauma) causes large stress forces between and within alveoli, resulting in mucosal injury with oedema and segmental collapse.

Barotrauma (e.g. pneumothorax or subcutaneous emphysema) results from high pressures in the respiratory system.

A number of ventilator settings may minimise the risk of VILI. They should be used in all ventilated patients, including those undergoing major surgery [5] (Table 39.3).

Biotrauma is the proinflammatory process that develops in response to alveolar damage in all regions due to both the primary injury and induced by mechanical ventilation. These cytokines are believed to contribute to multiple organ failure and mortality. It has also been shown that surfactant function is decreased during mechanical ventilation.

Oxygen toxicity

High FiO_2 can lead to direct damage of pulmonary tissue (e.g. through oxygen free radicals) and reabsorption atelectasis [4].

Protective mechanical ventilation strategies

Refer to Table 39.3.

TABLE 39.3 Initial ventilator settings in ALI

Parameter	Ventilator setting
Tidal volume	≤6 mL per kg predicted body weight
Plateau pressure	≤30 cmH_2O
Positive end expiratory pressure	≥5 cmH_2O
FiO_2	Minimum to maintain SpO_2 90–96%

Ventilator pressures

- Minimise to prevent barotrauma.
- Plateau pressure (Pplat), <30 cmH$_2$O, lower if possible.
- Tidal volumes, commence at 6 mL/kg, decrease to 4 mL/kg to ensure Pplat <30 cmH$_2$O.
- Pressure control ventilation is a commonly preferred mode (ensures safe pressure limits with deteriorating lung compliance).

Positive end expiratory pressure (PEEP)

- May limit atelectrauma, prevent alveoli collapse, improve oxygenation.
- Optimal level unclear.
- 5 cmH$_2$O minimum, 10–17 cmH$_2$O commonly for moderate to severe ARDS.

Fluid management

The stress response to the illness associated with ALI results in increased antidiuretic hormone (ADH) release and fluid retention, compounding pulmonary oedema. Critically ill patients often have unintended positive fluid balances after primary fluid resuscitation is complete. Although studies of conservative fluid management have not found a mortality benefit, results have shown an improvement in gas exchange and a decreased time of mechanical ventilation [6]. The aim in ALI should be to initially administer enough fluid to maintain haemodynamic stability and organ perfusion, but to avoid or treat unplanned positive fluid balances.

Rescue therapies

In refractory hypoxaemic states associated with established ARDS, a number of rescue therapies are commonly utilised. Unlike protective ventilator strategies which primarily focus on reducing VILI in lung zones 1 and 2 (Figure 39.1), some of these

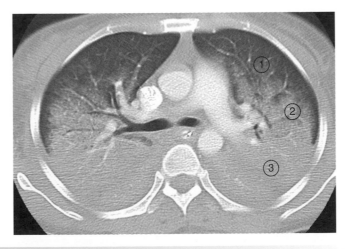

FIGURE 39.1 **CT scan in ARDS.** Zone ① represents areas of the lung that are inflated and at risk of overdistension. Zone ② represents areas of the lung that repetitively collapse and re-expand. Zone ③ represents areas of the lung that remain collapsed throughout tidal ventilation.

TABLE 39.4 Common rescue therapies used in ALI/ARDS

Modality	Brief explanation	Proposed effect
Inhaled pulmonary dilator	Inhaled nitric oxide or prostacyclin via ventilation circuit	Improve V/Q matching by dilating pulmonary vessels in ventilated lung regions, thereby diverting more blood flow to these regions
Recruitment manoeuvres	Administration of high airway pressures for a period of time (e.g. 30–120 seconds)	Aim to open atelectatic lung segments which can then be maintained open by lower airway pressures
Prone positioning	Rotating patient from supine to prone position	Shifts dependent lung zones, facilitates recruitment of collapsed segments and reduces overall shunt
HFOV	High mean airway pressures with rapid respiratory rate and very low tidal volumes	Recruit and maintain recruitment of atelectatic lung segments. Minimise VILI with delivery of minimal tidal volumes
ECMO	Oxygenation and CO_2 removal performed outside the patient via a mechanical oxygenator	Provides adequate extrapulmonary gas exchange. Allows ventilation settings to be minimised to limit VILI. Enables survival in patients with unventilatable lungs

ECMO, extracorporeal membrane oxygenation; HFOV, high-frequency oscillatory ventilation; VILI, ventilator-induced lung injury.

rescue therapies can be used to specifically address zone 3 (Table 39.4). All improve oxygenation, but only prone positioning [7] and ECMO [8] have been shown to improve mortality.

References

1. Ranieri VM, Rubenfeld GD, Thompson BT, et al. Acute respiratory distress syndrome: the Berlin Definition. *JAMA*, 2012;**307**(23):2526–2533. doi:10.1001/jama.2012.5669

2. Lumb AB. Acute lung injury. In: *Nunn's Applied Respiratory Physiology*, 7th edn. Oxford: Elsevier, 2012.

3. Gattinoni L, Caironi P, Pelosi P, Goodman LR. What has computerised tomography taught us about the acute respiratory distress syndrome? *American Journal of Respiratory and Critical Care Medicine*, 2001;**164**:1701–1711. doi:10.1164/ajrccm.164.9.2103121

4. Aboab J, Jonson B, Kouatchet A, Taille S, Niklason L, Brochard L. Effect of inspired oxygen fraction on alveolar derecruitment in acute respiratory distress syndrome. *Intensive Care Medicine*, 2006;**32**(12):1979–1986. doi:10.1007/s00134-006-0382-4

5. Futier E, Constantin JM, Paugam-Burtz C, et al. A trial of intraoperative low-tidal-volume ventilation in abdominal surgery. *New England Journal of Medicine*, 2013;**369**(5):428–4237. doi:10.1056/NEJMoa1301082

6. Wiedemann HP, Wheeler AP, Bernard GR, et al. Comparison of two fluid-management strategies in acute lung injury. *New England Journal of Medicine*, 2006;**354**(24):2564–2575. doi:10.1056/NEJMoa062200

7. Guerin C, Reignier J, Richard JC, et al. Prone positioning in severe acute respiratory distress syndrome. *New England Journal of Medicine*, 2013;**368**(23):2159–2168. doi:10.1056/NEJMoa1214103

8. Peek GJ, Mugford M, Tiruvoipati R, et al. Efficacy and economic assessment of conventional ventilatory support versus extracorporeal membrane oxygenation for severe adult respiratory failure (CESAR): a multicentre randomised controlled trial. *Lancet*, 2009;**374**(9698):1351–1363. doi:10.1016/S0140-6736(09)61069-2

40 Obstructive sleep apnoea

Matthew Naughton

The Alfred Hospital and Monash University, Australia

Introduction and definitions

Apnoeas during sleep are pauses to ventilation of >10 seconds duration. Hypopnoeas are a partial reduction in airflow associated with a fall in SpO_2 (usually ≥3%) or electroencephalographic arousal from sleep.

Sleep apnoea is quantified by the Apnoea Hypopnoea Index (AHI), which is the total number of apnoeas and hypopnoeas during sleep divided by hours of sleep.

Sleep apnoea syndrome is defined by AHI >5 events per hour (or >1 event per hour in children) associated with symptoms (e.g. daytime sleepiness).

Sleep apnoea can be further subdivided into:

* obstructive sleep apnoea (OSA), due to upper airway instability, usually with snoring
* central sleep apnoea (CSA), due to episodic loss of respiratory drive and secondary hypoventilation.

Central sleep apnoea can be further subdivided into:

* *continuous* hypoventilation and an elevated $PaCO_2$ (e.g. kyphoscoliosis or motor neurone disease) or
* *cyclic* hypoventilation – hyperventilation with elevated $PaCO_2$ (e.g. narcotics) or reduced $PaCO_2$ (e.g. heart failure with Cheyne Stokes respiration).

Epidemiology

In adults, snoring, OSA (AHI >5) and symptomatic OSA (AHI >5) are more common in men than women and have increased over the past 20 years by 14–55% due to increasing population age, obesity and co-existent medical problems [1]. The severity of OSA can be graded (Table 40.1).

* *Hypercapnic* CSA is common in patients with chest wall or neuromuscular diseases when the lung volumes (e.g. forced vital capacity on spirometry) drop to <50% or with narcotic ingestion.
* *Hypocapnic* CSA is common in patients with advanced heart failure (LVEF <35%).

Perioperative Medicine for the Junior Clinician, First Edition. Edited by Joel Symons, Paul Myles, Rishi Mehra and Christine Ball.
© 2015 John Wiley & Sons, Ltd. Published 2015 by John Wiley & Sons, Ltd.
Companion website: www.wiley.com/go/perioperativemed

TABLE 40.1 Severity of obstructive sleep apnoea

	AHI (episodes per hour)	Minimum SpO$_2$ (%)	Cardiovascular disease
Normal	<5	>92	Nil
Mild	5–15	88–92	Mild (hypertension on 1 drug)
Moderate	15–30	80–88	Modest (hypertension on 2 drugs, TIA)
Severe	30–120	50–80	Severe (hypertension on 3 or more drugs, HF)

AHI, Apnoea Hypopnoea Index; HF, heart failure; TIA, transient ischaemic attack.

Pathophysiology

Snoring and OSA are due to sleep-related loss of upper airway dilator muscle tone (e.g. genioglossus) in the oropharynx [2]. Airway collapse results in hypoxaemia and hypercapnia with large negative intrathoracic pressures until terminated by an arousal from sleep. Physiological changes result in the clinical sequelae of wide swings in systemic and pulmonary vascular pressure, tachy-bradycardia and other arrhythmias, increased myocardial oxygen demands and ischaemia, heart failure and cerebrovascular disease [3].

Central sleep apnoea with hypercapnia occurs due to loss of respiratory drive or inability of the respiratory pump. Sleep-related hypoventilation occurs, particularly during REM sleep when upper airway and intercostal muscle activity is switched off and ventilation relies purely on diaphragmatic activity.

Central sleep apnoea with episodic or periodic respiratory drive occurs in stages 1 and 2 non-REM sleep when ventilation is under CO_2 control. It is worsened by low cardiac output or pulmonary oedema as seen in heart failure, typically with an apnoea-hyperpnoea cycle length of ~60 seconds. Patients on narcotics present with a similar pattern but with elevated PaCO$_2$ level and a shorter apnoea–hyperpnoea cycle length (~30 seconds).

Perioperative complications of OSA are detailed in Box 40.1.

BOX 40.1 Perioperative complications of obstructive sleep apnoea

- Untreated OSA is associated with greater postoperative complications [4,6]
- A difficult airway is common in OSA [7]
- Atelectasis is common in obese patients
- Hypoxia and poor sleep lead to poor healing and diabetic control, and greater risk of infections
- Sensitivity to analgesics and sedatives increases the risk of hypercapnic acidosis
- Hyperoxia increases the risk of hypercapnic acidosis

BOX 40.2 The STOP-Bang questionnaire for assessing the presence of obstructive sleep apnoea

1. *Snoring*
   Do you snore loudly (louder than talking or loud enough to be heard through closed doors)?
   Yes No
2. *Tired*
   Do you often feel *tired*, fatigued, or sleepy during daytime?
   Yes No
3. *Observed*
   Has anyone *observed* you stop breathing during your sleep?
   Yes No
4. *Blood pressure*
   Do you have or are being treated for high blood *pressure*?
   Yes No
5. *BMI*
   BMI more than 35 kg/m^2?
   Yes No
6. *Age*
   Age over 50 yr old?
   Yes No
7. *Neck circumference*
   Neck circumference greater than 40 cm?
   Yes No
8. *Gender*
   Gender male?
   Yes No

   High risk of OSA: answering yes to 3 or more items

   Low risk of OSA: answering yes to less than 3 items

   Source: Chung et al. [4]. Reproduced with permission of Wolters Kluwer Health.

Preoperative management of OSA

Patients with known OSA should bring their own continuous positive pressure airway (CPAP) machine to the hospital. Ensure the pump is labelled with their name. Adherence can be measured objectively from the pump's digital memory or by the patient volunteering usage >4 hours per night.

Obstructive sleep apnoea can be suspected based upon a history of snoring (audible in other rooms and despite absence of alcohol), objective questionnaires (Positive STOP-Bang [Box 40.2] [4] or Berlin [5] questionnaires) or a likely body habitus (e.g. 'difficult airway', neck circumference >43 cm, BMI >30 kg/m^2).

Elective surgery

A suspected diagnosis of OSA can be confirmed with ambulatory cardiopulmonary or attended polysomnography (Video 40.1).

www.wiley.com/go/perioperativemed

VIDEO 40.1 **Polysomnography. An overnight sleep study can provide a variety of useful measures about sleep-related disorders, including a diagnosis of sleep apnoea and severity of sleep apnoea if present.**

The need for treatment depends on AHI, symptoms and the patient's cardiovascular risk profile.

Treatment options include lifestyle modification, mandibular advancement splints, surgery and CPAP via a nasal or oronasal mask. CPAP can be delivered in fixed and auto-titrating pressure with or without heated humidification.

Bilevel CPAP (inspiratory and expiratory pressures with back-up respiratory rate) is often used in acute respiratory failure and is often referred to as non-invasive ventilatory support (NIV). Most CPAP and NIV devices have detailed built-in digital usage meters. Many mask types are available and include nasal, nasal 'pillow', oronasal, oral and helmet (Figure 40.1; Video 40.2).

Emergency surgery

If severe OSA is suspected based upon clinical assessment, institute treatment (usually with CPAP) under close clinical observation.

Postoperative management of OSA

The management of OSA postoperatively depends on:

- type of surgery and associated anaesthesia
- severity of OSA
- treatment for OSA.

Patients with moderate-to-severe OSA should continue CPAP postoperatively in a general ward with experienced nursing staff. If the patient has severe untreated OSA and has undergone major abdominal or thoracic surgery, HDU monitoring and NIV may be required.

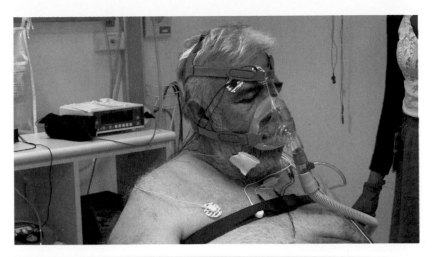

FIGURE 40.1 A variety of CPAP masks are available including nasal, oral and helmet. Shown here is a patient with an oronasal CPAP mask.

www.wiley.com/go/perioperativemed

VIDEO 40.2 Continuous positive airway pressure (CPAP) is an effective method for preventing airway collapse in patients with obstructive sleep apnoea.

Contraindications to CPAP include:

- craniofacial surgery or trauma
- base of skull fracture
- nasopharyngeal resection of pituitary tumour
- severe epistaxis (contraindication to nasal CPAP).

In patients with mild sleep apnoea, or those with moderate OSA who are intolerant of CPAP, positional therapy is crucial, ideally in the upright or lateral recovery position.

> Use supplemental oxygen cautiously (e.g. SpO_2 92–95%) to avoid hyperoxia and resultant CO_2 retention and narcosis.

References

1. Peppard PE, Young T, Barnet JH, Palta M, Hagen E, Hla K. Increased prevalence of sleep-disordered breathing in adults. *American Journal of Epidemiology*, 2013;**177**(9): 1006–1014. doi:10.1093/aje/kws342

2. Hamilton GS, Naughton MT. Impact of obstructive sleep apnoea on diabetes and cardiovascular disease. *Medical Journal of Australia*, 2013;**199**(8):S27–30. doi:10.5694/mja13.10579

3. Shamsuzzaman AS, Gersh BJ, Somers VK. Obstructive sleep apnea: implications for cardiac and vascular disease. *JAMA*, 2003;**290**(14):1906–1914. doi:10.1001/jama.290.14.1906

4. Chung F, Yegneswaran B, Liao P, et al. STOP questionnaire: a tool to screen patients for obstructive sleep apnea. *Anesthesiology*, 2008;**108**(5):812–821. doi:10.1097/ALN.0b013e31816d83e4

5. Netzer NC, Stoohs RA, Netzer CM, Clark K, Strohl KP. Using the Berlin Questionnaire to identify patients at risk for the sleep apnea syndrome. *Annals of Internal Medicine*, 1999;**131**(7):485–491. doi:10.7326/0003-4819-131-7-199910050-00002

6. Memtsoudis S, Liu SS, Ma Y, et al. Perioperative pulmonary outcomes in patients with sleep apnea after noncardiac surgery. *Anesthesia and Analgesia*, 2011;**112**(1):113–121. doi:10.1213/ANE.0b013e3182009abf

7. Hiremath AS, Hillman DR, James AL, Noffsinger WJ, Platt PR, Singer SL. Relationship between difficult tracheal intubation and obstructive sleep apnoea. *British Journal of Anaesthesia*, 1998;**80**(5):606–611. doi:10.1093/bja/80.5.606

Asthma

Alan Young

Eastern Health and Monash University, Australia

Asthma is common and, when uncontrolled, increases the risk of postoperative complications. This highlights the need for preoperative detection and intervention.

Perioperative complications of asthma

Airway hyper-responsiveness, airflow limitation and mucus hypersecretion predispose patients with asthma to perioperative respiratory complications. Additionally, tracheal intubation may result in bronchoconstriction [1]. Not surprisingly, asthma is a patient-related risk factor for [2]:

- bronchospasm
- atelectasis
- infection, pneumonia
- respiratory failure, hypoxaemia
- reintubation.

Postoperative pulmonary complications increase hospital length of stay [3] and respiratory failure is associated with increased mortality [4]. The postoperative pulmonary complication rate in asthmatic patients of 3% is similar to the rate for non-asthmatic patients [2] but the incidence doubles in patients with uncontrolled asthma. In the largest study of asthma patients undergoing general surgery, bronchospasm, laryngospasm and respiratory failure were more common in those with suboptimally controlled asthma (i.e. those patients with the need for medication or visit to emergency department/outpatient clinic) in the preceding month [5].

Preoperative assessment and management of asthma

The clinician's role in the preoperative assessment includes:

- detecting undiagnosed asthma
- assessing disease control in those with asthma
- identifying high-risk asthma patients
- optimising asthma control to reduce the risk of postoperative complications.

Perioperative Medicine for the Junior Clinician, First Edition. Edited by Joel Symons, Paul Myles, Rishi Mehra and Christine Ball.
© 2015 John Wiley & Sons, Ltd. Published 2015 by John Wiley & Sons, Ltd.
Companion website: www.wiley.com/go/perioperativemed

TABLE 41.1 Assessing asthma control

Characteristic (over 4-week period)	Controlled	Partly controlled	Uncontrolled
Daytime symptoms	None	> twice/week	≥3 features partly controlled asthma
Limitation activities	None	Any	
Nocturnal symptoms	None	Any	
Need reliever treatment	None	> twice/ week	
PEF or FEV$_1$	Normal	<80%	

Source: Adapted from GINA guidelines [7].
FEV, forced expiratory volume; PEF, peak expiratory flow.

Diagnosing asthma

Asthma is a chronic inflammatory disorder of the airways characterised by:

- recurrent episodes of breathlessness, wheezing, chest tightness and coughing (often nocturnal or exertional)
- airway hyper-responsiveness
- reversible airways obstruction.

A clinical diagnosis based on typical symptoms and response to treatment is appropriate in selected patients, but objective testing is often recommended. *Reversible airways obstruction* is defined as a significant bronchodilator (BD) response during spirometry (increase FEV$_1$ by 200 mL and 12% following inhaled salbutamol). Alternatively, diurnal variability in peak expiratory flow measurements of 20% can be used. If these investigations are non-diagnostic, *airway hyper-responsiveness* can be confirmed with challenge testing to inhaled mannitol or methacholine which induce a significant fall in FEV$_1$ of 15% and 20% respectively [6].

Assessing disease control

A key step in asthma management is to assess disease control and escalate treatment if required. Clinical features indicate whether optimal control has been achieved (Table 41.1) [7].

Identifying high-risk patients

Poor asthma control, frequent severe exacerbations, frequent use of a short-acting beta agonist and frequent hospital attendance for asthma are risk factors for future asthma exacerbations and fatal asthma attacks (Table 41.2). These are high-risk patients for surgery.

Optimising asthma management

Asthma management involves treating any underlying precipitating factors/ triggers (Table 41.3) and stepwise escalation of treatment to achieve optimal control (Table 41.4). Treatment begins with a short-acting beta-agonist as required (e.g. pre-exercise).

TABLE 41.2 Risk factors for future asthma exacerbation and fatal asthma attack

Asthma exacerbation	Fatal asthma attack
Poor clinical control	Previous severe exacerbation (intubation or ICU)
Frequent exacerbations in past year	≥ 2 hospitalisations for asthma in past year
Previous ICU admission for asthma	≥ 3 ED visits for asthma in past year
Low FEV_1	Hospitalisation or ED visit for asthma in past month
Cigarette smoker	Use of >2 canisters short-acting beta-2 agonist per month
High-dose asthma medications	Difficulty perceiving asthma symptoms or exacerbations
	Low socioeconomic status, illicit drug use, psychosocial issues
	Co-morbidities (e.g. cardiovascular, chronic lung, psychiatric)

Source: Adapted from GINA guidelines [7].
ED, emergency department; FEV, forced expiratory volume; ICU, intensive care unit.

TABLE 41.3 Common asthma triggers

Trigger	Clinical feature
Exercise	Often in cold air, after 15 minutes, persisting post exercise
Allergens	House dust mite, mould, pollen, grasses, animal dander
Infections	Viral most common
Cigarette smoking	Active or passive
Gastro-oesophageal reflux	Nocturnal or postprandial cough and wheeze
Medications	Aspirin, non-steroidal anti-inflammatory drugs, beta-blockers
Occupational	Dusts, chemicals, fumes

TABLE 41.4 Stepwise approach to asthma management

Step 1 →	Step 2 →	Step 3 →	Step 4 →	Step 5	Other
Inhaled SABA as required	Add ICS 400 mcg/d	Add LABA to ICS	Increase ICS 800 mcg/d with LABA	Add OCS. Specialist referral	LTRA Oral theophylline Anti-IgE

Source: Adapted from British Thoracic Society and Scottish Intercollegiate Guidelines Network [10].
ICS, inhaled corticosteroid (e.g. Pulmicort turbuhaler 200 mcg b.d. or flixotide MDI 250 mcg b.d. spacer);
LABA, long-acting beta-agonist (e.g. eformoterol 6 mcg b.d. or salmeterol MDI 50 mcg b.d.);
LTRA, leukotriene receptor antagonist (e.g. monteleukast 10 mg daily); MDI, metered dose inhaler;
OCS, oral corticosteroid (e.g. 10–40 mg prednisolone daily); SABA, short-acting beta-agonist
(e.g. salbutamol MDI 2 puffs p.r.n. via spacer).
Note that ICS/LABA combination inhalers are available (e.g. Symbicort tubuhaler or Seretide MDI).

Ongoing asthma symptoms or an exacerbation warrant introduction of inhaled corticosteroids. Ongoing suboptimal control leads to addition of a long-acting beta agonist (LABA), then an increase in the dose of inhaled corticosteroids. Systemic steroids are reserved for ongoing uncontrolled asthma and to treat severe exacerbations.

Preoperative screening for asthma and disease control

Identifying patients with uncontrolled asthma who are below their best allows more aggressive preoperative management to optimise airflow obstruction and reduce perioperative complications. Hence, all asthma patients should be assessed preoperatively.

History

To screen for and assess pre-existing asthma.

- *Episodic symptoms*: breathlessness, wheeze, chest tightness, coughing
- *Risk factors*: history of asthma during childhood, atopy, family history of asthma
- *Triggers* (Table 41.3): particularly current smoking, current infection
- *Control*: current control (Table 41.1), medication use, hospital or clinic visits in last 30 days
- *Medication*: current treatment, medications that worsen asthma (Table 41.3)

Examination

Signs of asthma on examination include breathlessness with talking, chest hyperexpansion, generalised expiratory wheezing and hypoxia on pulse oximetry.

Investigations

Perform in selected patients to (a) diagnose asthma or (b) assess suspected suboptimal control.

- *Peak flow measurement*: diurnal variability for diagnosis, suboptimal if <80% recent best
- *Spirometry*: BD response for diagnosis, suboptimal if BD response or FEV_1 <80% recent best
- *Challenge test*: fall in FEV_1 for diagnosis, suboptimal if fall in FEV_1 whilst on treatment

Preoperative asthma management

Well-controlled asthma patients (asymptomatic, not requiring reliever medications or medical attention last 12 months, peak flow >80% predicted) are at low risk for perioperative complications and require no additional intervention.

Patients with *active asthma* (current symptoms, uncontrolled asthma or significant BD response on spirometry) improve lung function in the preoperative period with ventolin and develop less postoperative wheezing if administered oral prednisolone 40 mg for five days preoperatively [8]. Patients should continue their regular asthma preventer medications. Inhaled corticosteroids should be commenced if not in use but may not reach maximal effect prior to surgery. For elective surgery, postponement until control is achieved and specialist referral should be considered. Upper abdominal and thoracic surgery are high-risk procedures due to postoperative

TABLE 41.5 Management of acute asthma exacerbation

Treatment	Dose
Oxygen therapy	For hypoxic patients, maintain SpO_2 ≥95%
Short-acting beta-agonist	Salbutamol MDI 100 mcg 4–6 puffs via spacer every 20 min 1st hour OR salbutamol nebulised 5 mg every 20 minutes 1st hour If improving, 2–4 puffs 4 hourly; not improving, 6 puffs 1–2 hourly*
Systemic corticosteroids	Prednisolone 40–60 mg orally daily, wean once stable Not improving, change to hydrocortisone 200 mg IV 6 hourly
Magnesium sulfate	2 g IV over 20 min

Source: Adapted from GINA guidelines [7].
*Monitor for side effects – tremor, tachycardia, hypokalaemia.

atelectasis and analgesic requirements [2]. Choice of appropriate anaesthetic agents and technique are important.

Triggers including current respiratory infection and reflux should be treated. Aspirin or NSAIDs should be avoided in those with aspirin sensitivity and nasal polyposis as they may precipitate an exacerbation. All patients should be screened for cigarette smoking and attempt cessation more than two months prior [2] to surgery where possible, but within two months of surgery is still beneficial.

Patients on long-term oral prednisolone can be administered IV hydrocortisone 100 mg 8 hourly perioperatively until the oral regimen can be resumed (refer to Chapter 27 Steroid medication) [1].

Postoperative management of an asthma exacerbation

Despite perioperative management, asthma exacerbations occur or, more commonly, asthma that has not been assessed worsens. Treatment is similar to that for any asthma exacerbation.

Conduct *rapid bedside assessment* – history, examination, peak flow measurement, pulse oximetry.

Detect clinical features of a *severe exacerbation* [9].

* Patient appears physically exhausted
* Talks in single words
* Pulse rate >120 beats per minute
* Palpable pulsus paradoxus
* Central cyanosis
* Quiet chest on auscultation
* Peak expiratory flow (PEF) <50% or 100 L/min
* SpO_2 <92%
* Hypoxia (PaO_2 <60 mmHg) or hypercapnia ($PaCO_2$ >45 mmHg) on arterial blood gas sample

Implement *stepwise management* [7] (Table 41.5), assessing response hourly.

* Short-acting beta-agonist, supplemental oxygen, treat underlying factors (sedation, infection)
* If not responding → systemic corticosteroids, IV magnesium

- If not responding and severe exacerbation → ICU referral/admission
- In ICU, consider IV glucocorticoids, IV beta-2 agonist, intubation and mechanical ventilation

Organise appropriate *follow-up* – GP or specialist, asthma management plan, peak flow monitoring, weaning systemic corticosteroids, ongoing inhaled corticosteroid and/or long-acting beta-agonist.

References

1. Su FW, Beckman DB, Yarnold PA, Grammer LC. Low incidence of complications in asthmatic patients treated with preoperative corticosteroids. *Allergy and Asthma Proceedings*, 2004;**25**(5):327–333.

2. Smetana GW, Lawrence VA, Cornell JE. Preoperative pulmonary risk stratification for noncardiothoracic surgery: systematic review for the American College of Physicians. *Annals of Internal Medicine*, 2006;**144**(8):581–595. doi:10.7326/0003-4819-144-8-200604180-00009

3. Lawrence VA, Cornell JE, Smetana GW. Strategies to reduce postoperative pulmonary complications after noncardiothoracic surgery: systematic review for the American College of Physicians. *Annals of Internal Medicine*, 2006;**144**(8):596–608. doi:10.7326/0003-4819-144-8-200604180-00011

4. Arozullah AM, Daley J, Henderson WG, Khuri SF. Multifactorial risk index for predicting postoperative respiratory failure in men after major noncardiac surgery. The National Veterans Administration Surgical Quality Improvement Program. *Annals of Surgery*, 2000;**232**(2):242–253. doi:10.1097/00000658-200008000-00015

5. Warner DO, Warner MA, Barnes RD, et al. Perioperative respiratory complications in patients with asthma. *Anesthesiology*, 1996;**85**(3):460–467. doi:10.1097/00000542-199609000-00003

6. Pellegrino R, Viegi G, Brusasco V, et al. Interpretative strategies for lung function tests. *European Respiratory Journal*, 2005;**26**(5):948–968. doi:10.1183/09031936.05.00035205

7. Global Initiative for Asthma (GINA). *Global Strategy for Asthma Management and Prevention*. 2012. www.ginasthma.org

8. Silvanus MT, Groeben H, Peters J. Corticosteroids and inhaled salbutamol in patients with reversible airway obstruction markedly decrease the incidence of bronchospasm after tracheal intubation. *Anesthesiology*, 2004;**100**(5):1052–1057. doi:10.1097/00000542-200405000-00004

9. National Asthma Council. *Asthma Management Handbook*. 2006. www.nationalasthma.org.au

10. British Thoracic Society and Scottish Intercollegiate Guidelines Network. British Guideline on the Management of Asthma. *Thorax*, 2008;**63**(Suppl 4):iv1–121. doi:10.1136/thx.2008.097741

Chronic obstructive pulmonary disease

Jeremy Wrobel[1] and Trevor Williams[2]

[1] Royal Perth Hospital, Australia
[2] The Alfred Hospital and Monash University, Australia

> The presence of chronic obstructive pulmonary disease (COPD) identifies a patient with increased perioperative morbidity (double) and mortality (four-fold increase at 30 days) who will require more intensive postoperative care and a longer hospital stay.

Although it is self-evident that the risk of postoperative pulmonary complications is greater in patients with COPD, the increased risk specifically relates to present smoking, smoking-related lung disease (including COPD) and the many associated medical conditions often identified in this patient group.

The presence of cough and dyspnoea in a past or present smoker should alert the physician to the possibility of COPD. The present Global Initiative for Chronic Obstructive Lung Disease (GOLD) guidelines include spirometric abnormalities (airflow obstruction with postbronchodilator $FEV_1/FVC < 70\%$) for the diagnosis [1].

The risk of postoperative pulmonary complications relates to the presence of airflow obstruction, chronic bronchitis and pulmonary parenchymal damage (emphysema), as well as the effects of cigarettes on mucociliary clearance. This leads perioperatively to:

- atelectasis
- infection, including bronchitis and pneumonia
- exacerbation of COPD including bronchospasm.

This contributes to postoperative respiratory failure (both hypoxic and hypercapnic), leading to increased length of ICU stay, increased overall length of hospital stay and a more than four-fold increase in 30-day mortality (of which a relative risk of 1.3 is directly attributable to COPD) compared with non-COPD patients [2].

Perioperative Medicine for the Junior Clinician, First Edition. Edited by Joel Symons, Paul Myles, Rishi Mehra and Christine Ball.
© 2015 John Wiley & Sons, Ltd. Published 2015 by John Wiley & Sons, Ltd.
Companion website: www.wiley.com/go/perioperativemed

Current smoking further increases the risk of postoperative complications. Ceasing smoking preoperatively for more than two months reduces this risk and ceasing more than six months preoperatively eliminates the additional smoking-related risk. The presence of co-existing pulmonary hypertension also adds to postoperative morbidity and mortality [3].

Effects of anaesthesia and surgery on lung function

Anaesthesia, the surgical procedure and the immediate postoperative period all have important effects on lung mechanics and function. The type of surgery (for example, thoracic and upper abdominal), anaesthesia management (general or regional anaesthesia) and the postoperative approach to analgesia all impact on postoperative pulmonary complications (Figure 42.1) [4,5]. The presence of any lung disease (including COPD) reduces ventilatory reserve and increases infection risk, which are significant risk factors for postoperative complications. Expiratory airflow limitation in COPD presents challenges during mechanical ventilation with gas trapping leading to dynamic hyperinflation and barotrauma (hypotension, pneumothorax and pneumomediastinum).

Chronic obstructive pulmonary disease co-morbidities

In western countries, smoking is the major risk factor for COPD but it is also a risk factor for many other diseases that increase perioperative risk. These include coronary artery disease, cerebrovascular disease, peripheral vascular disease, cancer, renal disease, venous thromboembolism and cachexia. Smokers tend to

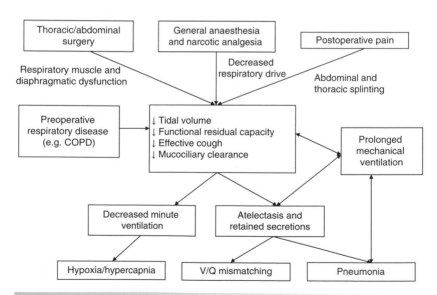

FIGURE 42.1 **Schematic of the pathophysiology of postoperative pulmonary complications.**

drink more alcohol, have higher rates of liver disease and diabetes, and have higher use of parenteral corticosteroids. These all contribute to increased perioperative complications including acute myocardial infarction, cardiac arrest, stroke, sepsis, renal failure and wound breakdown [2]. These co-morbidities, independent of pulmonary complications, also increase mortality and hospital length of stay [2,5,6]. These risks exist in smokers with even very mild COPD.

Preoperative assessment of COPD patients

Although the approach may differ in emergency versus elective surgery, the general principles of preanaesthetic assessment apply. First, assess the risk of surgery specifically to answer the following questions: (i) Does the benefit of surgery outweigh the risk? (ii) Can the risk be reduced? An issues and actions plan is outlined in Table 42.1.

Often our initial impression is that the risks are prohibitive (refer to Chapter 15 Pulmonary risk assessment). This is probably overly pessimistic as demonstrated by lung volume reduction surgery (via midline sternotomy) for severe emphysema. With careful selection and management, the majority of patients will be discharged from hospital despite complications along the way [2,7].

Although there is a paucity of data stratifying the risk of perioperative morbidity or mortality with severity of COPD, the impact on perioperative pulmonary mechanics and function is clear [7,8]. Assessment of anaesthetic risk, COPD severity and functional status (e.g. ASA physical status, GOLD stage [1] and NYHA functional class, respectively) will allow identification of 'at-risk' patients (Table 42.2). As there is substantial functional reserve in the lungs (patients with 50% lung function may have normal functional capacity, e.g. ASA I–II or NYHA I), spirometry (and diffusing capacity for carbon monoxide [DLCO] if available) should be performed to assess how much reserve is present. Those with severe COPD (FEV_1 < 50% predicted) warrant preoperative arterial blood gases as they may already be in respiratory failure. A chest X-ray is often poorly reflective of COPD severity but may show the presence of significant complications (cancer, pneumonia or pneumothorax).

Anaesthetic management of COPD patients

The exact approach to anaesthesia will be tailored to take into account patient factors and anaesthetist preference (see Table 42.1). The approach to monitoring, type of anaesthesia and postoperative pain management should be planned in advance, if possible. If the patient requires mechanical ventilation then strategies to reduce dynamic hyperinflation (rapid inspiratory flow, adequate expiratory time and permissive hypercapnia) should be considered.

Postoperative care

Postoperative care should be considered well in advance where possible. Those with severe COPD, certainly those in respiratory failure, should be managed in a high-dependency setting where low-flow oxygen, non-invasive ventilation or even reintubation and mechanical ventilation can be instituted quickly as appropriate. Careful postoperative analgesia (including regional anaesthesia) sufficient to allow deep breathing and expectoration with physiotherapist supervision and DVT prophylaxis are crucial. Continuation of inhaled bronchodilators and inhaled

TABLE 42.1 Surgery in chronic obstructive pulmonary disease (COPD) patients: the 'to do' list

Issue	Consider	Action
Preoperatively		
Is the patient high risk?	Respiratory failure risk. Does the patient have COPD? How severe?	Check spirometry, DLCO, ABGs
Is the patient a smoker?	Can surgery be delayed?	Smoking cessation advice, delay surgery
Is the procedure high risk?	Cardiothoracic/abdominal, laparoscopic/open surgery.	Understand the proposed procedure
Is the operation warranted?	Risk/benefit analysis	Get senior input
What can be done to alter the risk?	Patient management, preadmission, preoperative chest physiotherapy, optimise patient prior to surgery	Specialist referral, admit for preoperative management, defer elective surgery if unwell
Perioperatively		
What is the best anaesthetic strategy?	General versus regional anaesthesia	Discuss anaesthetic preference, cautious use of muscle relaxants
What is the best ventilation strategy?	Gas trapping, hyperinflation, barotrauma	Hypoventilation, permissive hypercapnia
How is the patient best monitored?	End-tidal CO_2, arterial line	Use extensive monitoring if high risk
Postoperatively		
Where is the patient best managed?	Recovery room, ICU, HDU, specialty or general ward	Move patient based on rate of recovery
When and how to extubate?	Non-invasive ventilation, O_2 mask or nasal O_2	Extubate early if tolerated
Are they getting too much oxygen?	Careful titration of O_2 flow	Keep SaO_2 88–92% if hypercapnic (refer to Chapter 40 Obstructive sleep apnoea)
Is pain control optimal?	Paracetamol, NSAID, opioid, other, regional anaesthesia	Aim to keep patient pain free and alert. Consult pain team early
Is postoperative care optimal?	DVT prophylaxis, bronchodilators, corticosteroids, antibiotics	Chemical or mechanical DVT prophylaxis. Regular bronchodilators, corticosteroid replacement, antibiotics if indicated
Have physiotherapy been alerted?	Deep breathing, coughing, early ambulation	Refer to physiotherapy, early mobilisation paramount

ABG, arterial blood gas; DLCO, diffusing capacity for carbon monoxide; DVT, deep vein thrombosis; HDU, high-dependency unit; ICU, intensive care unit; NSAID, non-steroidal anti-inflammatory drug.

Descriptor	ASA classification	GOLD stage	Functional class (FC) (adapted from NYHA)
Normal	ASA 1 A normal healthy patient	GOLD stage 1 Mild COPD: FEV_1/FVC <70% and FEV_1 ≥80% predicted	NYHA FC I No limitation of physical activity
Mild impairment	ASA 2 A patient with mild systemic disease	GOLD stage 2 Moderate COPD: FEV_1/FVC <70% and 50% ≤ FEV_1 <80% predicted	NYHA FC II Slight limitation of physical activity
Moderate impairment	ASA 3 A patient with severe systemic disease	GOLD stage 3 Severe COPD: FEV_1/FVC <70% and 30% ≤ FEV_1 <50% predicted	NYHA FC III Marked limitation of physical activity, but comfortable at rest
Severe impairment	ASA 4 A patient with severe systemic disease that is a constant threat to life	GOLD stage 4 Very severe COPD: FEV_1/FVC <70% and FEV_1 <30% predicted	NYHA FC IV Cannot perform any physical activity without discomfort. Symptoms may be present at rest
Moribund	ASA 5 A moribund patient who is not expected to survive without the operation	GOLD stage 4 as above	NYHA FC IV as above
Brain dead	ASA 6 A declared brain-dead patient whose organs are being removed for donor purposes	N/A	N/A

This table approximately correlates the ASA classification with two other important grading systems of functional impairment (and anaesthetic risk).
ASA, American Society of Anesthesiologists; GOLD Stage, Global initiative on Obstructive Lung Disease stage (COPD staging); NYHA FC, New York Heart Association Functional Class (heart disease functional staging).

corticosteroids may need augmentation with additional bronchodilators, parenteral corticosteroids (noting about 10% will be on oral corticosteroid now or recently) and antibiotics as appropriate. The patient should be sat out of bed and mobilised as soon as safe.

Conclusion

Chronic obstructive pulmonary disease will be present in nearly 5% of surgical patients [2]. Careful pre-, peri- and postoperative respiratory management will generally result in a good outcome. The greatest risk to the patient stems from the effects of cigarette smoking on almost all body systems and requires careful additional assessment and management.

References

1. Global Initiative for Chronic Obstructive Lung Disease (GOLD). Global Strategy for the diagnosis, management and prevention of chronic obstructive pulmonary disease. *American Journal of Respiratory and Critical Care Medicine*, 2013;**187**(4):347–365. doi:10.1164/rccm.201204-0596PP

2. Gupta H, Ramanan B, Gupta PK, et al. Impact of COPD on postoperative outcomes: results from a national database. *Chest*, 2013;**143**(6):1599–1606. doi:10.1378/chest.12-1499

3. Ramakrishna G, Sprung J, Ravi BS, Chandrasekaran K, McGoon MD. Impact of pulmonary hypertension on the outcomes of noncardiac surgery: predictors of perioperative morbidity and mortality. *Journal of the American College of Cardiology*, 2005;**45**(10):1691–1699. doi:10.1016/j.jacc.2005.02.055

4. Cellini C, Deeb AP, Sharma A, Monson JRT, Fleming FJ. Association between operative approach and complications in patients undergoing Hartmann's reversal. *British Journal of Surgery*, 2013;**100**(8):1094–1099. doi:10.1002/Bjs.9153

5. Mathis MR, Naughton NN, Shanks AM, et al. Patient selection for day case-eligible surgery: identifying those at high risk for major complications. *Anesthesiology*, 2013;**119**(6):1310–1321. doi:10.1097/ALN.0000000000000005

6. Easterlin MC, Chang DC, Wilson SE. A practical index to predict 30-day mortality after major amputation. *Annals of Vascular Surgery*, 2013;**27**(7):909–917. doi:10.1016/J.Avsg.2012.06.030

7. Saleh HZ, Mohan K, Shaw M, et al. Impact of chronic obstructive pulmonary disease severity on surgical outcomes in patients undergoing non-emergent coronary artery bypass grafting. *European Journal of Cardio-Thoracic Surgery*, 2012;**42**(1):108–113; discussion 13. doi:10.1093/ejcts/ezr271

8. Jeong O, Ryu SY, Park YK. The value of preoperative lung spirometry test for predicting the operative risk in patients undergoing gastric cancer surgery. *Journal of the Korean Surgical Society*, 2013;**84**(1):18–26. doi:10.4174/jkss.2013.84.1.18

43 Non-small cell lung cancer

Robert Stirling

Monash University, Australia

Lung cancer is currently the fourth most commonly diagnosed cancer, affecting over 10,000 people in Australia and 40,000 people in the United Kingdom each year [1]. Diagnosis is often achieved at a late age (71 years in men) and usually in those with significant smoking history. Disease presentation is often late, with approximately half of the patients presenting with metastatic disease and only a quarter with localised early disease potentially amenable to surgical resection. Survival remains poor, with 5-year relative survival of just 11% for males and 15% for females.

Surgical treatment

Surgical resection provides the greatest chance of long-term survival. For localised disease with no regional spread, lobectomy is the procedure of choice (Table 43.1) and has a low complication rate. Sublobar (wedge) resection provides similar early survival benefit but has increased rates of local recurrence and should therefore be restricted to those in whom poor lung function may contraindicate lobectomy. The use of the video-assisted thoracic surgery (VATS) approach for lobectomy significantly reduces intraoperative blood loss, chest drainage time, hospital stay and complications, with similar or better oncological control than open thoracotomy. For patients with localised (stage I and II) non-small cell lung cancer (NSCLC) (Table 43.2), systematic mediastinal lymph node dissection at the time of resection is recommended over selective or no sampling to improve pathological staging. For locally advanced disease, surgical approaches may potentially include lobectomy, sleeve lobectomy or pneumonectomy, all of which may be combined with adjuvant chemotherapy and or radiotherapy.

The preoperative assessment of suitability for surgical resection requires assessment of:

- suitability for resection
- fitness for surgery
- risk of perioperative complications and mortality
- pulmonary function to assess likelihood of pulmonary compromise (dyspnoea) following resection.

Perioperative Medicine for the Junior Clinician, First Edition. Edited by Joel Symons, Paul Myles, Rishi Mehra and Christine Ball.
© 2015 John Wiley & Sons, Ltd. Published 2015 by John Wiley & Sons, Ltd.
Companion website: www.wiley.com/go/perioperativemed

TABLE 43.1 Stage-dependent treatment for non-small cell lung cancer

Stage	Standard treatment	Survival
IA	Surgical resection	73%
IB		58%
IIA	Surgical resection	46%
IIB	± adjuvant chemotherapy	36%
IIIA	Surgery in selected patients and/or chemoradiotherapy	10–35%
IIIB	Chemoradiotherapy	5%
IV	Palliative chemo- or radiotherapy	<5%

TABLE 43.2 Lung function measures as predictors of postoperative respiratory compromise

	Risk		
	Low	Intermediate	High
FEV_1 (litres) Pneumonectomy Lobectomy	>2 >1.5	<2 <1.5	
$ppoFEV_1$	≥60%	≤60%	<0.8 L
$ppoDLCO$	≥60%	≤60%	
$ppoFEV_1 \times ppoDLCO$	>1650	<1650	
Shuttle walk test	>400 m	<400 m	
Stair walk	3 flights (22 m)	<3 flights	
VO_{2max} mL/kg/min	>20	10–20	<10

Suitability and fitness for surgery

Suitability for resection requires detailed preoperative assessment according to the TNM staging system [2]. Accurate staging requires the use of CT-positron emission tomography (PET) scanning with histological sampling of radiologically enlarged or PET-avid hilar and mediastinal lymph nodes. This can be performed by endobronchial ultrasound (EBUS) or at mediastinoscopy. If intracranial or bone pathology is suspected, these should be pursued with CT/MRI as indicated. For patients with T3N0-1M0 disease, radical treatment should be considered and the potential role of surgery decided by a multidisciplinary team with thoracic surgical input.

Optimal assessment of fitness for surgery requires multidisciplinary evaluation, with input from medical and radiation oncologists, physicians and surgeons [3,4]. A detailed history and examination is required.

An estimate of risk of postoperative cardiological events may be made using the thoracic Revised Cardiological Risk Score (tRCRI) [5]. Risk factors include pneumonectomy 1.5 points, previous ischaemic heart disease 1.5 points, previous stroke or TIA 1.5 points and creatinine >2 mg/dL 1 point. A tRCRI score ≥2 should prompt referral for preoperative cardiological evaluation.

The risk of perioperative mortality may be assessed using a risk stratification score such as the Thoracoscore which includes nine variables (www.sfar.org/scores2/thoracoscore2.php) (Table 43.3) [6]. Cardiovascular function is of key concern in this population where advanced age and high-dose cigarette exposure are usual. Examination should include history, physical examination and ECG. Any cardiac condition requiring medication, newly suspected cardiac condition or inability to climb two flights of stairs should prompt preoperative cardiological evaluation.

TABLE 43.3 Thoracoscore risk factors for prediction of perioperative mortality in thoracic surgery

Variable	Value	Code	β-coefficient
Age	<55 years	0	
	55–65 years	1	0.7679
	>65 years	2	1.0073
Sex	Female	0	
	Male	1	0.4505
ASA score	≤2	0	
	≥3	1	0.6057
Performance status	≤2	0	
	≥3	1	0.689
Dyspnoea score	≤2	0	
	≥3	1	0.9075
Priority of surgery	Elective	0	
	Urgent or emergency	1	0.8443
Procedure class	Other	0	
	Pneumonectomy	1	1.2176
Diagnosis group	Benign	0	
	Malignant	1	1.2423
Comorbidity score	0	0	
	≤2	1	0.7447
	≥3	2	0.9065
Constant			−7.3737

Thoracoscore online scoring algorithm available at: http://www.sfar.org/scores2/thoracoscore2.php#haut
Methods for using the logistic regression model to predict the risk of in-hospital death:
1. Odds are calculated with the patient values and the coefficients are determined from the regression equation:
Odds = exp[−7.3737 + (0.7679 if code of age is 1 or 1.0073 if code of age is 2) + (0.4505 × sex score) + (0.6057 × ASA score) + (0.6890 × performance status classification) + (0.9075 × dyspnoea score) + (0.8443 × code for priority of surgery) + (1.2176 × procedure class) + (1.2423 × diagnosis group) + (0.7447 if code of comorbidity is 1 or 0.9065 if code of comorbidity is 2)].
2. The odds for the predicted probability of in-hospital death are calculated: probability + odds/ (1 + odds).
ASA, American Society of Anesthesiologists.
Source: Falcoz et al. [6]. Reproduced with permission of Elsevier.

Assessment of pulmonary function and postoperative compromise

Preoperative pulmonary function may be assessed using a combination of spirometry (FEV_1), gas transfer (DLCO), exercise tests including shuttle walk test, stair climbing test, CPET (refer to Chapter 16 Preoperative cardiopulmonary exercise testing) and ABG (see Table 43.2).

Spirometry is predictive of low complication rates following pneumonectomy when preoperative FEV_1 >2 L, and lobectomy is well tolerated when preoperative FEV_1 >1.5 L. Spirometry is an imperfect sole predictor of postoperative lung function (especially in those with suspected interstitial lung disease and marked dyspnoea), so measurement of FEV_1 and DLCO is recommended in all preoperative surgical candidates.

> If both FEV_1 and DLCO are >80% predicted, resection candidates have low postoperative risk and no further preoperative pulmonary evaluation is required.

Arterial blood gas findings have not been shown to be strongly predictive of postsurgical risk. Hypoxaemia (oxygen saturation <90%) has been variably associated with postoperative complications, while hypercapnia ($PaCO_2$ >45 mmHg) has been traditionally described as a relative contraindication to pulmonary resection [7].

Prediction of postoperative lung function

Lung function outcomes may be combined to develop an algorithm for postoperative risk assessment (Figure 43.1). If postoperative risk is other than low (i.e. FEV_1 and/or DLCO <80% predicted) then estimation of postoperative pulmonary function should be made. This estimation can be made using either anatomical modelling or ventilation perfusion measures.

The anatomical model may be used to predict postoperative FEV_1 ($ppoFEV_1$).

$$ppoFEV_1 = \text{preoperative } FEV_1\% \text{ predicted}$$
$$\times(1-\text{number of resected segments / total functional segments})$$

There are 19 bronchopulmonary segments, (10 on the right – 3 upper, 2 middle and 5 lower; 9 on the left – 5 upper and 4 lower). If tumour involvement causes segmental obstruction, obstructed segments are subtracted from total segments. $ppoDLCO$ may be calculated similarly. A postoperative FEV_1 <0.8 L has been suggested as a lower threshold for tolerance of pulmonary resection; below this, pulmonary function may be severely compromised.

Alternative methods for estimation of $ppoFEV_1$ and DLCO include ventilation scintigraphy or perfusion scintigraphy, particularly where ventilation/perfusion mismatch is suspected (such as in emphysema) while newer techniques, including quantitative CT and MRI, await thorough validation in this task.

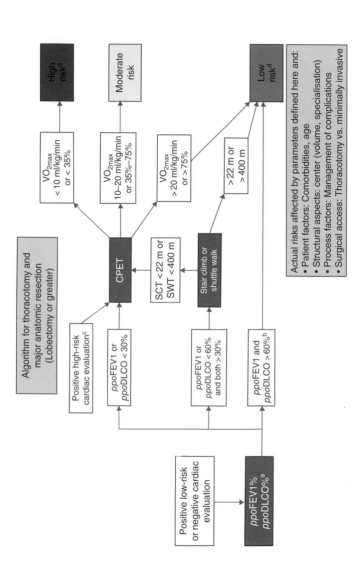

FIGURE 43.1 Pre-resection lung function testing algorithm. [a]For pneumonectomy candidates, perfusion scanning is recommended to calculate $ppoFEV_1$ or $ppoDLCO$. For lobectomy patients, segmental counting is indicated. [b]$ppoFEV_1$ or $ppoDLCO$ cut-off values of 60% predicted values have been chosen based on indirect evidence and expert consensus opinion. [c]For patients with a positive high-risk cardiac evaluation subsequently assessed as suitable for surgery, both pulmonary function tests and cardiopulmonary exercise test may more precisely define perioperative risk. [d]Definition of risk: Low risk: The expected risk of mortality is below 1%. Major anatomical resections can be safely performed in this group. Moderate risk: Morbidity and mortality rates may vary according to the values of split lung functions, exercise tolerance and extent of resection. Risks and benefits of the operation should be thoroughly discussed with the patient. High risk: The risk of mortality after standard major anatomical resections may be higher than 10%. Considerable risk of severe cardiopulmonary morbidity and residual functional loss is expected. Patients should be counselled about alternative surgical (minor resections or minimally invasive surgery) or non-surgical options. CPET, cardiopulmonary exercise testing; DLCO, diffusing capacity for carbon dioxide; FEV, forced expiratory volume; ppo, predicted postoperative; SCT, stair climb test; SWT, shuttle walk test [3]. Reproduced with permission of the American College of Chest Physicians.

TABLE 43.4 Comparison of complication rates following resection for early-stage NSCLC [9]. VATS conversion to open thoracotomy rate 17.6%

	VATS	Thoracotomy
Atrial fibrillation %	5.2	9.0
Pneumonia %	2.7	6.0
Persistent air leak %	5.0	8.8
Chest tube duration (d)	4.2*	5.7
Length of stay (d)	8.3*	13.3
Complication rate %	16.4*	31.2

Source: Adapted from Flores et al. [10].
*p <0.05.

A composite score of spirometry and gas transfer has been proposed as the predicted postoperative product (PPP) of ppoFEV$_1$% × ppoDLCO% [8]. A PPP <1650 is associated with significantly elevated risk of death.

Implications for postoperative care and complications

Lung cancer resection is associated with relatively low morbidity rates (Table 43.4) and 30-day mortality rates in the range 3–4%. However, these mortality rates may be double in the 30–90-day window, worsened by factors including procedure (pneumonectomy), male gender, increasing age and higher co-morbidity status.

References

1. Beckett P, Woolhouse I, Stanley R, Peake MD. Exploring variations in lung cancer care across the UK – the 'story so far' for the National Lung Cancer Audit. *Clinical Medicine*, 2012;**12**(1):14–18. doi:10.7861/clinmedicine.12-1-14

2. Mirsadraee S, Oswal D, Alizadeh Y, Caulo A, van Beek E Jr. The 7th lung cancer TNM classification and staging system: review of the changes and implications. *World Journal of Radiology*, 2012;**4**(4):128–134. doi:10.4329/wjr.v4.i4.128

3. Brunelli A, Kim AW, Berger KI, Addrizzo-Harris DJ. Physiologic evaluation of the patient with lung cancer being considered for resectional surgery. Diagnosis and management of lung cancer, 3rd ed: American College of Chest Physicians evidence-based clinical practice guidelines. *Chest*, 2013;**143**(5 Suppl):e166S–e190S. doi:10.1378/chest.12-2395

4. Lim E, Baldwin D, Beckles M, et al. Guidelines on the radical management of patients with lung cancer. *Thorax*, 2010;**65**(Suppl 3):iii1–27. doi:10.1136/thx.2010.145938

5. Ferguson MK, Celauro AD, Vigneswaran WT. Validation of a modified scoring system for cardiovascular risk associated with major lung resection. *European Journal of Cardio-Thoracic Surgery*, 2012;**41**(3):598–602. doi:10.1093/ejcts/ezr081

6. Falcoz PE, Conti M, Brouchet L, et al. The Thoracic Surgery Scoring System (Thoracoscore): risk model for in-hospital death in 15,183 patients requiring thoracic surgery. *Journal of Thoracic and Cardiovascular Surgery*, 2007;**133**(2):325–332. doi:10.1016/j.jtcvs.2006.09.020

7. Celli BR. What is the value of preoperative pulmonary-function testing? *Medical Clinics of North America*, 1993;**77**(2):309–325.

8. Pierce RJ, Copland JM, Sharpe K, Barter CE. Preoperative risk evaluation for lung cancer resection: predicted postoperative product as a predictor of surgical mortality. *American Journal of Respiratory and Critical Care Medicine*, 1994;**150**(4):947–955. doi:10.1164/ajrccm.150.4.7921468

9. Whitson BA, Groth SS, Duval SJ, Swanson SJ, Maddaus MA. Surgery for early-stage non-small cell lung cancer: a systematic review of the video-assisted thoracoscopic surgery versus thoracotomy approaches to lobectomy. *Annals of Thoracic Surgery*, 2008;**86**(6): 2008–2016; discussion 16–18. doi:10.1016/j.athoracsur.2008.07.009

10. Flores RM, Park BJ, Dycoco J, et al. Lobectomy by video-assisted thoracic surgery (VATS) versus thoracotomy for lung cancer. *Journal of Thoracic and Cardiovascular Surgery*, 2009;**138**(1):11–18. doi:10.1016/j.jtcvs.2009.03.030

43

44 Gastrointestinal disease

Lauren Beswick[1] and William Kemp[2]

[1] The Alfred Hospital, Australia
[2] The Alfred Hospital and Monash University, Australia

Surgery on the gastrointestinal tract is often high risk. A mortality rate of 4% after colorectal resection has been previously described by the American College of Surgeons National Surgical Quality Improvement Program [1]. Minimisation and management of the operative risk require four individual components to be addressed: the patient, the procedure, the provider and the anaesthetic [2]. A detailed review of each of these factors is beyond the scope of this chapter, but the principles of perioperative care will be highlighted through an examination of the surgical care of the patient with inflammatory bowel disease (IBD).

Definition and pathophysiology

Inflammatory bowel disease is a chronic disorder of the gastrointestinal tract and encompasses two major types – ulcerative colitis and Crohn's disease [3,4]. Ulcerative colitis is characterised by inflammation and ulceration in the superficial layers of the large intestine. Crohn's disease is a more complex disease process and can affect the gastrointestinal tract in any area from mouth to anus. The inflammation extends through the entire thickness of the bowel wall.

Epidemiology

One in five patients with ulcerative colitis will require surgery within 10 years of diagnosis whilst the overall 10-year incidence of surgery for Crohn's disease is 48%. For ulcerative colitis, this will usually be a protocolectomy with end ileostomy or subsequent formation of an ileal pouch anal anastomosis, which is a curative procedure. For Crohn's disease the type of operation varies but usually involves limited resection.

Preoperative assessment

Patients with IBD require a comprehensive preoperative review. Specific details should include the extent and severity of their disease, planned operation, usual IBD medications and patient expectations. This can sometimes be challenging in an

Perioperative Medicine for the Junior Clinician, First Edition. Edited by Joel Symons, Paul Myles, Rishi Mehra and Christine Ball.
© 2015 John Wiley & Sons, Ltd. Published 2015 by John Wiley & Sons, Ltd.
Companion website: www.wiley.com/go/perioperativemed

emergency situation when a patient with colitis requires an emergency colectomy for a complication such as toxic megacolon. In addition, the examination should include identification of potential complications such as fever, palpable abdominal masses (indicative of an inflammatory phlegmon or abscess), abdominal distension or peritonism.

Nutritional assessment is a key component of the preoperative assessment, for both elective and emergency operations. Another vitally important aspect of preoperative management is the utilisation of a multidisciplinary team meeting with the gastroenterologists, colorectal surgeons, dieticians, radiologists, pathologists and stomal therapists to discuss complex patients and optimisation of their care during the perioperative period.

Perioperative management of medications used in IBD

Medication management varies between individual patients depending on the type, extent and severity of disease and the type of surgery they are undergoing. For example, a patient undergoing a proctocolectomy for refractory ulcerative colitis will require no IBD medications postoperatively. However, a patient with complex fistulising small bowel Crohn's disease undergoing an ileocolic resection will require cessation of their usual IBD medications for a minimal period around the time of their operation and optimisation of their IBD management postoperatively to prevent disease recurrence.

Glucocorticoids are the main agent used for induction of remission in IBD. However, they are the most concerning drug in the perioperative period. A long-term follow-up study of Crohn's disease patients showed that the risk of infection and mortality was doubled when compared with patients not on steroids in the perioperative period, and the risk was higher if patients were on doses >40 mg daily [5]. Where possible, steroids should be ceased or tapered below 20 mg daily in the preoperative period. If patients remain on oral prednisolone, they should receive IV steroid maintenance therapy perioperatively. Whilst fasting, the patients should receive an equivalent dose of IV hydrocortisone and then be converted back to oral prednisolone once eating has resumed [6] (refer to Chapter 27 Steroid medication).

Aminosalicylates are safe in the perioperative period and should be continued when possible. The patient will usually be fasting for the first few days following a bowel resection so it is acceptable to withhold the aminosalicylates during this time. Care should be taken with adequate perioperative hydration if any underlying interstitial nephritis is present, a potential adverse effect of aminosalicylates.

There have been concerns previously regarding the risk of infection with the use of thiopurines, azathioprine and 6-mercaptopurine in the perioperative period. However, recent studies have not confirmed this risk and again the recommendations are that thiopurines should be continued in the perioperative period, unless the patient is fasting [6].

Anti-tumour necrosis factor (anti-TNF) agents, infliximab and adalimumab, are used for induction and maintenance of remission in IBD. The data regarding the use of these newer agents in the perioperative period are inconclusive, with some studies showing no increase in infection. In general, if there are no major complications with the surgery these agents should be administered two to four weeks postoperatively (with infliximab usually given eight-weekly and adalimumab being administered two-weekly). However, if there is an infective complication it would be reasonable to withhold the agents for a longer time but each case should be considered individually, depending on the disease severity, type of operation and significance of the infective complication.

Risk and prevention of thromboembolic events in the perioperative period

Venous thromboembolism (VTE) is more common in IBD patients. In the perioperative setting when IBD patients are generally less mobile, the risk of VTE events is thought to be even higher. Disease activity is the primary controllable risk factor for VTE in patients in IBD. It can be assumed from this that optimal medical management of IBD is the best strategy to reduce the risk of VTE in elective procedures. Prophylactic heparin and the use of thromboembolic deterrent (TED) stockings are recommended in all IBD patients perioperatively (refer to Chapter 24 Thromboprophylaxis). Concern regarding the use of heparin prophylaxis in the setting of rectal bleeding is probably unwarranted, as this does not significantly increase rectal bleeding in IBD patients.

References

1. Cohen ME, Bilimoria KY, Ko CY, Hall BL. Development of an American College of Surgeons National Surgery Quality Improvement Program: morbidity and mortality risk calculator for colorectal surgery. *Journal of the American College of Surgeons*, 2009;**208**(6):1009–1016. doi:10.1016/j.jamcollsurg.2009.01.043

2. Hendren SK, Morris AM. Evaluating patients undergoing colorectal surgery to estimate and minimize morbidity and mortality. *Surgical Clinics of North America*, 2013;**93**(1):1–20. doi:10.1016/j.suc.2012.09.005

3. Dignass A, van Assche G, Lindsay JO, et al. The second European evidence-based consensus on the diagnosis and management of Crohn's disease: current management. *Journal of Crohns and Colitis*, 2010;**4**(1):28–62. doi:10.1016/J.Crohns.2009.12.002

4. Dignass A, Lindsay JO, Sturm A, et al. Second European evidence-based consensus on the diagnosis and management of ulcerative colitis.Part 2: Current management. *Journal of Crohns and Colitis*, 2012;**6**(10):991–1030. doi:10.1016/J.Crohns.2012.09.002

5. Lichtenstein GR, Feagan BG, Cohen RD, et al. Serious infections and mortality in association with therapies for Crohn's disease: TREAT registry. *Clinical Gastroenterology and Hepatology*, 2006;**4**(5):621–630. doi:10.1016/J.Cgh.2006.03.002

6. Kumar A, Auron M, Aneja A, Mohr F, Jain A, Shen B. Inflammatory bowel disease: perioperative pharmacological considerations. *Mayo Clinic Proceedings*, 2011;**86**(8):748–757. doi:10.4065/mcp.2011.0074

Hepatic disease

Lauren Beswick[1] and William Kemp[2]

[1] The Alfred Hospital, Australia
[2] The Alfred Hospital and Monash University, Australia

Cirrhosis is a chronic disease of the liver and is defined histologically as a diffuse hepatic process characterised by fibrosis and the conversion of normal liver architecture into structurally abnormal nodules. Portal hypertension is the main complication of cirrhosis and is defined as a hepatic venous pressure gradient >5 mmHg. It can lead to the development of gastro-oesophageal varices and clinical decompensation of the liver characterised by encephalopathy, ascites or variceal bleeding.

Pathophysiology

Several mechanisms are believed to underlie the increased perioperative morbidity and mortality seen in patients with hepatic disease. Cirrhosis is associated with a hyperdynamic circulation characterised by a decrease in systemic vascular resistance and an increase in cardiac output, and the diseased liver is at particular risk of hypoxaemia and hypoperfusion. Patients with advanced liver disease are also more susceptible to increased bacterial translocation from the gut and ultimately bacterial infection, poor wound healing, bleeding due to coagulopathy, and altered drug metabolism.

Epidemiology

Operative mortality in cirrhotic patients exceeds 10%, with a perioperative complication rate of 30%. It has been estimated that approximately 10% of patients with cirrhosis will undergo an operation within the last two years of life [1]. Perioperative mortality has improved over the last 10 years, presumably because of improvements in the overall care of critically ill patients and possibly because of greater use of laparoscopic surgical techniques.

Assessment

The most useful and frequently used indicators of surgical risk are the Child Turcotte Pugh Score (CTP) (Table 45.1) and the Model for End-Stage Liver Disease (MELD) score (Box 45.1) which provide an assessment of the severity of the underlying liver

Perioperative Medicine for the Junior Clinician, First Edition. Edited by Joel Symons, Paul Myles, Rishi Mehra and Christine Ball.
© 2015 John Wiley & Sons, Ltd. Published 2015 by John Wiley & Sons, Ltd.
Companion website: www.wiley.com/go/perioperativemed

TABLE 45.1 Child Turcotte Pugh Score (CTP) and associated mortality

	1	2	3
Albumin (g/L)	>35	28–35	<28
Bilirubin (μmol/L)	<34	34–50	>50
Coagulation (INR)	<1.7	1.71–2.2	>2.2
Distension (ascites)	None	Mild (or controlled with diuretics)	Marked
Encephalopathy	None	Mild	Marked
CTP class	**A**	**B**	**C**
	<7	7–9	≥10
Survival 1 year	100%	81%	45%
Survival 2 years	85%	57%	35%
Operative mortality	10%	30%	76–82%

INR, international normalised ratio.

BOX 45.1 MELD score [1] and associated mortality

MELD	$(9.6 \times \log_e[\text{creatinine mg/dL}]) + (3.8 \times \log [\text{bili mg/dL}]) + (11.2 \times \log_e [\text{INR}]) + 6.4$ The maximum score is 40 (scores larger than 40 are assigned a value of 40). For any laboratory values less than 1.0, a value of 1.0 is used. The maximum creatinine concentration is 4.0 mg/dL (creatinine concentrations higher than 4.0 mg/dL are assigned a value of 4.0 mg/dL). If a patient has had dialysis twice within the previous week, the creatinine value is set as 4.0 mg/dL
Operative mortality	5.7% for MELD <8, >50% MELD >20. An approximation is a 1% increase in mortality for each MELD point below 20 and 2% for each point above 20 [4]

---

disease [2,3]. In addition, a useful online calculator is available (www.mayoclinic.org/meld/mayomodel9.html). These risk scores should be calculated in all patients with cirrhosis during the preoperative assessment. Each requires an appropriate physical examination looking for signs of chronic liver disease plus laboratory investigations including INR, creatinine and bilirubin.

In addition to using the above-mentioned scoring systems, there are a number of other variables that the clinician needs to be aware of and which will affect perioperative risk [4].

- *The type of surgery*: emergency abdominal and gastrointestinal surgery have the worst outcomes.
- *The hospital*: transplant centres generally have better outcomes.
- Portal hypertension increases risk.

In general, elective surgery can proceed in patients with CTP class A liver disease or a MELD < 10. For patients with CTP class B liver disease or a MELD 10–15, non-essential surgery should be postponed and the patient's condition optimised. In more advanced liver disease (CTP class C or MELD > 15), all non-essential surgery should be avoided [1].

Management

Preoperative phase

Advanced hepatic fibrosis and cirrhosis can be asymptomatic, often unrecognised until the time of surgery, and the risk is determined by the magnitude of hepatic dysfunction. A thorough preoperative evaluation is therefore particularly important in patients with chronic liver disease.

Preoperative management includes a detailed assessment for complications of cirrhosis: ascites, coagulopathy, nutritional assessment, cardiovascular evaluation, pulmonary evaluation, renal dysfunction and encephalopathy [2–5].

Converting a patient from a CTP class C to a CTP class B preoperatively improves survival and this underpins the importance of optimising the patient condition and liver disease management prior to surgical intervention.

Generally, elective surgery should be postponed in cirrhotic patients until a full assessment has been completed. Consider the operative environment and whether the hospital is adequately equipped to manage potential complications. Ideally, expertise in the management of liver failure should be onsite.

Vitamin K should be administered if the patient has an elevated INR. A gastroscopy may be needed to exclude or manage gastro-oesophageal varices. Ascites management is paramount. This may include dietary intervention with a low salt diet (< 80 mmol/day or < 2000 mg/day), diuretics and/or paracentesis. In some situations, patients with portal hypertension may benefit from a preoperative insertion of a transjugular intrahepatic portosystemic shunt. Early involvement of a hepatologist is advisable.

Intraoperative phase

The anaesthetist needs to be aware of the severity of the liver disease. Baseline blood pressure and serum sodium are often lower than in normal patients and are not easily corrected by administration of crystalloid. Intraoperative fluid management should be restrictive. Perioperative antibiotic prophylaxis needs to cover gram-negative bacteria (e.g. a third-generation cephalosporin such as ceftriaxone) if there is ascites to reduce the risk of bacterial peritonitis. Consider the need for a high-dependency bed for the first 24 hours postoperatively.

Postoperative phase

The clinician should avoid giving the patient excessive salt loads (including the use of saline) and nephrotoxins (antibiotics, NSAIDs, contrast agents). The patient should adhere to a low-salt diet (80 mmol/day). Early introduction of enteral feeding is preferable. The precipitants of encephalopathy should be minimised, i.e. electrolyte disturbance (particularly hyponatraemia), constipation, opioids, sedatives and gastrointestinal bleeding. Oral lactulose or enemas should be used to prevent constipation. Rifaximin can be useful in encephalopathy not responsive to lactulose.

Special consideration in patients with hepatic disease

Patients with acute hepatitis have a significant increase in surgical risk and surgery should be avoided until after resolution of the acute hepatitis. Likewise, for patients with CTP class C liver disease or MELD >15, surgery should be avoided and/or consideration for discussion with a liver transplant unit.

Perioperative mortality in patients with obstructive jaundice is high (8–28%) and therefore elective surgery should be postponed or avoided in this clinical setting.

References

1. Hanje AJ, Patel T. Preoperative evaluation of patients with liver disease. *Nature Clinical Practice Gastroenterology and Hepatology*, 2007;**4**(5):266–276. doi:10.1038/ncpgasthep0794

2. Muilenburg DJ, Singh A, Torzilli G, Khatri VP. Surgery in the patient with liver disease. *Medical Clinics of North America*, 2009;**93**(5):1065–1081. doi:10.1016/j.mcna.2009.05.008

3. Muir AJ. Surgical clearance for the patient with chronic liver disease. *Clinics in Liver Disease*, 2012;**16**(2):421–433. doi:10.1016/j.cld.2012.03.008

4. Bhangui P, Laurent A, Amathieu R, Azoulay D. Assessment of risk for non-hepatic surgery in cirrhotic patients. *Journal of Hepatology*, 2012;**57**(4):874–884. doi:10.1016/j.jhep.2012.03.037

5. Nicoll A. Surgical risk in patients with cirrhosis. *Journal of Gastroenterology and Hepatology*, 2012;**27**(10):1569–1575. doi:10.1111/j.1440-1746.2012.07205.x

Oliguria

Paul Myles

The Alfred Hospital and Monash University, Australia

Oliguria is a urine output that is less than 1 mL/kg/h in infants, less than 0.5 mL/kg/h in children, and less than 400 mL daily in adults.

The kidneys regulate water, salt and acid–base homeostasis; they also excrete nitrogenous and other waste products. In clinical settings, the kidneys are essential for clearance of most drug metabolites. Each of these roles has particular importance in the perioperative period.

The functional unit of the kidney is the nephron (refer to Chapter 47 Acute kidney injury), with its activity regulated by glomerular ultrafiltration, tubular secretion and selective reabsorption. In a healthy adult male about 180 litres of fluid are filtered by the glomerulus every day, producing about 2 litres of urine, but this will vary according to fluid and salt intake, environmental temperature, co-morbidity and medication usage. Renal function is in part co-ordinated by a variety of hormones including the renin-angiotensin-aldosterone system, atrial natriuretic peptide and ADH. ADH secretion is stimulated by angiotensin II in response to hypotension and hypovolaemia. Atrial natriuretic peptide inhibits ADH secretion.

Antidiuretic hormone acts via aquaporins, or water channels, in the apical membrane of the distal tubule and collecting duct epithelial cells of the nephron, thus facilitating water reabsorption. ADH also increases peripheral vascular resistance, which in turn increases arterial blood pressure. Although oliguria is an appropriate response to dehydration and hypovolaemia, it may also exist in euvolaemia if there is limited fluid intake or in an inflammatory state with vasodilation (Figure 46.1; Video 46.1).

> Oliguria is not necessarily an indicator of renal perfusion or function, and may not indicate or exacerbate acute kidney injury (AKI).

Disorders of sodium and water balance are commonly encountered in surgical and critically ill patients [1]. High levels of ADH secretion may lead to hyponatraemia. This may be an appropriate response to hypovolaemia, or inappropriate due to diseases (lung carcinoma and other tumours, heart failure, hypothyroidism) or drugs (opioids, antidepressants, anticonvulsants and antibiotics) [1]. Patients with the syndrome of inappropriate ADH secretion (SIADH) are typically euvolaemic or mildly volume expanded with a decreased capacity for free water excretion [1]. This syndrome is

Perioperative Medicine for the Junior Clinician, First Edition. Edited by Joel Symons, Paul Myles, Rishi Mehra and Christine Ball.
© 2015 John Wiley & Sons, Ltd. Published 2015 by John Wiley & Sons, Ltd.
Companion website: www.wiley.com/go/perioperativemed

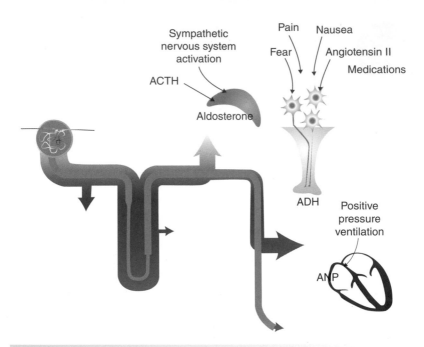

FIGURE 46.1 **Oliguria has a number of causes. ACTH, adrenocorticotrophic hormone; ADH, antidiuretic hormone; ANP, Atrial natriuretic peptide.**

www.wiley.com/go/perioperativemed

VIDEO 46.1 **Oliguria is an appropriate sign of hypovolaemia, but it may exist in euvolaemia if there is limited fluid intake or in an inflammatory state with vasodilation.**

the most common cause of acquired hyponatraemia in hospitalized patients, but is probably not the main cause of perioperative oliguria. The diagnostic criteria for the SIADH include evidence of serum hypo-osmolality (<275 mOsm/kg) and less than maximally dilute urine.

Non-steroidal anti-inflammatory and selective cyclo-oxygenase inhibitor drugs promote fluid retention and tissue oedema, increasing the likelihood of perioperative oliguria and potentially placing patients at risk of AKI. The renal effects of these drugs are unlikely to be mitigated by supplemental IV fluids.

There are two commonly used definitions of AKI, both derived from the critical care setting in which renal failure is much more common, and both definitions include a sustained period (6–12 hours) of oliguria as a key criterion [2]. The diagnostic utility of the oliguric component of these definitions has been questioned [2,3].

Most episodes of oliguria are not followed by kidney injury, even in the critical care setting.

Oliguria has a modest predictive ability for AKI defined only by creatinine criteria. In a study of 239 patients from seven intensive care units, the area under a receiver operating characteristic curve was only 0.75 (95% confidence interval [CI] 0.64–0.85). Oliguria persisting for at least four hours provided the best discrimination (sensitivity 52%, specificity 86%). However, only 30 of 487 individual episodes of oliguria preceded the new occurrence of AKI in the days that followed.

A low urine output is common during surgery, irrespective of the amount of IV fluid given [4]. Oliguria may not therefore be a marker of AKI [2–4]. Oliguria, of itself, seems to have no relationship with mortality, renal replacement therapy or duration in hospital stay after surgery [2]. The kidney is adapted to conserving sodium and water in times of fasting and limited water supply; it is not able to excrete an excess

BOX 46.1 A practical guide for the management of postoperative oliguria

1. A bedside clinical review of the patient that includes previous history of renal impairment or heart failure, patient thirst, fasting times, blood loss and other fluid losses, fever, blood pressure and estimated cardiac output.
2. Consider stopping NSAID or COX-2 inhibitor therapy.
3. Evaluate fluid responsiveness if such a monitor (e.g. arterial pressure analyser or oesophageal doppler) is available.
4. If any clinical evidence or suspicion of hypovolaemia, then administer a fluid challenge, say IV crystalloid 200 mL, and then review again.
5. If there is clinical evidence or suspicion of euvolaemia or hypervolaemia with a low cardiac output, consider admission to a critical care area for inotropic support and more invasive monitoring.
6. If otherwise clinically stable, accept oliguria as a normal response to surgery and review in 6 hours.
7. If oliguria persists beyond 6–12 hours, consider admission to a critical care area for possible inotropic support and more invasive monitoring.
8. Repeat serum creatinine, and perhaps potassium, lactate and/or C-reactive protein, measurements daily until resolved.
9. Exclude or treat sepsis.

of either water or salts over hours (or even days). Caution should therefore be exercised when considering administration of supplemental IV fluids. A practical guide for the management of postoperative oliguria can be found in Box 46.1.

Hypovolaemia is an uncommon cause of perioperative AKI. For many elderly and high-risk surgical patients, the most likely mechanism underlying oliguria is poor renal perfusion caused by a low cardiac output state. Other mechanisms include the vasodilation associated with anaesthesia, and the inflammatory response accompanying surgery and/or sepsis. Following surgery, factors such as hypotension, pain and tissue injury activate the sympathetic nervous and renin–angiotensin systems, as well as increasing secretion of ADH. These can override normal homeostatic mechanisms and trigger sodium and water retention.

Oliguria has been traditionally treated with additional IV fluids, with a belief that this should promote a diuresis, dilute tubular toxins and attenuate tubular obstruction from casts. The relationship between fluid input and natriuresis is weak, and the administration of IV fluid to maintain urine output will only lead to salt and water accumulation (5).

Recent observational studies have shown a consistent relationship between fluid overload and AKI (6, 7). Excessive IV fluid therapy can worsen tissue oedema, including renal capsular oedema, which may do no more than impair glomerular perfusion pressure and so limit its own resolution. Activation of the renin–angiotensin system will further limit urine flow. Fluid overload cannot be easily reversed and may result in inappropriate therapies such as diuretics.

There is no evidence that diuretics prevent AKI and they may even cause further complications (8).

Modern goal-directed IV fluid therapy is likely to decrease the risk of postoperative AKI, particularly if IV fluids are otherwise restricted, and perhaps with the addition of perioperative inotropic support (9).

Liberal fluids do not protect the kidneys. Although oliguria can be a marker of renal, cardiovascular or other problems in the perioperative period, its evaluation needs direct patient review to look for signs of heart failure, sepsis and hypovolaemia. In most cases oliguria is a normal response of the body to attempt to conserve fluid in times of physiological stress. It is common in the first 24 to 48 hours after surgery. It is not harmful in the short term, is unlikely to indicate kidney injury, and should not be treated with additional IV fluids unless hypovolaemia or fluid responsiveness can be demonstrated.

References

1. Bagshaw SM, Townsend DR, McDermid RC. Disorders of sodium and water balance in hospitalized patients. *Can J Anaesth*. 2009;**56**(2):151–67. Epub 2009/02/28. 10.1007/s12630-008-9017-2

2. McIlroy DR, Argenziano M, Farkas D, Umann T, Sladen RN. Incorporating oliguria into the diagnostic criteria for acute kidney injury after on-pump cardiac surgery: impact on incidence and outcomes. *Journal of cardiothoracic and vascular anesthesia*. 2013;**27**(6):1145–52. Epub 2013/06/06. 10.1053/j.jvca.2012.12.017

3. Prowle JR, Liu YL, Licari E, Bagshaw SM, Egi M, Haase M, et al. Oliguria as predictive biomarker of acute kidney injury in critically ill patients. *Crit Care*. 2011;**15**(4):R172. Epub 2011/07/21. 10.1186/cc10318

4. Matot I, Paskaleva R, Eid L, Cohen K, Khalaileh A, Elazary R, et al. Effect of the volume of fluids administered on intraoperative oliguria in laparoscopic bariatric surgery: a randomized controlled trial. *Arch Surg*. 2012;**147**(3):228–34. Epub 2011/11/23. 10.1001/archsurg.2011.308

5. Prowle JR, Echeverri JE, Ligabo EV, Ronco C, Bellomo R. Fluid balance and acute kidney injury. *Nature reviews Nephrology*. 2010;**6**(2):107–15. Epub 2009/12/23. 10.1038/nrneph.2009.213

6. Liu KD, Thompson BT, Ancukiewicz M, Steingrub JS, Douglas IS, Matthay MA, et al. Acute kidney injury in patients with acute lung injury: impact of fluid accumulation on classification of acute kidney injury and associated outcomes. *Critical care medicine*. 2011;**39**(12):2665–71. Epub 2011/07/26. 10.1097/CCM.0b013e318228234b

7. Bellomo R, Cass A, Cole L, Finfer S, Gallagher M, Lee J, et al. An observational study fluid balance and patient outcomes in the Randomized Evaluation of Normal vs. Augmented Level of Replacement Therapy trial. *Critical care medicine*. 2012;**40**(6):1753–60. Epub 2012/05/23. 10.1097/CCM.0b013e318246b9c6

8. Zacharias M, Conlon NP, Herbison GP, Sivalingam P, Walker RJ, Hovhannisyan K. Interventions for protecting renal function in the perioperative period. *Cochrane Database Syst Rev* 2008: CD003590 10.1002/14651858.CD003590.pub3

9. Prowle JR, Chua HR, Bagshaw SM, Bellomo R. Clinical review: Volume of fluid resuscitation and the incidence of acute kidney injury – a systematic review. *Crit Care* 2012;**16**: 230. 10.1186/cc11345

47 Acute kidney injury

Lloyd Roberts[1] and Owen Roodenburg[2]

[1] The Alfred Hospital, Australia
[2] The Alfred Hospital and Monash University, Australia

Acute kidney injury (AKI) is common [1] and associated with increased morbidity and mortality, even with small, transient increases in serum creatinine (>1.5 × baseline, >6 hours) [2].

Risk assessment and patient optimisation before, during and after surgery are important to minimise the frequency and severity of perioperative AKI (refer to Chapter 19 Risk assessment for perioperative renal dysfunction). Sepsis is the most common cause of AKI in the critically ill. Oliguria commonly occurs postoperatively and may be normal or a sign of impending or established AKI (refer to Chapter 46 Oliguria). This chapter considers issues of assessment and management, including the role of fluid and diuretic therapy.

Risk factors for perioperative acute kidney injury (Box 47.1)

Though of prognostic importance when informing patients about risks, many of these factors are non-modifiable. Modifiable causes to consider before, during and after surgery include the following.

Toxins

Aminoglycosides as surgical prophylaxis increase AKI. Diabetes, anaemia, high trough levels and prolonged courses probably increase this risk.

Imaging contrast should be avoided where possible (e.g. replace CT with ultrasound). If contrast is necessary [5], steps should be taken to:

- minimise dose
- avoid scans <48 hours apart
- ensure the patient is volume replete
- avoid other toxins, e.g. NSAIDs
- ensure an adequate interval between contrast procedure and surgery where surgical urgency permits
- consider N-acetylcysteine and bicarbonate in high-risk patients, although evidence of benefit is poor and use is decreasing.

Perioperative Medicine for the Junior Clinician, First Edition. Edited by Joel Symons, Paul Myles, Rishi Mehra and Christine Ball.
© 2015 John Wiley & Sons, Ltd. Published 2015 by John Wiley & Sons, Ltd.
Companion website: www.wiley.com/go/perioperativemed

BOX 47.1 Risk factors for perioperative AKI

Non-cardiac surgery [3]

Patient

Increasing age
ASA status IV/V (RR 3.94)
↑ BMI (24% ↑ per 5 kg/m²)
Baseline renal impairment -↑ serum urea (OR 2.1) or creatinine, or creatinine
clearance < 60 mL/min/m² (OR 5.8)
Chronic hypertension
Diabetes mellitus (OR 1.9–2.77)
Coronary artery disease (OR 2.07)
Heart failure (RR 2.34)
Stroke/TIA
Peripheral vascular disease (OR 4.4)
Anaemia

Surgery

Emergency surgery
High-risk surgery: intraperitoneal, intrathoracic or suprainguinal vascular
procedures (RR 3.34)

Toxins

Number of baseline antihypertensive medications
Preoperative ACEI, preoperative ARBs (OR 2.2)
NSAIDs (OR 3.2 with 7-day course)
Perioperative blood transfusion
Intraoperative starch administration (OR 1.5)
Gentamicin, contrast

Cardiac surgery (a major risk factor in itself, with up to 5% requiring temporary dialysis postoperatively) [4]

Patient

Age > 70 years
Preoperative serum creatinine > 90 micromol/L
Diabetes mellitus
Proteinuria
↓ left ventricular function (LVEF < 40%, ↑ BNP)
Atrial fibrillation
Vascular disease

Surgery

Emergency surgery
Valve surgery
Long duration of CPB

Interventions

Excessive haemodilution on CPB
Circulatory support devices (e.g. intra-aortic balloon pumps)

ACEI, angiotensin converting enzyme inhibitor; ARB, angiotensin receptor blocker; ASA, American Society of Anesthesiologists; BMI, Body Mass Index; BNP, brain natriuretic peptide; CPB, cardiopulmonary bypass; IV, intravenous; LVEF, left ventricular ejection fraction; NSAID, non-steroidal anti-inflammatory drug; OR, odds ratio; RR, relative risk; TIA, transient ischaemic attack

Cessation of ACE inhibitors/ARB is controversial (refer to Chapter 10 Perioperative medication management) with evidence of benefits and harms. NSAIDs and coxibs should be avoided, especially where risk is increased such as in the elderly, with loss of >10% of blood volume, and in combination with other nephrotoxins. If NSAIDs/coxibs are used, minimise the duration by writing a cessation date. Note that preoperative planning of pain management may help avoid the need for NSAIDs.

Starch solutions should be avoided (e.g. Voluven®) as there is accumulating evidence suggesting worsened renal outcomes [6]. Also consider avoiding high chloride solutions such as 0.9% saline, although evidence is preliminary [7] (refer to Chapter 19 Risk assessment for perioperative renal dysfunction).

Rhabdomyolysis

Rhabdomyolysis should be suspected in trauma patients, those with devascularised limbs and prolonged immobility (e.g. fractured hips where a prolonged period may be spent on the floor before the patient is discovered), and with severe metabolic derangements.

Check creatine kinase (CK) in crushed patients, assess for compartment syndrome and obtain an orthopaedic consult if required. With suspected or confirmed rhabdomyolysis, maintain urine output >100–300 mL/hr. If CK >5000 IU/L, obtain specialist advice and consider urinary alkalinisation or potentially dialysis. Avoid furosemide, which acidifies the urine.

Urinary tract obstruction

Flank or testicular pain suggests acute obstruction, whereas chronic obstruction is commonly painless. Note that urination does not exclude unilateral or partial obstruction. If obstruction is relieved in less than a week, substantial renal recovery is likely.

Abdominal compartment syndrome [8]

Severe increases in intra-abdominal pressures can reduce perfusion of intra-abdominal organs, including the kidneys. Risk factors include abdominal surgery, major trauma, positive fluid balance and shock. If suspected, obtain senior review. Treatment may include nasogastric (NG) or rectal tubes, enemas, percutaneous drainage of collections or even decompressive laparotomy.

Consider an oliguric patient 3 days postoperatively, with BP 110/70 mmHg, serum Cr 180 micromol/L and K$^+$ 4.2 mmol/L.

Important assessments include the following.

- *Is a BP 110/70 mmHg normal for that patient – or relative hypotension?* The patient's usual blood pressure should be maintained unless contraindicated.
- *Is the patient hypovolaemic, and what is the fluid balance?* If uncertain and the patient is not hypervolaemic, fluid challenge is reasonable – however, in the absence of a response or clear-cut hypovolaemia, senior consultation is more appropriate than repeated, large fluid boluses.

After confirming the usual BP is maintained and the patient is not hypovolaemic, furosemide is commonly used to produce urine, and senior doctors often have strongly held opinions either for or against its use. Currently, there is no clear evidence of overall benefit or harm in most AKI settings [9]. With hypervolaemia, short-term use of furosemide is reasonable, provided it is effective. However, oliguria can be a normal consequence of perioperative ADH release.

Sepsis and acute kidney injury

About 50% of AKI in critically ill patients is due to sepsis. Hypotension in septic AKI commonly requires a combination of fluid and vasopressor therapy [5] such as noradrenaline ± vasopressin, requiring ICU consultation (refer to Chapter 82 Sepsis and the inflammatory response to surgery).

Investigation and treatment of underlying sepsis may involve urgent:

- cultures (blood, urine, sputum, with others as appropriate, e.g. wound) and imaging (e.g. CT scan)
- antibiotics
- source control (eg. drainage).

Other measures

Conventional glucose control, targeting glucose ≤ 10 mmol/L (≤ 180 mg/dL) is appropriate in critically ill patients at risk of AKI.

References

1. Kellum JA, Bellomo R, Ronco C. The concept of acute kidney injury and the RIFLE criteria. *Contributions to Nephrology*, 2007;**156**:10–16. doi:10.1159/0000102010

2. Hoste EA, Clermont G, Kersten A, et al. RIFLE criteria for acute kidney injury are associated with hospital mortality in critically ill patients: a cohort analysis. *Critical Care*, 2006;**10**(3):R73. doi:10.1186/cc4915

3. Abelha FJ, Botelho M, Fernandes V, Barros H. Determinants of postoperative acute kidney injury. *Critical Care*, 2009;**13**(3):R79. doi:10.1186/cc7894

4. Mehta RH, Grab JD, O'Brien SM, et al. Bedside tool for predicting the risk of postoperative dialysis in patients undergoing cardiac surgery. *Circulation*, 2006;**114**(21):2208–2216; quiz. doi:10.1161/CIRCULATIONAHA.106.635573

5. Kidney Disease: Improving Global Outcomes (KDIGO) Acute Kidney Injury Work Group. KDIGO clinical practice guideline for acute kidney injury. *Kidney International*, 2012;**2**(Suppl):1–138.

6. Myburgh JA, Finfer S, Bellomo R, et al. Hydroxyethyl starch or saline for fluid resuscitation in intensive care. *New England Journal of Medicine*, 2012;**367**(20):1901–1911. doi:10.1056/NEJMoa1209759

7. Yunos NM, Bellomo R, Hegarty C, Story D, Ho L, Bailey M. Association between a chloride-liberal vs chloride-restrictive intravenous fluid administration strategy and kidney injury in critically ill adults. *JAMA*, 2012;**308**(15):1566–1572.

8. Kirkpatrick AW, Roberts DJ, de Waele J, et al. Intra-abdominal hypertension and the abdominal compartment syndrome: updated consensus definitions and clinical practice guidelines from the World Society of the Abdominal Compartment Syndrome. *Intensive Care Medicine*, 2013;**39**(7):1190–1206. doi:10.1007/s00134-013-2906-z

9. Ho KM, Power BM. Benefits and risks of furosemide in acute kidney injury. *Anaesthesia*, 2010;**65**(3):283–293. doi:10.1007/s00134-013-2906-z

Renal transplantation

Solomon Menahem

The Alfred Hospital, Australia

The treatment of choice for patients with dialysis-dependent renal failure or progressive and irreversible chronic kidney disease is renal transplantation. Despite advances in the care of dialysis-dependent patients, outcomes remain poor [1]. In patients with few major co-morbidities and good functional status, renal transplantation can significantly improve life expectancy and, by abrogating the need for regular dialysis, quality of life as well [2].

Added to the usual perioperative complications are the unique risks of acute graft rejection, plus the short- and long-term complications of immunosuppressive drugs.

Types of renal transplantation

Live donor renal transplantation

A live donor, often a family member, donates a kidney. The donor needs to be evaluated to ensure excellent physical and mental health, and normal kidney function and anatomy.

Deceased donor renal transplantation

Kidneys can be donated after brain death or cardiac death (refer to Chapter 78 Organ donation).

Pre-emptive renal transplantation

Renal transplantation occurring prior to the recipient requiring dialysis (in Australia, live donor usually).

Combined organ renal transplantation

Occasionally renal transplantation may be combined with another organ from the same deceased donor, e.g. kidney and pancreas for people with type 1 diabetes and advanced kidney failure.

Perioperative Medicine for the Junior Clinician, First Edition. Edited by Joel Symons, Paul Myles, Rishi Mehra and Christine Ball.
© 2015 John Wiley & Sons, Ltd. Published 2015 by John Wiley & Sons, Ltd.
Companion website: www.wiley.com/go/perioperativemed

Preoperative renal transplant recipient assessment

Potential transplant recipients undergo extensive evaluation to ensure they are suitable and fit for renal transplant surgery. As they are at increased risk of cardiovascular disease, assessment often involves screening for ischaemic heart disease, pelvic vessel calcification and peripheral vascular disease.

Assessment for end-organ disease is essential as this will impact on the perioperative risk of transplant surgery, the risks of long-term immunosuppressive therapy and the patient's long-term survival. Patient education and informed consent are critical to ensure patient compliance post transplantation.

> When a deceased donor kidney becomes available at short notice it is important to ensure that the recipient has not developed significant intercurrent illness since last review. It is also critical to establish if dialysis is required prior to surgery, the main indications being significant hyperkalaemia and/or fluid overload.

Human leucocyte antigen matching and cross-matching

The degree of matching between donor and recipient with respect to the genetically determined human leucocyte antigen (HLA) predicts rejection rates and graft outcome [3]. Prior to transplantation, the HLA subclasses of donor and recipient are established. At a minimum, the two alleles for class I HLA-A and HLA-B as well as the two for class II HLA-DR are determined for the donor and recipient. The degree of mismatch is then calculated, ranging from 6 for a complete mismatch to 0 for a perfect match.

Human leucocyte antigen antibodies can develop in the recipient prior to transplantation, causing acute graft rejection post transplant if the antibodies are to mismatched donor HLA. To detect recipient antibodies prior to transplantation, recipient serum is mixed with donor leucocytes in a 'cross-match'. If in the presence of complement there is donor cell lysis, the antibodies are thought to be of significance, rejection of the kidney is highly likely and transplantation should not proceed.

Immunosuppression

Without the early introduction of immunosuppression in the recipient, acute rejection could result in graft loss within hours of surgery. Where possible, immunosuppression is commenced immediately prior to transplant surgery and continued for the life of the kidney allograft. Modern immunosuppressive agents are successful at keeping acute rejection rates very low [4] but are also associated with significant side effects (Table 48.1).

Standard care includes the use of steroids, initially IV then oral, a calcineurin inhibitor (tacrolimus or cyclosporine), an antiproliferative agent (azathioprine or

TABLE 48.1 Immunosuppressive agents used after renal transplantation

Immunosuppressive agent	Effect on immune system	Usual dose	Common side effects
Antithymocyte globulin	Depletes T cells	3–5 mg/kg IV for 7–14 days	Anaphylaxis, cytopenia
Azathioprine	Blocks B and T cell proliferation	2 mg/kg daily	Nausea and vomiting, cytopenia
Basiliximab	Inhibits T cell proliferation	20 mg IV 2 doses	Fevers, chills
Cyclosporine	Inhibits T cell activation	3 mg/kg b.d.	Tremor, gum hypertrophy, nephrotoxicity, hirsutism
Everolimus	Inhibits B and T cell activation	0.75 mg b.d.	Impaired wound healing, oedema, proteinuria
IV immunoglobulin	Reduces circulating antibodies and tissue injury	1–2 g/kg IV	Anaphylaxis, thrombosis
Mycophenolate mofetil	Blocks B and T cell proliferation	1000 mg b.d.	Diarrhoea, cytopenia
Prednisolone	Suppresses cytokine release and inflammatory cells	20 mg daily	Hypertension, diabetes, peptic ulcers, weight gain
Rituximab	Depletes B cells	375 mg/m^2 IV 2–4 doses	Fevers, chills
Sirolimus	Inhibits B and T cell activation	3 mg daily	Impaired wound healing, oedema, proteinuria
Tacrolimus	Inhibits T cell activation	0.1 mg/kg b.d.	Tremor, diabetes, alopecia, nephrotoxicity

b.d., twice a day; IV, intravenous.

mycophenolate mofetil), and often induction therapy with an antibody to interleukin-2 receptors (basiliximab) or T cell-depleting antibody (antithymocyte globulin [ATG]).

Surgery

The transplanted kidney is usually implanted in the recipient's right or left iliac fossa. There are three surgical anastomoses:

- allograft renal artery to recipient's external or internal iliac artery
- allograft renal vein to recipient's external iliac vein
- allograft ureter to the recipient's bladder.

During surgery, a central line and urinary catheter are usually inserted to allow for accurate measurement of CVP and urine output. Blood pressure should be maintained during surgery to ensure adequate renal transplant perfusion following the arterial anastomosis. Care should be taken not to volume overload the patient, as delayed graft function and poor urine output postoperatively, especially when combined with poor LV function, may precipitate pulmonary oedema.

Principles of postoperative care

> In the initial post-transplant period, meticulous care must be applied to monitoring fluid balance. It is vital to ensure that the transplanted kidney is well perfused in order to avoid exacerbating or precipitating acute kidney injury.

Blood pressure must be regularly measured and IV fluid administered (crystalloid, colloid or, where needed, packed cells) cautiously to maintain CVP and BP within an acceptable range. Urine output can be highly variable post transplant. Regular review is vital to avoid fluid overload or dehydration. Nephrotoxic drugs, including NSAIDs, must be avoided.

Post-renal transplantation complications

Early

Along with the usual complications of major abdominal surgery, delayed graft function can also occur. It is not uncommon for the transplanted kidney to function poorly in the immediate postoperative period. Urine output may be minimal such that fluid loading can be hazardous to the patient. Depending on the severity, delayed graft function can last weeks and the patient may remain dialysis dependent for this period.

In the early post-transplant period, renal function is monitored closely to enable early detection and treatment of acute rejection. Acute rejection is suggested by a deterioration in renal function and is diagnosed by renal biopsy. It usually responds to pulsed therapy with methylprednisolone and increased immunosuppression, but may require the use of more potent (and toxic) agents such as ATG.

New-onset diabetes after renal transplantation is very common (up to 25% of patients) in the setting of high-dose steroid therapy as well as other diabetogenic agents [5]. It is usually managed with attention to diet and oral hypoglycaemic agents, but often insulin therapy is required.

Late

Profound immunosuppression of the recipient to prevent graft rejection increases the risk of opportunistic infection with organisms such as Cytomegalovirus and *Pneumocystis jiroveci*.

Cancers occur with significantly increased frequency, mainly skin cancers such as squamous cell carcinoma and basal cell carcinoma, as well as some forms of lymphoma [6].

References

1. McDonald S. Deaths. In: McDonald S, Clayton P, Hurst K, editors. *ANZDATA Registry Report 2012*. Adelaide, South Australia: Australia and New Zealand Dialysis and Transplant Registry, 2012, pp. 1–9.

2. Clayton P, Campbell S, Hurst K, McDonald S, Chadban S. Transplantation. In: McDonald S, Clayton P, Hurst K, editors. *ANZDATA Registry Report 2012*. Adelaide, South Australia: Australia and New Zealand Dialysis and Transplant Registry, 2012, pp. 10–27.

3. Lim WH, Chadban SJ, Clayton P, et al. Human leukocyte antigen mismatches associated with increased risk of rejection, graft failure, and death independent of initial immunosuppression in renal transplant recipients. *Clinical Transplantation*, 2012;**26**(4):E428–437. doi:10.1111/j.1399-0012.2012.01654.x

4. Ekberg H, Tedesco-Silva H, Demirbas A, et al. Reduced exposure to calcineurin inhibitors in renal transplantation. *New England Journal of Medicine*, 2007;**357**(25):2562–2575. doi:10.1056/NEJMoa067411

5. Pham PT, Pham PC, Lipshutz GS, Wilkinson AH. New onset diabetes mellitus after solid organ transplantation. *Endocrinology and Metabolism Clinics of North America*, 2007;**36**(4):873–890; vii. doi:10.1016/j.ecl.2007.07.007

6. Kasiske BL, Snyder JJ, Gilbertson DT, Wang C. Cancer after kidney transplantation in the United States. *American Journal of Transplantation*, 2004;**4**(6):905–913. doi:10.1111/j.1600-6143.2004.00450.x

Diabetes mellitus

David Story

The University of Melbourne, Australia

Incidence

Over 25% of surgical inpatients aged over 60 years have diabetes, half undiagnosed on admission [1,2]. In developed countries about 90% of patients with diabetes will have type 2 diabetes. However, many of these patients will also require insulin therapy.

Diagnosis

While diagnosis based on a random blood sugar of >11 mmol/L or a fasting blood sugar >7 mmol/L is still valid, there is increasing use of the glycosylated haemoglobin (HbA$_1$c) to not only measure longer term glucose control but also to diagnose type 2 diabetes. An HbA$_1$c >6.5% (48 mmol/mol) is diagnostic of diabetes. This test is easily added to routine preoperative blood tests (fasting not required) in higher risk patients, including those aged over 60 years, and patients with vascular disease or obesity.

Known diabetes

HbA$_1$c is a measure of long-term glucose control. Patients with an HbA$_1$c >8% (54 mmol/L) are at increased risk of perioperative complications and mortality [2]. Glucose control should be optimised where possible, particularly for elective non-cancer surgery. This can be done collaboratively with physicians and general practitioners. The nature, severity and optimal management of other conditions associated with diabetes should be addressed including ischaemic heart disease, renal impairment, neuropathy, obstructive sleep apnoea and obesity.

Treatment of diabetes

Community management of patients with type 1 diabetes (no endogenous insulin production) is always with insulin plus lifestyle changes. Insulin therapy has evolved [3] with newer, genetically modified human insulin that allows more rapid release after subcutaneous injection (aspart and lispro) or delayed release with a flat profile (glargine). This combination of boluses of rapidly acting insulin with meals, combined with basal insulin, provides a more physiological profile. A related approach is

Perioperative Medicine for the Junior Clinician, First Edition. Edited by Joel Symons, Paul Myles, Rishi Mehra and Christine Ball.
© 2015 John Wiley & Sons, Ltd. Published 2015 by John Wiley & Sons, Ltd.
Companion website: www.wiley.com/go/perioperativemed

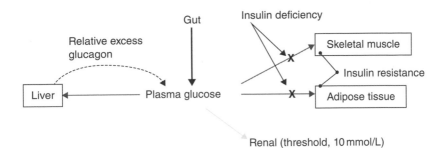

FIGURE 49.1 **Metabolic changes in type 2 diabetes.**

continuous subcutaneous rapid-acting insulin with basal and bolus infusions. However, if the pump is stopped or disconnected, the patient may rapidly become hyperglycaemic and ultimately ketotic. All patients taking insulin will have strategies to deal with hypoglycaemia (glucose) and hyperglycaemia (corrective insulin). This basal/nutritional/corrective insulin regime (basal-bolus) is one good option for inpatient management [4]. The traditional sliding scale of insulin is corrective only and constitutes poor care [5].

Many patients with type 2 diabetes will be on insulin in the community or will require insulin in hospital [6]. One approach is to treat all patients on insulin (type 1 and type 2) in a similar manner. There is considerable variation in hospital protocols because evidence is limited. For junior doctors, the best strategy is to know the protocol of the hospital or unit you are working in, the important points being the approach to basal, nutritional and corrective insulin. Many patients with type 2 diabetes will be managed with lifestyle change alone or with oral diabetes drugs [7]. Importantly, management between patients and for individuals over time will vary considerably because the (multiple) mechanisms for hyperglycaemia in patients with type 2 diabetes vary (Figure 49.1). Subsequently, there are numerous oral diabetes drugs (refer to Chapter 26 Diabetes medication), with metformin having the best supporting evidence and widespread use. Metformin has a minimal risk of hypoglycaemia while sulfonylureas (glibenclamide and glicazide) share a risk of hypoglycaemia comparable to that of therapeutic insulin.

> Perioperative management of blood sugar can be viewed as similar to managing blood pressure. Like blood pressure, the key is to *measure the blood sugar* at individualised intervals and *respond appropriately*.

Perioperative management

While *hyperglycaemia* is important, it is rarely an emergency, like hypertension, for surgical inpatients but *hypoglycaemia*, like hypotension, is more serious and more likely to be an emergency. Hypoglycaemia can lead to significant brain injury [2].

The plan

Managing diabetes for patients undergoing the physiological stress of anaesthesia and surgery, including the challenges of fasting, is not easy and has limited evidence for guidance [2,8,9]. Perioperative management should involve an individualised plan developed or at least agreed to by the anaesthesia, internal medicine and surgical teams. Inpatient management can involve co-management with internal medicine and diabetes educators.

A patient with diabetes, particularly on insulin, should ideally be first on a morning list; management becomes more complex as the day progresses. The most conservative approach for morning day of surgery admissions is for patients not to take any diabetes medication before admission.

On the day

* *Measure the blood sugar level* frequently and respond appropriately.
* Have an adaptable plan for glucose management (refer to Chapter 26 Diabetes medication).
* Aim for a blood sugar level of 8 mmol/L, with a range of 5–10 mmol/L.
* Have plans for hypoglycaemia and hyperglycaemia.
* Consider antiemetics; beware of the glycaemic effect of dexamethasone.

The optimal blood sugar range during the perioperative period is unclear but a reasonable option is to aim for 5–10 mmol/L and treat blood sugars outside this range [6,10]. The *first* dose of sugar for hypoglycaemia can be 10 g; this can be given orally if time allows (two barley sugars or 200 mL of apple juice) or 5% dextrose 200 mL IV (10 g glucose) or 50% dextrose 20 mL (10 g glucose) IV. The reason for hypoglycaemia should be considered and managed.

Hyperglycaemia can be treated with corrective insulin as per Chapter 26 but the underlying causes should be addressed. One simple formula for corrective insulin is:

Measured blood sugar (mmol/L) – 10 = rapid-acting insulin dose in units

Postoperative

* *Measure the blood sugar level* frequently and respond appropriately.
* Have an insulin plan. Beware of oral diabetes drugs and mixed insulins.
* Return to out-of-hospital management of diabetes as soon as possible.
* Intraoperative stay, co-managed with endocrine or general medicine.
* Monitor electrolytes with insulin therapy; dextrose and insulin infusions have a risk of hyponatraemia and hypokalaemia.

References

1. Valentine NA, Alhawassi TM, Roberts GW, Vora PP, Stranks SN, Doogue MP. Detecting undiagnosed diabetes using glycated haemoglobin: an automated screening test in hospitalised patients. *Medical Journal of Australia*, 2011;**194**(4):160–164. doi:10.5694/mja11.10534c

2. Russo N. Perioperative glycemic control. *Anesthesiology Clinics*, 2012;**30**(3):445–466. doi:10.1016/j.anclin.2012.07.007

3. Killen J, Tonks K, Greenfield J, Story DA. New insulin analogues and perioperative care of patients with type 1 diabetes. *Anaesthesia and Intensive Care*, 2010;**38**(2):244–249. www.ncbi.nlm.nih.gov/pubmed/20369755

4. Wesorick D, O'Malley C, Rushakoff R, Larsen K, Magee M. Management of diabetes and hyperglycemia in the hospital: a practical guide to subcutaneous insulin use in the non-critically ill, adult patient. *Journal of Hospital Medicine*, 2008;**3**(5 Suppl):17–28. doi:10.1002/jhm.353

5. Umpierrez GE, Palacio A, Smiley D. Sliding scale insulin use: myth or insanity? *American Journal of Medicine*, 2007;**120**(7):563–567. doi:10.1016/j.amjmed.2006.05.070

6. Lipshutz AK, Gropper MA. Perioperative glycemic control: an evidence-based review. *Anesthesiology*, 2009;**110**(2):408–421. doi:10.1016/j.anclin.2012.07.007

7. Rodbard HW, Jellinger PS, Davidson JA, et al. Statement by an American Association of Clinical Endocrinologists/American College of Endocrinology consensus panel on type 2 diabetes mellitus: an algorithm for glycemic control. *Endocrine Practice*, 2009;**15**(6):540–559. doi:10.4158/EP.15.6.540

8. Kadoi Y. Anesthetic considerations in diabetic patients. Part II: intraoperative and postoperative management of patients with diabetes mellitus. *Journal of Anesthesia*, 2010;**24**(5):748–756. doi:10.1007/s00540-010-0988-0

9. Kadoi Y. Anesthetic considerations in diabetic patients. Part I: preoperative considerations of patients with diabetes mellitus. *Journal of Anesthesia*, 2010;**24**(5):739–747. doi:10.1007/s00540-010-0987-1

10. Keegan MT, Goldberg ME, Torjman MC, Coursin DB. Perioperative and critical illness dysglycemia – controlling the iceberg. *Journal of Diabetes Science and Technology*, 2009;**3**(6):1288–1291. doi:10.1177/193229680900300608

49

Thyroid disorders

Shane Hamblin

The Alfred Hospital, Western Health, Monash University and
The University of Melbourne, Australia

Thyroid disorders are common (Table 50.1). Hypothyroidism and hyperthyroidism both present challenges in the perioperative period. Goitre and nodular thyroid disease are also common. It is important to deal with these issues carefully before elective surgery is undertaken. However, emergency surgery may be required at a time when the patient is not euthyroid or when an enlarged gland has not been adequately investigated. Changes in thyroid function tests associated with non-thyroidal illness in the perioperative period also need careful interpretation and assessment.

Thyroid disorders

Clinical findings of thyroid overactivity or underactivity, while still important, are now generally considered subservient to the results of thyroid function tests (TFTs).

Hypothyroidism

Most cases are due to primary thyroid failure caused by autoimmune thyroid disease (Table 50.2), thyroidectomy or radioactive iodine. Lithium or amiodarone may also cause hypothyroidism. TFTs confirm the diagnosis with elevated thyroid-stimulating hormone (TSH) and low free thyroxine (FT4) and tri-iodothyronine (FT3) levels. Secondary hypothyroidism due to pituitary or hypothalamic disease is much less common. In secondary hypothyroidism, TSH is inappropriately normal or low, despite low FT4 and FT3.

Hyperthyroidism

Graves' disease is an autoimmune disorder associated with TSH receptor-stimulating antibodies. It is more common in younger women. 'Toxic' or hyperfunctioning nodules are more likely in older people and are also more common in women. Only 5% of solitary nodules are hyperfunctioning. Toxic multinodular goitre involves one or more hyperfunctioning nodules within a heterogeneous gland.

Subclinical thyroid disease

The availability of reliable rapid biochemical testing has led to many patients being detected with low or high TSH but normal FT4 and FT3 levels. Although a biochemical diagnosis, ironically it is termed 'subclinical' thyroid disease, even if the patient has clinical features.

Perioperative Medicine for the Junior Clinician, First Edition. Edited by Joel Symons, Paul Myles, Rishi Mehra and Christine Ball.
© 2015 John Wiley & Sons, Ltd. Published 2015 by John Wiley & Sons, Ltd.
Companion website: www.wiley.com/go/perioperativemed

TABLE 50.1 The prevalence of thyroid disease in the population

Palpable goitre	Thyroid nodules	Hypothyroidism	Hyperthyroidism
Iodine insufficiency 3–4% (women 6%, men 1%)	Palpable 5% Ultrasound 25%	Clinical (women 2%, men 0.16%)	Clinical 0.5% (70% due to Graves' disease)
Previously iodine deficient now supplemented: 10%	Much higher in older age groups	Up to 20% subclinical disease in older women	Subclinical 0.7%
Currently iodine deficient: 30%	Much higher in iodine-deficient areas	Hashimoto's increases with age	Toxic nodular disease increases with age

TABLE 50.2 The prevalence of thyroid antibodies in health and disease

Population	Antithyroid peroxidase	Thyroglobulin antibodies	TSH receptor antibody
General population	11% (no thyroid disease history) 27% (thyroid disease history)	5% (no thyroid disease history) 20% (thyroid disease history)	1–2% (significance uncertain)
Graves' disease	50–80%	50–70%	90–99%
Hashimoto's thyroiditis	90–100%	80–90%	10–20%

TSH, thyroid-stimulating hormone.

Thyroid nodules and goitre

The widespread use of ultrasound has revealed that thyroid nodules are far more prevalent than previously thought from clinical examination alone [1]. Areas of iodine deficiency are associated with a higher prevalence of thyroid nodularity. If TFTs are normal, the presence of most nodules will not affect perioperative management.

Goitre (enlarged thyroid gland) may be due to a variety of causes. It may be diffuse (e.g. Graves' disease) or multinodular. It may be asymmetrical. A retrosternal goitre may cause tracheal deviation which may be concerning for anaesthetists. Large goitres may cause venous obstruction, especially with the arms elevated (Pemberton's sign). Thyroidectomy for long-standing large retrosternal goitre may be associated with tracheomalacia in the immediate postoperative period. This rare complication can occasionally lead to respiratory compromise.

Iodine and amiodarone

Iodine exposure (e.g. iodinated contrast agents) may precipitate hyperthyroidism in someone with nodular disease, especially if TSH is already suppressed. Think carefully before requesting a CT scan with contrast. TFTs should be rechecked in the six-week period following the scan.

Amiodarone deserves special mention as its unintended thyroid effects are numerous. Amiodarone-induced thyroid dysfunction occurs in 15–20% of

TABLE 50.3 **Alterations in thyroid hormone and TSH levels in various conditions**

Diagnosis	FT4	FT3	TSH
Primary hypothyroidism	↓	↓	↑
Secondary hypothyroidism	↓	↓	↓ →
Hyperthyroidism	↑	↑	↓
Non-thyroidal illness ('sick euthyroid')	↑ ↓ →	↓ →	↑ ↓ →

FT3, tri-iodothyronine; FT4, thyroxine; TSH, thyroid-stimulating hormone.

amiodarone-treated patients [2]. Hypothyroidism may occur and is easily treated with thyroxine therapy. Hyperthyroidism may be due to the Jod-Basedow effect (similar to that seen with iodinated contrast) or a chemical thyroiditis, which can be very difficult to treat. Such patients present considerable risk perioperatively and specialist advice should be sought.

Non-thyroidal illness ('sick euthyroidism')

Interpretation of TFTs is important and at times challenging. Many factors influence these tests, not all of which are well understood. In particular, the effects of severe non-thyroidal illness need to be taken into account, especially in the postoperative period. Several TFT patterns may occur, including low TSH, low FT4 and low FT3 suggesting pituitary/hypothalamic dysfunction or low FT4, low FT3 with high TSH during the recovery phase, suggesting primary hypothyroidism (Table 50.3).

The key is to recognise the possibility of illness effect and repeat the tests over a period of days to see if there is a trend. 'Non-steady state' tests are frequently seen in hospitalised patients.

Perioperative management

Hypothyroidism

The main issues in hypothyroidism relate to reduced clearance of drugs and water, along with altered respiratory, thermoregulatory and cardiovascular responses [3]. It is essential to reduce the dose of drugs prescribed (especially opioids) because of their reduced clearance. Care should be taken to limit the use of 5% dextrose, as hyponatraemia can readily develop due to reduced free water clearance, especially in severe hypothyroidism (myxoedema). In myxoedema, close monitoring of respiratory rate is required postoperatively. Patient warming measures (passive and sometimes active) are required. IV tri-iodothyronine may be given judiciously, with continuous ECG monitoring. IV hydrocortisone 50–100 mg is usually also given in case there is co-existing cortisol deficiency. Postoperative management of the patient with myxoedema should take place in an ICU.

Hyperthyroidism

Surgery in an inadequately treated or untreated hyperthyroid patient (usually with Graves' disease) may precipitate 'thyroid storm'. This is associated with severe worsening of thyrotoxicosis. Features include marked tachycardia, tremor, fever (above 40°C), agitation, delirium or coma. Management should take place in the ICU.

The principles of management of thyroid storm
- Block thyroid hormone synthesis
- Block thyroid hormone release
- Decrease conversion of FT4 to FT3
- Control tachycardia and rate-dependent heart failure
- Restore hydration
- Sedation

Specific drug treatment of thyroid storm includes the following [4].

Antithyroid drugs
- Propylthiouracil 200 mg orally 4–6 hourly preferred as it blocks both hormone formation and FT4 to FT3 conversion.
- Alternatively, carbimazole 20 mg 8 hourly orally (blocks hormone formation, but not FT4 to FT3 conversion).

Other therapy
- Lugol's iodine solution 0.5 mL orally t.d.s. to block hormone release.
- Dexamethasone 4 mg IV 12 hourly to block FT4 to FT3 conversion.
- Beta-blockade (e.g. IV metoprolol or esmolol or oral propranolol).

Conclusion

Safe perioperative management of patients with thyroid disorders requires careful clinical and biochemical assessment. Correction of hyperthyroidism or hypothyroidism well in advance of surgery is recommended. In emergency surgery, an understanding of the physiology of thyroid hormone action helps guide the management of the rare emergencies of myxoedema or thyroid storm.

References

1. Guth S, Theune U, Aberle J, Galach A, Bamberger CM. Very high prevalence of thyroid nodules detected by high frequency (13 MHz) ultrasound examination. *European Journal of Clinical Investigation*, 2009;**39**(8):699–706. doi:10.1111/J.1365-2362.2009.02162.X

2. Bogazzi F, Tomisti L, Bartalena L, Aghini-Lombardi F, Martino E. Amiodarone and the thyroid: a 2012 update. *Journal of Endocrinological Investigation*, 2012;**35**(3):340–348. doi:10.3275/8298

3. Kohl BA, Schwartz S. Surgery in the patient with endocrine dysfunction. *Medical Clinics of North America*, 2009;**93**(5):1031. doi:10.1016/J.Mcna.2009.05.003

4. Treating thyroid storm. In: *Therapeutic Guidelines*. Melbourne: Therapeutic Guidelines Ltd. www.tg.org.au/etg_demo/desktop/tgc.htm#tgc/edg51/11469.htm

Parathyroid disorders

Shane Hamblin

The Alfred Hospital, Western Health, Monash University and The University of Melbourne, Australia

Perioperative management of parathyroid disorders is important, as severe disturbances of plasma calcium constitute medical emergencies. Acute changes in calcium are more likely to be associated with significant symptoms than chronically stable low or high calcium states.

Calcium homeostasis

Only 2% of calcium circulates in blood, with the rest in bone. Plasma calcium is regulated by both parathyroid hormone (PTH) and calcitriol (1,25 $(OH)_2$, vitamin D). PTH mobilises calcium from bone into the bloodstream and also reduces calcium loss in urine. It stimulates the synthesis of calcitriol in the kidney which in turn increases calcium absorption from the gut. PTH also promotes phosphate loss from the kidneys. Magnesium is required for normal parathyroid function.

Calcium is present in the plasma in three forms:

- free ionised calcium (Ca^{2+}) which makes up 50% of the total: the physiologically active component
- protein bound (predominantly to albumin)
- complexed (mostly with phosphate).

Traditionally, free Ca^{2+} is called ionised calcium but this is only partly true, as protein-bound calcium is also ionised. Plasma albumin concentration changes will affect the measured total plasma calcium, while the free ionised calcium may be normal. Laboratories attempt to adjust for this by reporting 'corrected' calcium levels.

A common formula used to correct plasma calcium for albumin is:

$$\text{measured calcium concentration} + 0.02(40 - \text{albumin concentration}).$$

However, corrected calcium measurements cannot be relied upon in the following circumstances:

- plasma albumin less than 25 g/L
- abnormal globulin concentrations (as they also bind calcium)

Perioperative Medicine for the Junior Clinician, First Edition. Edited by Joel Symons, Paul Myles, Rishi Mehra and Christine Ball.
© 2015 John Wiley & Sons, Ltd. Published 2015 by John Wiley & Sons, Ltd.
Companion website: www.wiley.com/go/perioperativemed

- abnormal blood pH
- jaundice
- high free fatty acid concentrations.

In these circumstances free ionised calcium should be measured directly.

Hyperparathyroidism

The age- and sex- adjusted incidence of hyperparathyroidism has been reported to be 21.6 per 100,000 person-years (and declining) in a white population [1]. However, in a racially mixed population, the overall incidence was much higher at 24.7 in men and 65.5 in women, rising to 196 in older women [2].

Most cases are due to single parathyroid adenomas but rarely multiple adenomas can be present. About 5% of hyperparathyroidism is due to parathyroid hyperplasia of all four glands.

Symptoms of hyperparathyroidism are variable, with many patients being asymptomatic or only mildly affected (e.g. tiredness may be the only symptom). Milder cases may require no intervention, apart from periodic calcium monitoring and bone mineral density assessment. Marked hypercalcaemia may be associated with thirst, dehydration, constipation, nausea, vomiting, coma and possibly death.

Chronic kidney disease is also a cause of hyperparathyroidism. The calcimimetic Cinacalcet, a calcium sensing receptor (CaSR) agonist, is useful in earlier stages of renal parathyroid disease. When tertiary hyperparathyroidism develops, parathyroidectomy is usually required.

Other situations where PTH is high include normocalcaemic hyperparathyroidism, where plasma calcium is normal, and vitamin D deficiency where elevation of PTH is physiologically appropriate. The former causes no perioperative issues and the latter is a perioperative problem only in severe deficiency.

Calcium sensing receptor

The parathyroid and kidney both express the CaSR. Under normal circumstances, calcium binds to this receptor and reduces PTH secretion while increasing calcium loss in the urine.

Inactivating mutations of CaSR gene lead to hypercalcaemia and hypocalciuria. The most well-known condition is familial hypocalciuric hypercalcaemia.

Hypoparathyroidism

Most cases of hypoparathyroidism are due to inadvertent damage to the parathyroid glands or their blood supply at the time of neck surgery (e.g. thyroidectomy). Less common causes include autoimmune parathyroid damage, activating CaSR mutations leading to hypercalciuria and low PTH secretion (known as autosomal dominant hypocalcemia), and a genetic condition affecting chromosome 22 known as DiGeorge syndrome.

Treatment of permanent hypoparathyroidism is imperfect. Calcitriol and oral calcium are used to increase calcium, but the phosphate elevation seen with hypoparathyroidism is not helped with this treatment. The therapeutic aim is for calcium to be in the lower part of the normal range to minimise the risk of nephrocalcinosis. Clinical trials of PTH injections or subcutaneous PTH infusions have shown promise.

Perioperative management

Hypocalcaemia

Hypocalcaemia may cause paraesthesiae, muscle cramps, tetany and, rarely, seizures. The patient may become very distressed, with hyperventilation worsening symptoms (due to respiratory alkalosis lowering ionised calcium). The most common time for acute perioperative hypocalcaemia is in the first 24–48 hours after thyroid surgery.

It can also occur after parathyroidectomy for hyperparathyroidism (especially where there is co-existent vitamin D deficiency) or where increased bone ALP is present preoperatively, suggesting accelerated bone turnover. Postoperatively, calcium and phosphate flood back into bone, causing acute hypocalcaemia ('hungry bones').

Patients with tertiary hyperparathyroidism due to chronic kidney disease are prone to marked hypocalcaemia after parathyroidectomy.

Mild cases of acute hypocalcaemia can be treated with oral calcium and calcitriol. Hypomagnesaemia should also be corrected.

If the patient develops tetany or very low plasma calcium (e.g. less than 1.80 mmol/L), 10 mL calcium gluconate 10% (i.e. 1 g or 2.2 mmol) should be given intravenously over 10 minutes [3]. For recurrent severe hypocalcaemia, an IV calcium infusion is used: 100 mL calcium gluconate 10% in 900 mL 0.9% saline at 50 mL per hour. The infusion rate is titrated to achieve plasma calcium concentrations of 2.0–2.3 mmol/L [4]. Plasma calcium should be checked three to four times daily during IV calcium infusion.

Oral calcitriol and calcium should also be started to enable weaning from the calcium infusion over one to two days. Postoperative hypocalcaemia associated with 'hungry bones' may require calcium infusion for a number of days. Specialist management is recommended in those cases.

Hypercalcaemia

Occasionally a patient with significant hyperparathyroidism requires emergency surgery for another condition (e.g. coronary artery bypass grafting) before parathyroidectomy has occurred. The mainstay of management is IV hydration with 0.9% saline. If the calcium remains very high, IV bisphosphonate is usually beneficial as a temporary measure [5]. Parathyroidectomy is the definitive treatment but, depending on the clinical circumstances, may need to be delayed.

Conclusion

Table 51.1 summarises the aetiology, biochemical changes and perioperative management of patients with parathyroid disorders.

Most calcium disorders will not interfere with the patient's perioperative course. Severe hypocalcaemia and hypercalcaemia, however, are medical emergencies requiring prompt treatment and close biochemical monitoring.

TABLE 51.1 Aetiology, biochemistry and perioperative management of patients with parathyroid disorders

Disorder	Aetiology	Parathyroid hormone	Calcium	Phosphate	Perioperative management
Primary hyperparathyroidism	Adenoma (95%), Hyperplasia (5%)	↑	↑	↑↓	IV fluids (0.9% NaCl), IV bisphosphonates in selected cases
Tertiary hyperparathyroidism	Chronic kidney disease	↑↑↑	↑	↑	Specialist nephrology input essential
Hypoparathyroidism	Post neck surgery, Autoimmune, Activating CaSR mutations, Genetic syndromes	↓	↓	↑	Oral calcium ± calcitriol, IV calcium bolus in selected cases, IV calcium infusion in selected cases
Familial hypocalciuric hypercalcaemia	Inactivating CaSR mutations	↑↓	↑	↑↓	No special management required

CaSR, calcium sensing receptor; IV, intravenous.

51

References

1. Wermers RA, Khosla S, Atkinson EJ, et al. Incidence of primary hyperparathyroidism in Rochester, Minnesota, 1993–2001: an update on the changing epidemiology of the disease. *Journal of Bone and Mineral Research*, 2006;**21**(1):171–177. doi:10.1359/Jbmr.050910

2. Yeh MW, Ituarte PHG, Zhou HC, et al. Incidence and prevalence of primary hyperparathyroidism in a racially mixed population. *Journal of Clinical Endocrinology and Metabolism*, 2013;**98**(3):1122–1129. doi:10.1210/Jc.2012-4022

3. Tohme JF, Bilezikian JP. Hypocalcemic emergencies. *Endocrinology and Metabolism Clinics of North America*, 1993;**22**(2):363–375.

4. Acute treatment of symptomatic hypocalcaemia. In: Therapeutic Guidelines. Molbourne: Therapeutic Guidelines Ltd. www.tg.org.au/

5. Phitayakorn R, McHenry CR. Hyperparathyroid crisis: use of bisphosphonates as a bridge to parathyroidectomy. *Journal of the American College of Surgeons*, 2008;**206**(6):1106–1115. doi:10.1016/J.Jamcollsurg.2007.11.010

Adrenal disorders

Jonathan Serpell

The Alfred Hospital and Monash University, Australia

Conditions affecting the adrenal gland include:

- adrenal incidentalomas, which are not hyperfunctioning
- adrenal tumours and hyperplasias which produce excess adrenal hormones
- syndromes of subclinical hormone excess
- adrenocortical cancer
- Addison's disease (adrenal insufficiency) (refer to Chapter 102 Case Study 7 Addisonian crisis).

Therefore, the adrenal pathologies and surgical approach will vary considerably. Adrenalectomies are usually undertaken laparoscopically, either transabdominally or retroperitoneoscopically. Open adrenalectomy is still required on occasion, involving a transverse upper abdominal incision, a midline incision, a thoracoabdominal incision or a posterior approach via a vertical incision in the back, with the patient prone.

Varying pathology, hormonal excesses and complex surgery require excellent communication between the surgical and anaesthetic teams.

Investigation of an adrenal lesion

Assessment should establish the involvement of adjacent structures and whether the tumour is producing excess hormones [1].

All adrenal tumours require imaging, which may be a combination of ultrasound, CT or MRI scanning. It is critically important to establish the presence of a contralateral normal adrenal gland. Imaging cannot diagnose histopathology but will be a helpful pointer to the diagnosis. The tests listed in Box 52.1 are useful for the exclusion and diagnosis of adrenal disease.

Phaeochromocytoma

Phaeochromocytomas are rare tumours producing catecholamines, including noradrenaline, adrenaline and dopamine. They arise from the chromaffin cells of the adrenal medulla. Less commonly, they arise from other extra-adrenal sites, anywhere from the neck to the pelvis. These tumours only produce noradrenaline because

Perioperative Medicine for the Junior Clinician, First Edition. Edited by Joel Symons, Paul Myles, Rishi Mehra and Christine Ball.
© 2015 John Wiley & Sons, Ltd. Published 2015 by John Wiley & Sons, Ltd.
Companion website: www.wiley.com/go/perioperativemed

the enzyme for conversion to adrenaline is not present in extra-adrenal chromaffin tissue. Phaeochromocytomas may produce sustained or paroxysmal hypertension, causing sudden death in up to one-third of cases [2]. Treatment is urgent, both in terms of controlling BP and safely removing the tumour.

Preoperatively, hypertensive crises should be avoided by appropriate treatment of BP and avoiding interventions which may precipitate hypertensive crises (e.g. iodinated contrast in CT scans, percutaneous biopsies of the tumour). The excess catecholamines cause intense vasoconstriction, tachycardia and hypertension and, secondarily, reduce intravascular volume.

Aims of treatment, therefore, are to optimise cardiovascular status by normalising BP and restoring intravascular volume. An important component of this is to avoid surgically induced hypertensive crises.

Preoperative blockade

The aim of preoperative blockade is to reduce the incidence and magnitude of fluctuations in BP and the incidence of arrhythmias. The duration of blockade should be at least 7–14 days, with many endocrinologists recommending up to 28 days preoperatively [3]. Phenoxybenzamine, a long-acting alpha-adrenergic antagonist, is commenced at 10 mg twice daily, increasing gradually under the supervision of an endocrinologist to control BP. Orthostatic hypotension is often the limiting factor in the dosage. A reflex tachycardia inevitably occurs which can be treated with a beta-blocker.

A beta-blocker should never be introduced prior to alpha-blockade as a beta-blocker will block the vasodilatory action of adrenaline, precipitating severe vasoconstriction and possibly a hypertensive crisis.

Volume repletion

Phenoxybenzamine blocks catecholamine-induced vasoconstriction, and so intravascular blood volume will expand following initiation of therapy. Patients may benefit from a high salt and fluid diet, and be given 1–2 L of IV crystalloid preoperatively.

Intraoperative management

Optimal monitoring requires insertion of an arterial and central venous catheter, and probably a monitor of fluid responsiveness.

Vasoactive infusions of noradrenaline, nitroprusside and/or nitroglycerine (GTN) should be available before induction of anaesthesia. Magnesium may also be efficacious [4].

It may be necessary for the anaesthetist to request the surgeon to stop operating for a period whilst normalisation of BP occurs. It is also essential the surgeon informs the anaesthetist when the adrenal vein is clamped or ligated because a precipitous fall in BP may occur.

Postoperative management

There are two main risks in the postoperative period.

- Decreased BP due to hypovolaemia, residual effect of alpha-blockade or haemorrhage. Close monitoring of BP in a high-dependency setting is therefore required for 24 hours postoperatively.
- Hypoglycaemia. Catecholamines induce alpha-2 receptor inhibition of insulin secretion, resulting in hyperglycaemia. Removal of the phaeochromocytoma results in a rebound increase in insulin secretion which may cause hypoglycaemia. Patients therefore need regular glucose monitoring and a prophylactic dextrose infusion in the postoperative period.

Conn's syndrome

Conn's syndrome is due to small (< 1 cm diameter) solitary adenomas and, less commonly, bilateral adrenal hyperplasia. The distinction is important as the treatment for a solitary adenoma is surgery whereas hyperplasia will usually be treated medically. There is often a long history of difficult-to-control hypertension, with patients on combination antihypertensives. One-third of patients are hypokalaemic.

Apart from localisation studies to accurately define which adrenal requires removal, the preoperative management is directed towards controlling BP and correcting hypokalaemia. Spironolactone, a mineralocorticoid receptor blocker, achieves both aims.

Most solitary Conn's adenomas can be removed laparoscopically. Intra- and postoperatively, monitoring of potassium and BP is important. Postoperatively, the number and doses of antihypertensives can usually be reduced; at six months some patients will no longer require treatment.

Cushing's syndrome

The causes of Cushing's syndrome are:

- pituitary disease
- adrenal adenoma
- ectopic ACTH-secreting tumours
- adrenocortical cancer.

52

Investigations include a combination of low- then high-dose dexamethasone suppression tests, ACTH assay and imaging studies, which may involve both the pituitary and the adrenals.

Cushing's syndrome leads to metabolic syndrome with central adiposity, hypertension, insulin resistance, hyperlipidaemia, a thrombotic tendency and a four-fold increased risk in mortality. DVT prophylaxis, blood glucose and BP control are important.

Post adrenalectomy, a relative deficiency in cortisol due to suppression of the contralateral gland will require replacement, initially with hydrocortisone, then prednisolone for up to six months. Bilateral adrenalectomy patients require permanent replacement of glucocorticoid and mineralocorticoid.

Adrenocortical cancers

These often require more extensive, usually open surgery. Preoperative preparation includes imaging to assess the site and extent of the tumour, and potential invasion and/or tumour embolus. Hormonal screening (commonly cortisol but often others), electrolytes and blood cross-matching are required.

References

1. Roy R, Lee, J.A. Adrenal Incidentaloma In: Sippel RS, Chen H, editors. *The Handbook of Endocrine Surgery 2012*. New Jersey: World Scientific, 2012, pp. 279–286.

2. Sutton MG, Sheps SG, Lie JT. Prevalence of clinically unsuspected pheochromocytoma. Review of a 50-year autopsy series. *Mayo Clinic Proceedings*, 1981;**56**(6):354–360. www.ncbi. nlm.nih.gov/pubmed/6453259

3. Pacak K. Approach to the patient – preoperative management of the pheochromocytoma patient. *Journal of Clinical Endocrinology and Metabolism*, 2007;**92**(11):4069–4079. doi:10.1210/Jc.2007-1720

4. James MFM. Use of magnesium-sulfate in the anaesthetic management of pheochromocytoma – a review of 17 anaesthetics. *British Journal of Anaesthesia*, 1989;**62**(6):616–623. doi:10.1093/Bja/62.6.616

53

Carcinoid syndrome

Alexandra Evans

The Alfred Hospital, Australia

Definitions

- *Neuroendocrine tumour (NETs)*: tumour arising from hormone-producing neuroendocrine cells, in the distribution of the embryological fore-, mid- and hindgut. NETs are usually described according to their organ of origin, their secretory status or the presence of symptoms/clinical syndrome.
- *Serotonin (5-HT) secreting NETs*: most commonly found in the gastrointestinal tract (particularly the midgut) and bronchi. Other secretory NETs of gut embryology include insulinoma, glucagonoma, gastrinoma, somatostatinoma, VIPoma and pancreatic polypeptidoma.
- *Carcinoid syndrome*: a constellation of symptoms and signs produced by the release of mediators from a well-differentiated serotonin-secreting NET, directly into the systemic circulation (bypassing hepatic first-pass metabolism). Misdiagnosis and delayed diagnosis are common.
- *Carcinoid crisis*: a life-threatening expression of the syndrome due to the release of large quantities of mediator into the systemic circulation. Triggers include a catecholamine surge (stress, exercise, surgery and anaesthesia), certain foods and alcohol, or direct physical stimulation of the tumour.

Mediators of carcinoid syndrome

The mediators of carcinoid syndrome are listed in Box 53.1.

Serotonin: production, metabolism and action

Serotonin is produced from dietary tryptophan (an essential amino acid). It is stored within secretory granules containing chromogranin A (CgA) in the CNS, enterochromaffin cells and platelets. Serotonin does not cross the blood–brain barrier. Its site of action is the 5-hydroxytryptamine (5HT) receptor. It undergoes hepatic metabolism to 5-hydroxyindoleacetic acid (5HIAA), via monoamine oxidase and aldehyde dehydrogenase. 5HIAA is excreted in the urine.

Perioperative Medicine for the Junior Clinician, First Edition. Edited by Joel Symons, Paul Myles, Rishi Mehra and Christine Ball.
© 2015 John Wiley & Sons, Ltd. Published 2015 by John Wiley & Sons, Ltd.
Companion website: www.wiley.com/go/perioperativemed

TABLE 53.1 **Presentation of carcinoid syndrome**

System		Symptoms
Cardiovascular system	Inotrope and chronotrope	Palpitations
	Vasoconstriction and	Flushing
	vasodilation	Hypotension
		Hypertension
	Valvular heart disease	RVF, LVF
Gastrointestinal tract	Increased motility	Abdominal pain
	Increased secretion water/	Diarrhoea
	electrolytes	
Respiratory	Bronchoconstriction	Wheeze

LVF, left ventricular failure; RVF, right ventricular failure.

Presentation

IF YOU DON'T SUSPECT IT, YOU CAN'T DETECT IT

Patients with a serotonin-secreting NET may present in a variety of ways.
- Carcinoid syndrome (Table 53.1)
- Mass effect or pain from a primary within the GI tract, lung or other rare locations, e.g. gonadal, or secondaries within liver, bone
- Fibroblastic reaction due to retroperitoneal extension/fibrosis, mesenteric ischaemia or carcinoid heart disease (see below)
- Tryptophan depletion resulting in hypoproteinaemia and niacin deficiency
- Incidental finding, particularly with gastric and rectal tumours

Carcinoid heart disease [1]

Up to 20% of patients with carcinoid syndrome will have cardiac involvement.

Fibrosis within the endocardium and valvular tissue creates reduced compliance of the right ventricle and tricuspid and pulmonary regurgitation (predominates) and stenosis. Left-sided disease, usually mitral regurgitation, may also occur if the patient has a patent foramen ovale, endobronchial tumour or very high tumour activity. Plaques may also occur within the vena cava, pulmonary arteries and coronary sinus.

Medical management has a 3-year 30% survival.

Cognitive impairment [2]

Cognitive impairment is more common in cancer patients with carcinoid syndrome compared with those without the syndrome.

Diversion of tryptophan to serotonin production peripherally may result in niacin deficiency and depletion of CNS serotonin. Niacin deficiency may rarely present with pellagra (4Ds: diarrhoea, dementia, dermatitis and death). Correction of niacin deficiency is with niacin or nicotinamide, not tryptophan, which may cause the life-threatening eosinophilic myalgia syndrome.

Mandatory perioperative investigations [3,4]

- Plasma CgA – usually elevated in the presence of a NET
- 24 hr urinary 5HIAA – 30 mg/day is diagnostic for a serotonin-secreting NET
- Full blood examination (FBE) – detection of anaemia
- Urea and electrolytes (U&E) – electrolyte disturbances secondary to diarrhoea, glucose homeostasis (secondary to disease or treatment)
- Live function tests (LFTs) – protein depletion
- Transthoracic echocardiography and N-terminal pro-brain natriuretic peptide (a marker of heart failure) – if these are abnormal consider further cardiac assessment with transoesophageal echocardiography or cardiac MRI.

Management of the patient with carcinoid syndrome [3,4]

A multidisciplinary team approach in a tertiary referral centre, with experience managing these patients, is a fundamental requirement. The team may encompass the services of surgeon, anaesthetist, cardiologist, oncologist, endocrinologist and interventional radiologist, with the support of intensive care and cardiothoracic services.

Medical management

The aims of medical management include symptom control with somatostatin analogue therapy, correction of dehydration and electrolyte imbalances, stabilisation of valvular heart disease and dietary assessment and correction of nutritional deficiencies.

Somatostatin analogue therapy

Somatostatin is an inhibitory regulatory peptide with a short duration of action. It inhibits the endocrine and exocrine secretion of most hormones within the GI tract, decreases blood flow, GI tract motility and gallbladder contractility, and inhibits the action of circulating peptides.

Somatostatin analogues are the mainstay of therapy for symptom control in serotonin-secreting NETs. They have a high affinity for two of the five receptor subtypes (sst2 and sst5) at which somatostatin exerts its action. However, 20% of 'carcinoids' do not express sst2 and may not respond well to treatment with somatostatin analogues. Receptor expression is identified with somatostatin receptor scintigraphy (SSRS or octreoscan). Somatostatin analogues also exhibit an antiproliferative effect.

Three somatostatin analogues are currently in clinical use (Table 53.2).

The approach to initiating somatostatin analogue therapy depends on the urgency of the surgery and the availability and cost of the formulations. Patients are initially stabilised on short-acting octreotide. Long-acting therapy is commenced after two weeks of octreotide SC therapy. Octreotide SC is then discontinued two weeks later, at the peak effect of the long-acting preparation. This is the ideal timing for surgery.

Side effects of somatostatin analogues are summarised in Table 53.3.

Surgical management

Staging
Specific imaging tests will be required to determine the site and extent of the primary tumour and assess for the presence of secondaries. Specialised imaging may involve gallium PET/CT and SSRS.

Surgery
Surgery may be required to resect or debulk primary or secondary NETs or to relieve a bowel obstruction.

Cardiac surgery may be indicated to improve functional state if there is severe symptomatic valve dysfunction, stable carcinoid tumour and syndrome, and an otherwise reasonable life expectancy [1].

Interventional radiology
Non-operative techniques may involve radiofrequency ablation (RFA), cryoablation or transarterial chemoembolisation (TACE).

TABLE 53.2 Somatostatin analogues currently in clinical use

Preparation	Onset	Route	Dosing
Octreotide	Rapid	IV SC	0.5–2 mcg/kg/hr 100–600 b.d.–q.i.d.
Octreotide acetate Sandostatin LAR	Slow release	IM	20–60 mg monthly
Lanreotide	Slow release	Deep SC	60–120 mg monthly

IM, intramuscular; IV, intravenous; SC, subcutaneous.

TABLE 53.3 Side effects of somtatostatin analogues

System	Effect
Inhibition of pancreatic secretions	Hyper- and hypoglycaemia Diarrhoea and abdominal pain
Thyroid function	Hypothyroidism
Gallbladder	Cholelithiasis
Cardiovascular system	Bradydysrhythmias with large/rapid dosing

Perioperative management [5]

> The aim of perioperative management is to prevent mediator release and hence a carcinoid crisis
>
> As the occurrence, severity and presentation of carcinoid crisis are unpredictable, no given regime is totally reliable

Continue standard octreotide therapy. Commence octreotide infusion 1–2 hr preoperatively at 0.5–2 mcg/kg/hr and continue for 48 hr postoperatively.

Premedicate with:

- H1 blocker – promethazine 12.5 mg IV
- H2-blocker – ranitidine 50 mg IV
- 5HT3 blocker – ondansetron
- inhibit bradykinin release – dexamethasone
- anxiolytic – benzodiazepine.

Avoid the use of tramadol, selective serotonin reuptake inhibitors (SSRIs), MAOIs and ketamine.

Postoperative patients should be monitored in the HDU or ICU.

Carcinoid crisis management

> - Call for help.
> - Cease precipitating event, if known.
> - Administer octreotide bolus 0.5–2 mcg/kg IV.
> - Use standard therapies for bronchospasm and haemodynamic instability if poor response to octreotide.

References

1. Raja SG, Bhattacharyya S, Davar J, Dreyfus GD. Surgery for carcinoid heart disease: current outcomes, concerns and controversies. *Future Cardiology*, 2010;**6**(5):647–655. doi:10.2217/fca.10.87

2. Pasieka JL, Longman RS, Chambers AJ, Rorstad O, Rach-Longman K, Dixon E. Cognitive impairment associated with carcinoid syndrome. *Annals of Surgery*, 2014;**259**(2):355–359. doi:10.1097/SLA.0b013e318288ff6d

3. Modlin IM, Moss SF, Oberg K, et al. Gastrointestinal neuroendocrine (carcinoid) tumours: current diagnosis and management. *Medical Journal of Australia*, 2010;**193**(1):46–52. www.ncbi.nlm.nih.gov/pubmed/20618115

4. Clinical Oncology Society of Australia (COSA). Clinical Oncology Society of Australia (COSA) NETs Guidelines: guidelines for the diagnosis and management of gastroenteropancreatic neuroendocrine tumours (GEP NETs). http://wiki.cancer.org.au/australia/COSA:NETs_guidelines/Histopathology

5. Mancuso K, Kaye AD, Boudreaux JP, et al. Carcinoid syndrome and perioperative anesthetic considerations. *Journal of Clinical Anesthesia*, 2011;**23**(4):329–341. doi:10.1016/j.jclinane.2010.12.009

53

54 Intracranial surgery

Hilary Madder

Oxford University Hospitals NHS Trust, United Kingdom

This chapter focuses on the perioperative management of elective intracranial surgery where there is scope for preoperative optimisation. However, the principles involved apply equally to emergency surgery. Understanding intracranial pathology and cerebral physiology is essential to the perioperative management of neurosurgical patients.

Preoperative assessment

Comprehensive preoperative assessment guides intraoperative and postoperative management. In addition to routine assessment and optimisation of co-morbidities, there are specific requirements for intracranial surgery, and communication with the neurosurgeon is essential.

Understand the neurosurgical lesion

The pathology and the degree of urgency of the intracranial pathology should be determined. This will include a careful history, physical examination and review of all imaging. The pathology of the lesion will determine specific issues to be addressed (Table 54.1). For all lesions, determine:

- site and size
- focal neurological deficit
- systemic effects
- history of seizures
- perioperative anticonvulsant requirement
- Glasgow Coma Score (GCS) (refer to Chapter 59 Traumatic brain injury)
- pupil size and reactivity
- adequacy of cough and swallow functions
- vital signs to determine blood pressure targets for intraoperative and postoperative management
- blood glucose control, particularly for patients receiving dexamethasone.

For space-occupying lesions, estimate where the patient sits on the intracranial pressure–volume curve (Figure 54.1). Signs and symptoms of raised intracranial pressure (ICP) include headache, nausea, vomiting and confusion [1].

Perioperative Medicine for the Junior Clinician, First Edition. Edited by Joel Symons, Paul Myles, Rishi Mehra and Christine Ball.
© 2015 John Wiley & Sons, Ltd. Published 2015 by John Wiley & Sons, Ltd.
Companion website: www.wiley.com/go/perioperativemed

TABLE 54.1 Factors specific to pathology of lesion

Neurosurgical lesion	Specific issues
Meningioma	Potential for blood loss? • Revision procedure • Proximity to venous sinuses • Arterial supply • Need for preoperative embolisation Raised intracranial pressure? Superficial or deep? • Deep lesion means prolonged surgery with brain retraction Potential for seizures?
Arteriovenous malformation	Need for preoperative embolisation? Raised intracranial pressure? Superficial or deep? Seizures? Large enough to cause postresection changes in cerebral blood flow? Define blood pressure targets
Cerebral aneurysm	Ruptured or unruptured? Conformation • Simple or complex, giant Local effects? Potential for delayed cerebral ischaemia? Potential for hydrocephalus? Presence of other unruptured aneurysms? Define blood pressure targets
Pituitary surgery	Approach • Transnasal or craniotomy? Pituitary function? Potential difficult intubation? • Acromegaly Endocrine review essential
Intracerebral haematoma	Raised intracranial pressure? Underlying vascular anomaly? • Computed tomography angiography Potential for hydrocephalus? Poorly treated hypertension? Systemic disturbance? • Coronary artery disease • Renal dysfunction
Cerebral metastasis	Local effects of primary • Mediastinal involvement? Systemic effects of primary? Reason for surgery • To obtain tissue biopsy • To treat effects cerebral metastasis
Intracerebral tumour	Raised intracranial pressure? Superficial or deep? Seizures? Response to dexamethasone? Gastric ulcer prophylaxis?

54

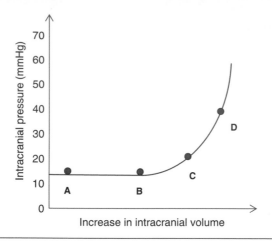

Point A. Normal ICP with buffering reserve for an increase in intracranial volume. Spatial compensation occurs within venous capacitance and CSF spaces.

Point B. Normal ICP but compensatory mechanisms have been exhausted and there is no reserve for further increase in intracranial volume.

Point C. ICP is now elevated. Intracranial elastance is the tangent to the curve (dP/dV). As the curve becomes steeper, elastance increases and there is a greater increase in ICP for a given increase in volume.

Point D. ICP is markedly elevated. A minimal increase in volume will cause further marked increase in ICP.

FIGURE 54.1 **Intracranial pressure–volume curve.**

Intraoperative positioning

The site of lesion determines the neurosurgical approach and patient positioning. Patients with cardiac or respiratory disorders tolerate prone and sitting positions poorly so these must be optimised prior to surgery or an alternative approach discussed with the neurosurgeon.

Potential for blood loss

This is determined by the pathology, site and size of the lesion. Revision procedures are associated with increased bleeding. Preoperative embolisation may reduce bleeding potential. Antiplatelet agents and anticoagulants should be stopped before surgery. Timing of cessation and postoperative reintroduction requires liaison with haematology, cardiology and the neurosurgeon.

Preoperative investigations

These are determined by the nature of the lesion and co-morbidities. Routine investigations include:

• baseline haemoglobin
• coagulation profile, including platelet count
• electrolytes, urea, creatinine and glucose
• blood group and antibody screen.

Electrocardiogram changes are often associated with neurosurgical lesions and need to be distinguished from primary cardiac pathology.

Need for postoperative critical care

Prolonged surgery requires planned allocation of a critical care bed. Patients with reduced level of consciousness, or altered cough or swallow function risk pulmonary aspiration and also require postoperative critical care.

Premedication

Patients with intracranial lesions, particularly in the posterior fossa, are sensitive to sedative drugs so the mainstay of premedication is explanation and reassurance.

Intraoperative management

Neuroanaesthesia

The principles of neuroanaesthesia focus on maintenance of the cerebral oxygen demand–supply balance and provision of optimal operating conditions.

Reduction of cerebral metabolic rate (CMR) is achieved through anaesthesia, seizure prophylaxis and temperature control. Adequate oxygenation and prevention of hypoglycaemia support metabolic supply. Maintenance of cerebral blood flow is critical. The anaesthetist should avoid hyperventilation and aim for normocapnia. Cerebral autoregulation is altered by anaesthesia so predefined BP targets are important.

Good neurosurgical conditions are provided by minimising cerebral volume. Prevention of hypercapnia and optimisation of cerebral venous drainage are the mainstay. Further measures include mannitol, dexamethasone and cerebrospinal fluid (CSF) drainage.

Intraoperative adverse events include major haemorrhage, seizures, cerebral swelling and venous air embolism (VAE). Prevention and early detection are central to the management of these.

Intraoperative monitoring

Intraoperative monitoring is determined by patient co-morbidities as well as the procedure. Routine monitoring includes:

- intra-arterial BP
- intermittent ABG for CO_2, glucose, Hb and electrolyte measurements
- temperature to maintain normothermia
- hourly urine output as a guide to intravascular volume.

Central venous pressure measurement is not routine unless major blood loss, lengthy procedure or haemodynamic instability is anticipated. CVP may be useful where administration of mannitol means urine output is a poor guide to intravascular volume. Electroencephalogram (EEG) and evoked potentials may be a guide to cerebral metabolism and functional integrity but are not routine. Transoesophageal echocardiography is sometimes used in sitting position surgery to assist detection of VAE. Electromyography (EMG) is routine in cerebellopontine angle tumour resection to identify the anatomy of cranial nerves and preserve their integrity during dissection.

Patient positioning

Patient positioning is crucial. Head elevation 10–15° above the heart balances optimal venous drainage against risk of VAE. Sitting and prone positions require an experienced team for avoidance and early management of associated complications.

Anaesthetic agents

The choice of agents is less important than the principles which guide their use. Muscle relaxant at induction ensures tracheal intubation without cough. Cough with an open craniotomy is disastrous but deep anaesthesia without muscle relaxant means a generalised seizure may be seen and treated.

Fluid management

Fluid management is according to physiological requirements for normovolaemia. Blood and blood products should be used where indicated. Hypo-osmolar and dextrose-containing fluids should be avoided as they may exacerbate cerebral oedema.

Postoperative care

Emergence is a critical period where close observation of airway, ventilation and circulation is paramount. Patients should steadily return to their preoperative neurological state. Failure to emerge or deterioration post emergence should be addressed promptly with ABG to exclude systemic causes such as hypoxia or hypoglycaemia followed by CT brain. Postoperative seizure may be a cause of failure to emerge.

Postoperative complications include haematoma, cerebral oedema, seizures, pneumocephalus, hydrocephalus, CSF leak and infection.

For postoperative analgesia, opioids are generally required in combination with non-opioids such as paracetamol [2]. Careful titration of opioids avoids sedation and respiratory depression. Antiplatelet effects of NSAIDs should be considered. Tramadol has been associated with seizures and is generally avoided in intracranial surgery [3]. Persistent headache may indicate a postoperative complication.

Postcraniotomy hypertension must be watched for closely. Treat causative factors such as pain or nausea promptly (refer to Chapter 79 Postoperative nausea and vomiting). Marked hypertension should be controlled with pharmacological agents such as IV labetolol or hydralazine (refer to Chapter 32 Hypertension). Aggressive treatment risks deleterious reduction in cerebral blood flow.

Postoperative disturbance of sodium and water balance may occur secondary to diabetes insipidus (DI), cerebral salt wasting syndrome (CSWS) or SIADH [4]. Serum sodium and fluid balance should be monitored for at least 48 hours postoperatively. Both DI and CSWS are associated with intravascular volume depletion and require fluid replacement (refer to Chapter 76 Electrolyte abnormalities).

Cerebrospinal fluid drainage via external ventricular or lumbar drain may be implemented to prevent CSF leak or hydrocephalus (Figure 54.2; Video 54.1). This requires an understanding of management instructions such as set height or target hourly drainage.

Postoperative review is targeted towards early detection of complications. Ensure that there are clear plans for analgesia, antiemetics, fluid management and anticonvulsant and steroid regimens.

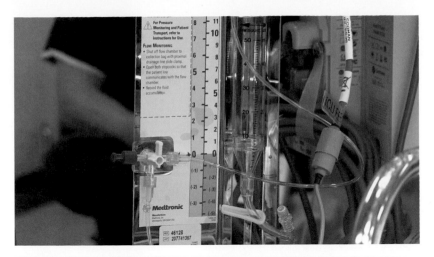

FIGURE 54.2 **External ventricular drain.** An external ventricular drain is a method of removing CSF to relieve intracranial pressure, or alternatively to allow serial sampling of CSF for microbiology.

www.wiley.com/go/perioperativemed

VIDEO 54.1 **Intracranial pressure monitoring.** There are a number of methods of measuring intracranial pressure, including placement of an external ventricular drain (EVD) or use of a fibreoptic pressure monitor.

References

1. Dunn LT. Raised intracranial pressure. *Journal of Neurology, Neurosurgery and Psychiatry*, 2002;**73**(Suppl 1):i23–27. doi:10.1136/jnnp.73.suppl_1.i23

2. Talke PO, Gelb AW. Postcraniotomy pain remains a real headache! *European Journal of Anaesthesiology*, 2005;**22**(5):325–327. doi:10.1017/s0265021505000542

3. Kahn LH, Alderfer RJ, Graham DJ. Seizures reported with tramadol. *JAMA*, 1997;**278**(20):1661. doi:10.1001/jama.278.20.1661b

4. Bradshaw K, Smith, M. Disorders of sodium balance after brain injury. *Continuing Education in Anaesthesia, Critical Care and Pain*, 2008;**8**(4):129–133. doi:10.1093/bjaceaccp/mkn019

Carotid surgery

Matthew Claydon

The Alfred Hospital, Australia

Cerebrovascular accident (CVA) is the second most common cause of death worldwide [1] and approximately 15% is due to atherosclerotic disease of the extracranial carotid arteries [2]. This chapter focuses on atherosclerotic stenosis of the carotid artery – the most common indication for carotid surgery.

Pathology

The blood supply of the brain is through four main vessels (two internal carotid arteries and two vertebral arteries) variably collateralised through the circle of Willis.

Atherosclerosis has numerous causative influences including hypertension, hyperlipidaemia, smoking and diabetes. Atherosclerotic plaques are complex, active lesions whose effects are usually mediated by emboli of platelet aggregates, thrombus and atherosclerotic material released into the cerebral circulation.

Clinical manifestations

These include transient ischaemic attack (TIA), CVA, amaurosis fugax and retinal artery occlusion causing monocular blindness. The carotid stenosis may also be asymptomatic and the first presentation may be a major CVA. For this reason, asymptomatic lesions may still warrant treatment. Crescendo TIA and stroke-in-evolution are emergency conditions. Several scoring systems now exist to assess the risk of a major recurrent event after initial symptomatic manifestations. Many recurrent events occur in the first six weeks [2,3].

There are a number of common concomitant conditions present in patients with atherosclerotic carotid disease which can impact on the perioperative care of the patient. These are listed in Table 55.1.

Investigations

Duplex ultrasound is the primary and usual initial investigation for atherosclerotic carotid stenosis. This may be the only investigation required prior to operative treatment, other than routine perioperative work-up. However, other investigations

Perioperative Medicine for the Junior Clinician, First Edition. Edited by Joel Symons, Paul Myles, Rishi Mehra and Christine Ball.
© 2015 John Wiley & Sons, Ltd. Published 2015 by John Wiley & Sons, Ltd.
Companion website: www.wiley.com/go/perioperativemed

TABLE 55.1 Specific investigations used in planning carotid procedures

Focus of investigation	Investigation/s utilised	Information required	Implications for treatment
Lesion anatomy	Duplex ultrasound CT angiogram MRI angiogram Digital subtraction catheter angiogram (DSA)	**Degree** of stenosis (% of normal lumen) **Level** of stenosis, i.e. proximal or distal ICA **Number** of stenoses, e.g. synchronous CCA stenoses Plaque morphology and calcification Evidence of recanalisation of previous occlusion Intracranial arterial aneurysms and anatomy Collateral supply status. (e.g. vertebral and contralateral carotid disease)	Usually treat >70% stenosis Distal ICA lesion – inaccessible during CEA Heavy calcification, soft atheroma or thrombus – relative C/I for CAS Aneurysm – neurosurgical review Contralateral carotid or vertebral artery disease – higher chance of shunt dependence
Cerebral ischaemia and anatomy	CT brain MRI brain	Previous CVAs Size recent CVA including evidence of cerebral oedema or haemorrhage Mass lesion	Exclude differential diagnosis (mass, haemorrhage, etc.) Sensitive ischaemic penumbra – ⇑ need shunt Large recent infarct – ⇑ risk periprocedural bleed Cerebral haemorrhage – C/I to procedure
Procedural planning considerations	Duplex US CT angiogram carotid arteries CT angiogram aortic arch	Level of carotid bifurcation, ? high bifurcation Aortic arch anatomy (CAS)	High carotid bifurcation – relative C/I to CEA under local anaesthetic Very high carotid bifurcation – may need ENT assistance for CEA, or CAS Heavily diseased arch/tortuous or difficult arch – relative C/I to CAS Extensive loose thrombus or atheroma in lesion – relative C/I to CAS

(continued)

TABLE 55.1 (Continued)

Focus of investigation	Investigation/s utilised	Information required	Implications for treatment
Vocal cord function	ENT – direct endoscopic visualisation	In selected patients with possible or previous vocal cord palsy, e.g. previous contralateral CEA	Contralateral cord palsy – risk of airway loss on extubation if new ipsilateral recurrent laryngeal nerve palsy
Specific pathology investigations – selected patients only	HITTS screen Thrombophilia screen Vasculitis screen	Thrombophilia/thrombocytosis Coagulopathy Heparin allergy Vasculitis	HITTS screen – heparin contraindicated Platelet disorders – need treatment. Affect antiplatelet med cation use Coagulopathy – needs Rx perioperatively Vasculitis – procedure may be C/I if active

CAS, carotid angioplasty and stenting; common carotid artery; CCA; CEA, carotid endarterectomy; C/I, contraindication; CT, computed tomography; CVA, cerebrovascular accident; ENT, ear, nose and throat; HITTS, heparin-induced thrombotic thrombocytopenia syndrome; ICA, internal carotid artery; MRI, magnetic resonance imaging; Rx, medical therapy; US, ultrasound.

may also be used, including investigations for cerebral ischaemia and contrast imaging of the extra- and intracranial circulation and great vessels. In selected patients, investigations for thrombophilia, platelet disorders, hyperhomocysteinaemia and hyperlipidaemia may be indicated. It is important to understand the aim of these investigations and their potential ramifications. These specific investigations and their implications for treatment are presented in Table 55.1.

Of course, all patients having carotid surgery need the routine minimum preoperative work-up.

Treatment

The management of carotid disease is broadly divided into risk factor modification, medical treatment and procedural treatment. The first two should be optimised in all patients whenever possible. Medical therapy usually includes an antiplatelet agent and may include antihypertensive therapy, anticoagulation and statin therapy [4].

The treatment of atherosclerotic carotid stenosis usually includes an antiplatelet agent (e.g. aspirin, asasantin, clopidogrel). Less frequently, anticoagulation, either alone or in combination with an antiplatelet agent, may be used when there are co-existing conditions requiring anticoagulation.

Many carotid lesions are managed without procedural intervention. In severe stenosis (i.e. >70%), a procedure to relieve the stenosis may be indicated.

For many years, the main treatment for carotid artery atherosclerotic stenosis has been carotid endarterectomy (CEA). More recently, carotid angioplasty and stenting (CAS) has been introduced and is applicable in selected cases [5]. This chapter will concentrate on carotid endarterectomy.

Carotid endarterectomy is an operative procedure performed under local or general anaesthetic. During the procedure, the intima and two-thirds of the medial layers of the carotid artery containing the atherosclerotic plaque are removed while the artery is clamped. There are several techniques for this procedure. When required, internal carotid blood flow is maintained with a diversionary shunt. The vessel is often closed with a patch.

Carotid artery stenting is a percutaneous procedure during which the lesion is accessed via a femoral artery, carefully crossed with a wire and then angioplastied

55

BOX 55.1 Common co-morbidities associated with CEA patients

- Hypertension
- Diabetes
- Hyperlipidaemia/hypercholesterolaemia
- Peripheral vascular disease
- Coronary artery disease
- Age >65
- Renal impairment
- Chronic obstructive pulmonary disease

and stented to return it to the normal diameter. Carotid artery stenting is done in the radiology suite under local anaesthetic and consciousness-altering medications should be avoided preoperatively.

Multiple factors influence the choice between CEA and CAS [5].

Preoperative management

In the emergency setting, the patient would usually be on an antiplatelet agent, anticoagulation or both. The absence of one of these agents should be brought to the attention of the surgeon.

In other patients there is an opportunity to optimise their medical state. Alterations of the antihypertensive medication should be measured, with care taken to avoid precipitous drops in the blood pressure, and undertaken in combination with the patient's usual physician. Smoking cessation and dietary change should be encouraged where applicable.

The patient would usually be on an antiplatelet agent unless anticoagulated [4]. If the patient is anticoagulated, this should be 'crossed over' to a shorter acting agent such as enoxaparin or IV heparin perioperatively which is ceased shortly before the procedure. It is important that the antiplatelet agent should *not* be stopped before the procedure as this increases the risk of perioperative stroke. The absence of one of these agents should be brought to the attention of the surgeon.

A routine work-up for a carotid procedure is outlined in Box 55.2.

Patients with carotid disease usually have multiple co-morbidities. Co-existing severe conditions should be looked for as they may represent a contraindication to the carotid procedure (Box 55.3); the presence of these 'red flags' should be discussed with the treating surgeon and anaesthetist.

BOX 55.2 Perioperative work-up and management

- Pathology: FBE, U&E, coagulation profile, group and hold
- ± CXR ± ECG as indicated or per local protocol
- Ensure imaging available: Duplex, ± CTA, ± DSA, CT/MRI brain if performed
- For *carotid endarterectomy*, continue antiplatelet agent unless otherwise instructed. Check with the surgeon if not prescribed
- For *carotid stenting,* patient should be on clopidogrel before the procedure. Check with the surgeon if not prescribed
- Oral anticoagulation changed to short-acting agent unless otherwise instructed
- ± Vocal cord examination if cord palsy suspected, or if previous contralateral major neck/carotid surgery

CT, computed tomography; CTA, CT angiogram; CXR, chest X-ray; DSA, digital subtraction angiography; ECG, electrocardiogram; FBE, full blood examination; MRI, magnetic resonance imaging; U&E, urea and electrolytes.

BOX 55.3 'Red flags' – conditions which may warrant deferring carotid surgery

Newly diagnosed life-threatening conditions

- Malignancy
- Unstable or severe CAD
- Severe lung disease/respiratory failure
- Dense CVA
- Significant untreated cardiac arrhythmia
- Generalised sepsis
- Other major organ failure

Anatomical/operative site conditions

- Infection or injury at the operative site – neck (CEA)/groin (CAS)

Changed physiological state

- Severe uncontrolled hypertension
- Significant symptomatic hypotension
- Significant dehydration
- Significant electrolyte disturbance

Changed pathology results

- Severe anaemia
- New severe renal impairment or renal failure
- New coagulopathy/coagulation disorder

Patient factors

- Patient refusal

CAD, coronary artery disease; CAS, carotid angioplasty and stenting; CEA, carotid endarterectomy; CVA, cerebrovascular accident.

Postoperative management

Postoperatively, the vital signs, operative site and neurological observations should be closely monitored. Both hypotension and hypertension need to be avoided and the surgeon will usually request tight blood pressure parameters. Hypotension may promote carotid thrombosis, while hypertension may promote bleeding and hyperperfusion syndrome. The pulse rate and cardiac rhythm should be monitored. The operative site/s should be carefully monitored for swelling or bleeding – the neck after open surgery or the groin after carotid stenting. After carotid stenting, intermittent lower limb vascular observations should be included.

Oxygen should be administered as required. Antiplatelet agents are usually continued in the postoperative period indefinitely. In selected cases, the anticoagulation may also be continued or recommended. Several doses of antibiotics may be prescribed in the postoperative period, especially if a prosthetic patch has been used. There are complications of particular concern after carotid procedures (Table 55.2).

TABLE 55.2 **Early postoperative complications and their management**

Complication	Implication/ramification	Management
High drain output post CEA • e.g. >50 mL/hr, or >150 mL total in recovery with ongoing drainage	Potential major bleeding, which could progress to neck haematoma	Notify surgeon, anaesthetist and theatre about potential re-exploration Consider cessation of anticoagulation (e.g. heparin) or antiplatelet infusion (e.g. dextran) – discuss with surgeon Fast patient Ensure adequate IV access, group and hold, coagulation profile (or ACT), FBE
Neck haematoma/ swelling post CEA	Potential major vessel bleeding Potential loss of airway	Notify surgeon, anaesthetist and theatre Fast patient and transfer to theatre Ensure adequate IV access, group and hold, coagulation profile or ACT, FBE If imminent/actual airway loss and senior team unavailable – emergency removal of sutures to release haematoma with sterile dressing coverage
Acute neurological event/ deterioration <24 hours postoperatively	Possible embolic CVA Possible carotid artery thrombosis Possible exacerbation ischaemic penumbra of previous CVA	Notify surgeon, anaesthetist and theatre – possible need for re-exploration Fast patient Ensure adequate IV access and group and hold, coagulation profile, FBE Urgent CT brain and duplex/CTA *unless* immediate re-exploration chosen by surgeon – immediate restoration of flow may reverse the deficit
Suspected cardiac ischaemia	Possible myocardial infarction	Oxygen, analgesia, ensure adequate IV access ECG, cardiac enzymes, FBE, coagulation profile Notify anaesthetist and surgeon Urgent medical/cardiology review Refer to Chapter 85 Postoperative chest pain
Hyperperfusion syndrome. Unilateral headache ± seizure activity ± cerebral haemorrhage (2–3% cases)	Potential for cerebral haemorrhage (<1%) More often after procedure for very tight stenosis ~2–7 days post carotid procedure Uncontrolled hypertension – ↑ risk	MRI brain or CT brain to exclude major haemorrhage Neurology/neurosurgery urgent review if major cerebral haemorrhage Neurology review if seizure activity MRI may show oedema/microhaemorrhage – readmit for seizure precautions and neurology review Hypertension management – medical review Consider temporary cessation of antiplatelet agent/anticoagulation if confirmed hyperperfusion syndrome – discuss with surgeon

Sinus bradycardia and cardiovascular instability	Changed vessel wall properties stimulate the carotid sinus	Exclude other causes IV access, FBE, U&E Usually settles in 24 hours May need increased monitoring (e.g. HDU) and rhythmogenic and inotropic support
Cranial nerve palsy post CEA	Can be mistaken for CVA – greater auricular, marginal mandibular, glossopharyngeal, vagus, accessory, hypoglossal, recurrent laryngeal, superior laryngeal nerves	Commonly transient due to traction injury Most not immediately dangerous but rather inconvenient and source of anxiety Bilateral recurrent laryngeal nerve palsy can cause vocal cord palsy and threatened airway – anaesthetic and ENT review Glossopharyngeal nerve – loss of pharyngeal sensation and ability to protect the airway – fast, ENT review. If permanent, may need tracheostomy
Groin bleeding/retroperitoneal haematoma(post CAS)	Potential for massive blood loss – retroperitoneum Possible local complications – nerve, skin, venous compression	Lie flat, digital pressure over the arterial puncture (just proximal to the skin puncture site) Oxygen Fast patient Ensure adequate IV access, group and hold, coagulation profile, FBE Notify surgeon If severe haemodynamic instability – immediate transfer to theatre If possible retroperitoneal bleed without severe instability – non-contrast ± contrast CT if available
Acute limb ischaemia (post CAS)	Potential irreversible ischaemic damage due to femoral vessel thromboembolism	Notify surgeon Urgent duplex arteries +/– ankle pressure study to confirm diagnosis, level and severity IV access, group and hold, FBE, coagulation profile Fasting – may require thrombectomy, arterial reconstruction, fasciotomy

ACT, activated clotting time; CAS, carotid angioplasty and stenting; CEA, carotid endarterectomy; CT, computed tomography; CTA, CT angiogram; CVA, cerebrovascular accident; ECG, electrocardiogram; ENT, ear, nose and throat; FBE, full blood examination; HDU, high-dependency unit; IV, intravenous; MRI, magnetic resonance imaging; U&E, urea and electrolytes.

References

1. World Health Organization. WHO Fact Sheet – The Top 10 Causes of Death. www.who.int/mediacentre/factsheets/fs310/en/index3.html

2. Rothwell PM. Prediction and prevention of stroke in patients with symptomatic carotid stenosis: the high-risk period and the high-risk patient. *European Journal of Vascular and Endovascular Surgery*, 2008;**35**(3):255–263. doi:10.1016/j.ejvs.2007.11.006

3. Johnston SC, Rothwell PM, Nguyen-Huynh MN, et al. Validation and refinement of scores to predict very early stroke risk after transient ischaemic attack. *Lancet*, 2007;**369**(9558): 283–292. doi:10.1016/S0140-6736(07)60150-0

4. Constantinou J, Jayia P, Hamilton G. Best evidence for medical therapy for carotid artery stenosis. *Journal of Vascular Surgery*, 2013;**58**(4):1129–1139. doi:10.1016/j.jvs.2013.06.085

5. Carotid Stenting Guidelines Committee. Guidelines for patient selection and performance of carotid artery stenting. *Internal Medicine Journal*, 2011;**41**:344–347. doi:10.1111/j.1445-5994.2011.02445.x

Epilepsy

Richard Stark

The Alfred Hospital and Monash University, Australia

Patients with epilepsy may run an increased risk of seizures in the perioperative period for a number of reasons [1].

- Patients already well controlled on anticonvulsants may not be able to take oral medication during this time.
- There may be interactions between the anticonvulsants and other drugs which are required.
- There may be metabolic abnormalities arising in relation to surgery that increase the risk of seizures.
- Some anaesthetic drugs may have a proconvulsant effect.
- Certain neurosurgical procedures carry an intrinsic risk of seizures.

Patients with well-controlled epilepsy (refer to Chapter 10 Perioperative medication management)

> The degree of disruption to routine dosing of anticonvulsants should be minimised. This means that, unless there is a clear cut reason not to, patients should take their routine medications on the morning of surgery. Medication should be resumed as soon as possible postoperatively.

Some medications with long half-lives (such as phenytoin) will maintain satisfactory levels if the whole daily requirement is given as a single dose. If multiple doses are likely to be missed, then parenteral supplementation may be required. Phenytoin, valproate and levetiracetam are all available in IV form with IV dosing identical to oral formulations. If a patient's usual medication is not available in parenteral form, a decision must be made about drug substitution. This will depend on previous responses to various agents, the precise type of epilepsy (primary generalised versus secondary) and other factors, so input from the patient's usual treating neurologist will be vital.

There are particular problems with IV phenytoin. The need to inject slowly (<50 mg/min in adults) is well known. Interactions with other drugs causing precipitation mean

Perioperative Medicine for the Junior Clinician, First Edition. Edited by Joel Symons, Paul Myles, Rishi Mehra and Christine Ball.
© 2015 John Wiley & Sons, Ltd. Published 2015 by John Wiley & Sons, Ltd.
Companion website: www.wiley.com/go/perioperativemed

that phenytoin should preferably not be given in the same line as other agents, or, if drugs are to be mixed, compatibility should explicitly be confirmed. Extravasation may cause an intense reaction ('purple glove' phenomenon) [2], so particular care must be taken to avoid this. The related drug fosphenytoin is less irritant but is more expensive and not universally available.

Drug interactions

Because of their narrow therapeutic index and ability to interfere with a range of drug-metabolising enzymes, anticonvulsants are commonly implicated in important drug interactions. Failure to recognise these interactions and to take appropriate corrective measures can have life-threatening clinical consequences [3].

Many of the older anticonvulsants such as phenytoin, carbamazepine, phenobarb and primidone induce the hepatic cytochrome P450 system. This is likely to result in lowering of serum levels of other drugs metabolised by these enzymes including various antibiotics, beta-blockers, calcium channel blockers and warfarin. Oxcarbazepine and topiramate have similar but less dramatic effects. Valproate, on the other hand, inhibits hepatic microsomal enzyme systems and may reduce clearance and thus increase the serum levels of various drugs, including lamotrigine. As a rule of thumb, the dose of lamotrigine should be half the usual dose in patients on valproate. Gabapentin, lamotrigine and levetiracetam are not considered to produce significant hepatic enzyme induction. Some macrolide antibiotics, such as erythromycin, inhibit CYP3A4, which is involved in carbamazepine metabolism and this may result in carbamazepine toxicity. On the other hand, carbapenem antibiotics can reduce serum valproate levels.

Electrolyte disturbances

Many electrolyte disturbances have been associated with seizures, especially hypocalcaemia and hypernatraemia. Some anticonvulsants may affect electrolyte levels; carbamazepine and especially the related oxcarbazepine are notorious for causing hyponatraemia.

Proconvulsant effects of anaesthetic agents

In a person with epilepsy, the choice of anaesthetic agent may be influenced by the risk of provoking seizures.

Inhalational agents

There have been a number of case reports of seizure activity apparently provoked by sevoflurane (especially in children) and enflurane. Nitrous oxide may provoke seizures in animal models but there is no convincing evidence of a substantial risk in humans.

Opioids

In general, opioids appear to have proconvulsant properties [4]. Tramadol and pethidine may be the most potent in this respect but fentanyl, alfentanil, sufentanil and morphine have been reported to be the presumed cause of generalised seizures. Epilepsy surgery allows the effect of anaesthetic agents on susceptible cortex to be recorded directly; remifentanil and alfentanil both provoke spike activity in epileptogenic areas [5].

Intravenous hypnotic agents

In general, these are predominantly anticonvulsant in effect. There have been occasional reports of myoclonus or other excitatory activity on induction of anaesthesia with propofol, but this is not believed to be epileptogenic. Benzodiazepines are well recognised to be anticonvulsant in effect.

Local anaesthetic agents

Inadvertent intravascular injection of local anaesthesia may provoke seizures. The amount circulating systemically following local anaesthetic use should usually not be sufficient to cause concern.

Neuromuscular blocking agents

These are not known to be proconvulsant.

Anticholinergics

Atropine and scopolamine can produce a central anticholinergic syndrome with seizures.

References

1. Perks A, Cheema S, Mohanraj R. Anaesthesia and epilepsy. *British Journal of Anaesthesia*, 2012;**108**(4):562–571. doi:10.1093/bja/aes027

2. O'Brien TJ, Cascino GD, So EL, Hanna DR. Incidence and clinical consequence of the purple glove syndrome in patients receiving intravenous phenytoin. *Neurology*, 1998;**51**(4): 1034–1039. www.ncbi.nlm.nih.gov/pubmed/9781525

3. Patsalos PN, Perucca E. Clinically important drug interactions in epilepsy: interactions between antiepileptic drugs and other drugs. *Lancet Neurology*, 2003;**2**(8):473–481. doi:10.1016/s1474-4422(03)00409-5

4. Saboory E, Derchansky M, Ismaili M, et al. Mechanisms of morphine enhancement of spontaneous seizure activity. *Anesthesia and Analgesia*, 2007;**105**(6):1729–1735. doi: 10.1213/01.ane.0000287675.15225.0b

5. Gronlykke L, Knudsen ML, Hogenhaven H, Moltke FB, Madsen FF, Kjaer TW. Remifentanil-induced spike activity as a diagnostic tool in epilepsy surgery. *Acta Neurologica Scandinavica*, 2008;**117**(2):90–93. doi:10.1111/j.1600-0404.2007.00920.x

57 Neuromuscular disease

Erik Andersen and Andrew Kornberg

The Royal Children's Hospital, Australia

Neuromuscular diseases (NMDs) represent a broad range of disorders with many challenges in perioperative management. Malignant hyperthermia, rhabdomyolysis, respiratory failure, cardiovascular complications and medication sensitivity may be seen. This chapter will consider the implications of myopathies, diseases of the neuromuscular junction (NMJ), acquired/hereditary neuropathies, other prejunctional disorders and neurometabolic diseases in the perioperative context.

Classification

It is useful to consider NMDs by the site of involvement as a guide for consideration of perioperative issues. Disorders affecting structure or function proximal to the NMJ may cause weakness of respiratory muscles, dysregulation of the autonomic nervous system, cardiac dysfunction and denervation of muscles leading to hypersensitivity to medications due to upregulation of NMJ receptors.

Disorders of the NMJ may cause respiratory weakness, which can be exacerbated by factors accentuating neuromuscular blockade such as hypothermia, hypokalaemia, hypophosphataemia and many medications [1].

Myopathies may cause respiratory compromise and primary cardiac dysfunction.

Many patients with NMDs are at risk of life-threatening complications including malignant hyperthermia, rhabdomyolysis and severe hyperkalaemia with cardiac involvement [2].

The classification of NMD may be found in Table 57.1.

Preoperative assessment

Optimisation of preoperative care is the key to the successful management of patients with NMD. An accurate diagnosis is the vital first step. A thorough history, including questions asking about muscle cramping, weakness and fatigue, must be obtained and a careful examination should be performed, looking for signs of weakness, bulbar dysfunction, scoliosis and cardiac/ respiratory failure.

Perioperative Medicine for the Junior Clinician, First Edition. Edited by Joel Symons, Paul Myles, Rishi Mehra and Christine Ball.
© 2015 John Wiley & Sons, Ltd. Published 2015 by John Wiley & Sons, Ltd.
Companion website: www.wiley.com/go/perioperativemed

TABLE 57.1 Neuromuscular disease classifications

Peripheral nerve/ prejunctional	Hereditary	Charcot–Marie–Tooth	Acquired	Gullian–Barré syndrome
		Friedreich's ataxia		Chronic inflammatory demyelinating polyneuropathy
		Spinal muscular atrophy		
		Amyotrophic lateral sclerosis		
		Primary lateral sclerosis		
Neuromuscular junction	Hereditary	Congenital myasthenia gravis	Acquired	Myasthenia gravis
				Lambert–Eaton syndrome
Muscular	Hereditary	Dystrophinopathies	Acquired	Inflammatory myopathies
		Duchenne, Becker's, DMD-associated dilated cardiomyopathy		Critical care myopathy/ neuropathy
		Myotonias		
		Myotonic dystrophy, myotonia congenita		
		Periodic paralysis (PP)		
		Hypo/hyperkalaemic PP, paramyotonia congenita, Andersen–Tawil syndrome		
		Congenital myopathies		
		Central core/nemaline / multiminicore/ centronuclear disease, King Denborough syndrome		
		Metabolic myopathies		
		Glycogen/lipid storage diseases, mitochondrial diseases		

Simple baseline blood testing including an FBE (to screen for anaemia), renal function and U&E (to ensure normal preoperative glomerular filtration rate [GFR] and potassium homeostasis), and Vitamin D (important for wound healing and muscle strength) can all be useful tools in assessing perioperative safety.

Respiratory compromise is common in many NMDs, with initially a restrictive and then a mixed restrictive/obstructive pattern being seen. Pulmonary function testing is recommended to assess current function and physiological reserve. Other testing such as CXR, blood gases and overnight oximetry/polysomnography should be considered if indicated. Preoperative training in the use of non-invasive ventilation has been recommended for patients with a FVC <50% and is strongly suggested for NMD patients with a forced vital capacity (FVC) <30% [3]. For those with impaired cough, training with a mechanical insufflator-exsufflator device (MI-E) should be considered [4].

The degree of cardiac dysfunction may not be predictable, particularly for Duchenne muscular dystrophy-associated dilated cardiomyopathy, so an ECG should be routine, looking for cardiomyopathy (typically dilated but hypertrophic in Friedreich's ataxia) and arrhythmias. Echocardiography should also be done in most patients with primarily muscular diseases.

Optimisation of nutritional status is important as muscle strength, wound healing and respiratory function may be impacted. Periods of fasting should be treated with caution, particularly in patients with metabolic/mitochondrial NMDs, as many of these patients have increased energy requirements and lactate production in periods of physiological stress. Isotonic fluid containing dextrose should be considered during the fasting period [5].

Perioperative NMD medication needs consideration. Some patients, particularly those with dystrophinopathies, chronic inflammatory demyelinating polyneuropathy and myasthenia gravis, may be on long-term steroid treatment and 'stress steroid dosing' may be required (refer to Chapter 27 Steroid medication). Most treatments including steroid therapy and enzyme replacement therapy for metabolic myopathies should be continued throughout the surgical period, although anticholinesterase medications in myasthenia gravis may need to be omitted six hours prior to surgery due to potential interactions with neuromuscular blocking drugs.

Intraoperative period

Life-threatening complications of anaesthetic agents are one of the primary concerns in those with NMDs in the perioperative setting, so regional anaesthesia should be considered whenever practical.

Malignant hyperthermia is a rare inherited disorder where a hypermetabolic crisis is triggered by the use of halogenated agents or the depolarising neuromuscular blocking agent succinylcholine (refer to Chapter 91 Postoperative hyperthermia). This condition is linked to ryanodine receptor (RYR1) gene mutations, which are associated with an increasing spectrum of myopathic NMDs, including central core disease, centronuclear myopathy, multiminicore disease and King Denborough syndrome. A closely related entity of anaesthesia-related rhabdomyolysis caused by the same triggers has been associated with a broader range of NMDs (either trigger for muscular diseases and succinylcholine for any

NMDs). Life-threatening hyperkalaemia can occur with succinylcholine use in patients with muscle denervation as seen in prejunctional NMDs. Prevention of these complications is primarily through the use of appropriate 'trigger-free' anaesthesia.

Neuromuscular junction disorders do not lead to the above life-threatening complications, but as noted above, factors enhancing neuromuscular blockade should be avoided.

Mitochondrial function may be suppressed by thiopentone and propofol so a theoretical risk exists with their use in mitochondrial disorders. However, these agents have been used without problem in patients with these diseases so there is no compelling evidence for avoiding them [6].

Thermoregulation is important as both hyper- and hypothermia can have deleterious effects in NMDs. Myotonia, neuromuscular blockade, rhabdomyolysis, arrhythmias and bleeding may all be aggravated by poor thermoregulation.

Dysautonomic reactions occur with some NMDs, particularly those involving the peripheral nerves. These events can lead to hypotension and bradycardia and may require treatment with sympathomimetic drugs. Cautious use of these agents is recommended because of increased sensitivity.

BOX 57.1 Medications exacerbating neuromuscular blockade in NMJ disorders (myasthenia gravis)

Antibiotics	Aminoglycosides (gentamicin, tobramycin, etc.)
	Fluoroquinolones (ciprofloxacin, norfloxacin)
	Ketolides (telithromycin)
	Lesser extent macrolides, tetracyclines and penicillins
Quinolones	Quinine
	Quinidine
	Chloroquine

Theoretical/case reports of potential harm

Beta-blockers	Propranolol
	Atenolol
Calcium channel blockers	Verapamil
Anticonvulsants	Phenytoin
	Barbiturate
	Ethosuximide
	Carbamazepine
	Gabapentin

Postoperative period

Postoperative respiratory function remains an important consideration, and non-invasive ventilation and MI-E may be needed. Tracheal extubation and conversion to non-invasive ventilation in patients with FVC <30% should be strongly considered [3]. Adequate analgesia to prevent diaphragmatic and chest wall splinting and allow early mobilisation is key to management of patients with NMD as rapid deconditioning can occur [7].

Postoperative analgesia with opioids should be carefully titrated due to opioid sensitivity in patients with NMDs. Opioids should also be used cautiously in myotonic disorders as they may precipitate contractions.

There is a considerable list of medications that can exacerbate NMJ disorders that need to be considered (Box 57.1).

References

1. Hirsch NP. Neuromuscular junction in health and disease. *British Journal of Anaesthesia*, 2007;**99**(1):132–138. doi:10.1093/bja/aem144

2. Racca F, Mongini T, Wolfler A, et al. Recommendations for anesthesia and perioperative management of patients with neuromuscular disorders. *Minerva Anestesiologica*, 2013;**79**(4):419–433.

3. Birnkrant DJ, Panitch HB, Benditt JO, et al. American College of Chest Physicians consensus statement on the respiratory and related management of patients with Duchenne muscular dystrophy undergoing anesthesia or sedation. *Chest*, 2007;**132**(6):1977–1986. doi:10.1378/chest.07-0458

4. Marchant WA, Fox R. Postoperative use of a cough-assist device in avoiding prolonged intubation. *British Journal of Anaesthesia*, 2002;**89**(4):644–647. doi:10.1093/Bja/Aef227

5. Shipton EA, Prosser DO. Mitochondrial myopathies and anaesthesia. *European Journal of Anaesthesiology*, 2004;**21**(3):173–178. doi:10.1017/S0265021504003023

6. Driessen JJ. Neuromuscular and mitochondrial disorders: what is relevant to the anaesthesiologist? *Current Opinion in Anaesthesiology*, 2008;**21**(3):350–355. doi:10.1097/ACO.0b013e3282f82bcc

7. Bushby K, Finkel R, Birnkrant DJ, et al. Diagnosis and management of Duchenne muscular dystrophy, part 2: implementation of multidisciplinary care. *Lancet Neurology*, 2010;**9**(2):177–189. doi:10.1016/S1474-4422(09)70272-8

58 Trauma: pretheatre management

John Moloney

The Alfred Hospital and Monash University, Australia

The ideal management of a patient with major trauma requires a team of healthcare providers working in a co-ordinated manner, performing multiple tasks simultaneously. These tasks can be broadly categorised as diagnosis, resuscitation, co-ordination and communication.

Initial management

Advanced Trauma Life Support (ATLS) and Emergency Management of Severe Trauma (EMST) describe a systematic approach to the patient, using a **DR ABCE** approach. This is similar to that used in a cardiac arrest scenario, but with some additions.

In a prehospital environment, situational awareness of **D**angers, such as other vehicles or a nearby assailant, may seem obvious. Other hazards, such as fallen power lines and fuel spills, need to be managed. In the hospital, combative patients, weapons and blood-borne viruses are among the hazards.

Making efforts to obtain an appropriate escalated **R**esponse can be critical. The need for staff with appropriate skills must be appreciated early and the staff mobilised. This may include radiographers, blood bank scientists, surgeons and operating room staff.

Recent experience from warfare-related injuries has heightened an awareness of controlling exsanguinating haemorrhage. In soldiers with blast-related lower limb amputations, **C**irculation – control of haemorrhage – moved ahead of **A**irway in the management algorithm. Control can occur through the use of tourniquet or direct pressure on wounds or major arteries.

Perioperative Medicine for the Junior Clinician, First Edition. Edited by Joel Symons, Paul Myles, Rishi Mehra and Christine Ball.
© 2015 John Wiley & Sons, Ltd. Published 2015 by John Wiley & Sons, Ltd.
Companion website: www.wiley.com/go/perioperativemed

Classic teaching has **A**irway at the top of the treatment list. In the trauma scenario, cervical spine management is a vital component of airway management. Assessment and management occur simultaneously. Does the patient have a patent airway? Is there a foreign body, including vomitus and dentures, causing obstruction? Has the tongue fallen backwards in an unconscious patient, obstructing the airway? (Refer to Chapter 14 Airway assessment and planning.) Airway manoeuvres, such as chin lift and jaw thrust, implemented as needed, and oxygen can be applied. Head tilt is avoided due to concerns about the cervical spine. Airway adjuncts may be required, including a Guedel airway, laryngeal mask airway (LMA) or tracheal intubation. It should be recognised that this patient group is at risk of aspiration, and that facial and/or neck trauma may impede laryngoscopy.

Breathing (and ventilation) can be impaired due to injury along the neural or mechanical pathways. Head, spinal cord or phrenic nerve injury may occur. Likewise, pneumothorax (especially open or tension types), injuries to the diaphragm, chest wall (including flail chest) or lungs can prevent adequate ventilation (refer to Chapter 63 Chest injuries). Examination should look for equal and adequate chest expansion. Tracheal deviation may be a sign of tension pneumothorax. Surgical emphysema may indicate damage to the chest wall or lung. Inadequate ventilation should be managed when identified. This may include needle or tube thoracostomy, bag mask ventilation and/or tracheal intubation and positive pressure ventilation. A chest X-ray is a key initial adjunct to clinical assessment. Subsequently, arterial blood gases can guide further management.

Circulation, including haemorrhage control, is next in order of priority. Major trauma patients should have two large-bore IV cannulae placed. Heart rate and blood pressure can be used to assess volume status [1] (Table 58.1).

It is important to note that healthy younger patients may maintain blood pressure despite significant blood loss, and that heart rate response in some patients may be limited by medications (including beta-blockers) or underlying disease processes (e.g. pacemaker).

TABLE 58.1 **American College of Surgeons advanced trauma life support (ATLS) classification of blood loss based on initial patient presentation**

	Class 1	Class 2	Class 3	Class 4
Blood loss (mL)	Up to 750	750–1500	1500–2000	2000 or more
Blood loss (% blood volume)	Up to 15%	15–30%	30–40%	40% or more
Pulse rate	<100	>100	>120	140 or higher
Blood pressure	Normal	Normal	Decreased	Decreased
Capillary refill time	Normal	Increased	Increased	Increased
Urine output (mL/hr)	30 or more	20–30	5–15	Negligible
CNS-mental status	Slightly anxious	Anxious	Anxious – confused	Confused – lethargic

Source: American College of Surgeons Committee on Trauma [1]. Reproduced with permission from the American College of Surgeons.

Focused assessment with sonography in trauma (Video 58.1)

Focused assessment with sonography in trauma (FAST) can be used to assess blood volume, as well as examining for some sources of hypovolaemia. An examination of the heart, particularly a short axis view of the left ventricle, can assess cardiac preload (Figure 58.1). The pericardium can also be examined to exclude the diagnosis of a tamponade. The size of the IVC, in the liver, can be used as a guide to CVP. Three views of the abdomen – left and right upper quadrants (Figure 58.2, Figure 58.3) and lower abdomen – can show fluid around the kidneys, liver, spleen or in the pelvis (Figure 58.4) (refer to Chapter 64 Abdominal injuries). In a trauma patient, this fluid is most commonly blood but other sources, e.g. urine from

www.wiley.com/go/perioperativemed

VIDEO 58.1 **The focused assessment with sonography in trauma (FAST) scan allows rapid point-of-care testing to exclude major life-threatening haemorrhages. Ultrasound views allow examination of the heart, abdominal contents and pelvis to look for accumulation of fluid or blood.**

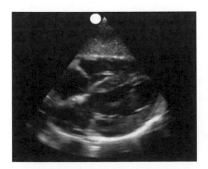

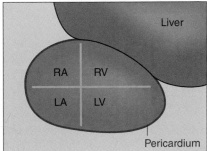

FIGURE 58.1 **FAST scan view of the heart allows both examination of ventricular function and assessment of fluid status.**

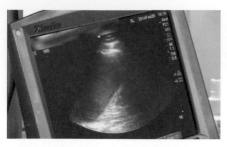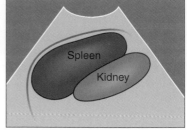

FIGURE 58.2 **FAST scan of the left upper quadrant allows identification of the spleen and left kidney.**

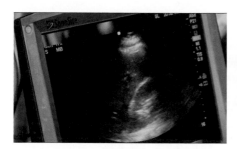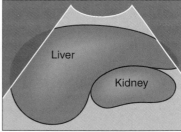

FIGURE 58.3 **FAST scan of the right upper quadrant allows identification of the liver and right kidney.**

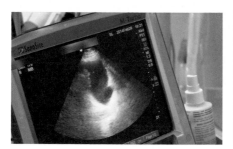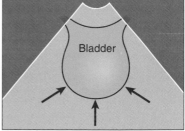

FIGURE 58.4 **FAST scan of the suprapubic region allows examination of the bladder and pelvis.**

bladder rupture or pre-existing ascites, cannot be excluded by FAST scanning. A pelvic X-ray is important in blunt trauma patients.

Fluid resuscitation

Appropriate fluid resuscitation of trauma patients is controversial. There is some evidence that in patients with *penetrating* truncal trauma, minimising fluid resuscitation until surgical haemorrhage control is achieved may be beneficial [2]. Fluid resuscitation goals in patients with *blunt* trauma are less clear. However, in patients with suspected or confirmed raised intracranial pressure, a higher blood pressure is probably appropriate.

The CRASH-2 trial demonstrated that tranexamic acid, an antifibrinolytic, administered to trauma patients with significant haemorrhage reduced all-cause mortality [3]. If used, it should be delivered as soon as possible, as it is much more effective when given within the first three hours following the injury. There is ongoing discussion and research about its role in complex trauma systems.

The use of packed red blood cells and procoagulant blood products should be guided by clinical assessment and laboratory investigations (refer to Chapter 77 Blood transfusion).

Further management

Prevention of secondary brain injury is vital. Surgical management of subdural and extradural haematoma as well as prevention of hypotension, hypoxia and hypercarbia are important (refer to Chapter 59 Traumatic brain injury).

Exposure of the patient to enable an accurate head-to-toe assessment is necessary. Environmental control, with maintenance of body temperature, can assist in maintenance of normal physiological functions, including blood clotting.

Early transfer to a major trauma centre may improve outcome. Major life-saving interventions may need to be performed prior to this, e.g. laparotomy to control haemorrhage, airway intervention. Early and effective communication with ambulance services, receiving hospitals and units is needed. Effective communication and co-ordination within an institution are also essential. The family of the injured should also be considered within a communication strategy.

References

1. American College of Surgeons Committee on Trauma. *Advanced Trauma Life Support for Doctors (ATLS) Student Course Manual*, 8th edn. Chicago, IL: American College of Surgeons, 2008.

2. Bickell WH, Wall MJ Jr, Pepe PE, et al. Immediate versus delayed fluid resuscitation for hypotensive patients with penetrating torso injuries. *New England Journal of Medicine*, 1994;**331**(17):1105–1109. doi:10.1056/NEJM199410273311701

3. Shakur H, Roberts I, Bautista R, et al. Effects of tranexamic acid on death, vascular occlusive events, and blood transfusion in trauma patients with significant haemorrhage (CRASH-2): a randomised, placebo-controlled trial. *Lancet*, 2010;**376**(9734):23–32. doi:10.1016/S0140-6736(10)60835-5

59 Traumatic brain injury

Winifred Burnett

The Alfred Hospital and Monash University, Australia

Traumatic brain injury (TBI) has a high morbidity and mortality. It is an injury that affects males more than females and mostly a younger population (less than 45 years), with motor vehicle accidents, falls, firearms and work-related injury being the main causes. However, as our population ages, TBI is increasingly seen in the elderly population as a result of falls.

The *primary injury* in TBI is the result of the direct impact of the trauma and may lead to extradural haematoma (Figure 59.1), acute subdural haematoma (Figure 59.2), chronic subdural haematoma, diffuse axonal injury, intracerebral haematoma (Figure 59.3) and traumatic subarachnoid haemorrhage (Video 59.1).

Secondary injury follows from the primary injury, progressing over hours and often days. It is often multifactorial but can eventually lead to impairment of the cerebral oxygen supply/demand balance, and ultimately brain ischaemia. These secondary factors may be intracranial or systemic. The treatment of TBI is essentially directed at management and prevention of the causes of secondary injury (Box 59.1).

The management of head-injured patients will be determined by the severity of the injury. This is usually classified using the Glasgow Coma Scale (Table 59.1) [1,2].

Management of mild head injury (GCS score 13–15)

The patient should be observed for four hours post injury with half-hourly observations of the GCS score, pupil size and vital signs. Patients who fail to improve clinically after four hours or have an abnormal CT head scan are usually admitted to hospital for a more extended period of observation. Confusion beyond four hours post injury requires referral to a neurosurgeon.

Beware – patients with mild head injury can deteriorate suddenly.

A CT head scan is usually performed on patients with minor head injury who fit the criteria outlined in the Canadian CT Head Rule (Box 59.2) [3].

Perioperative Medicine for the Junior Clinician, First Edition. Edited by Joel Symons, Paul Myles, Rishi Mehra and Christine Ball.
© 2015 John Wiley & Sons, Ltd. Published 2015 by John Wiley & Sons, Ltd.
Companion website: www.wiley.com/go/perioperativemed

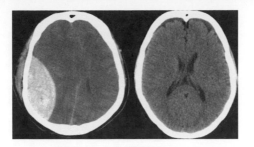

FIGURE 59.1 Acute extradural haemorrhage. A normal brain is shown on the right side for comparison. Note the characteristic 'lens' shape which indicates a bleed external to the dura. The bleed has caused a huge increase in intracranial pressure.

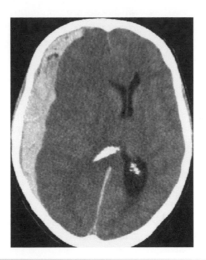

FIGURE 59.2 Acute subdural haemorrhage. The bleed is internal to the dura and hence exhibits a different pattern to that of an extradural haemorrhage.

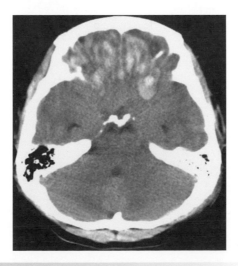

FIGURE 59.3 An example of intracerebral bleeding, particularly affecting the frontal lobes.

www.wiley.com/go/perioperativemed

VIDEO 59.1 **Principles of management of traumatic brain injury involve rapid diagnosis and prevention of secondary brain injury.**

BOX 59.1 Causes of secondary brain injury

Intracranial

Raised intracranial pressure/brain swelling
Haematoma extradural haemorrhage/subdural haemorrhage
Contusion/intracranial haemorrhage
Seizures
Infection
Cerebral vasospasm

Systemic

Hypoxaemia
Hypotension
Hypercarbia
Hypocarbia
Anaemia
Pyrexia/sepsis
Hyponatraemia
Hypoglycaemia
Hyperglycaemia
Coagulopathy
Acidosis

TABLE 59.1 Modified Glasgow Coma Scale (GCS) score

Feature	Point(s)
Eye opening	
Spontaneously	4
To verbal command	3
To pain	2
None	1
Best verbal response	
Oriented, conversing	5
Disoriented, conversing	4
Inappropriate words	3
Incomprehensible sounds	2
No verbal response	1
Best motor response	
Obeys verbal commands	6
Localises to pain	5
Flexion or withdrawal	4
Abnormal flexion (decorticate)	3
Extension (decerebrate)	2
No response	1

Source: Teasdale and Jennett [2].

BOX 59.2 Canadian CT Head Rule

Patients with minor head injury* with one of the following will require a CT brain

High risk (for neurological intervention)

- GCS score < 15 at 2 hours after injury
- Suspected open or depressed skull fracture
- Any sign of basal skull fracture (haemotympanum, 'racoon' eyes, CSF otorrhoea/rhinorrhoea, Battle's sign)
- Vomiting ≥ 2 episodes
- Age ≥ 65 years

Medium risk (for brain injury on CT)

- Amnesia before impact > 30 min
- Dangerous mechanism (pedestrian struck by motor vehicle, occupant ejected from motor vehicle, fall from height > 3 feet or five stairs)

Source: Stiell et al. [3]. Reproduced with permission from Elsevier Ltd.

*Minor head injury is defined as witnessed loss of consciousness, definite amnesia or witnessed disorientation in a patient with a GCS score of 13–15.

Management of moderate head injury (GCS score 9–12)

The patient with a moderate head injury is observed as above, being alert to the possibility that they may deteriorate suddenly. These patients all require a CT head scan and referral to a neurosurgeon.

Guidelines exist for the management and referral of head-injured patients [4,5]. Patients should be referred to a neurosurgeon for any of the following.

* Any significant abnormality on CT head scan
* Persisting coma (GCS score 8 or less) after initial resuscitation
* Unexplained confusion which persists for more than four hours
* Deterioration in GCS score after admission (greater attention should be paid to motor response deterioration)
* Progressive focal neurological signs
* A seizure without full recovery
* Definite or suspected penetrating injury
* A CSF leak

Management of severe head injury (GCS score ≤8) (Figure 59.4) [5,6]

Severe head injury often presents in the setting of other significant injuries. Initial resuscitation should be according to EMST/ATLS guidelines, adhering to DRABCE (refer to Chapter 58 Trauma: pretheatre management and Chapter 62 Cervical spine injuries).

Airway

Patients with traumatic head injury and a GCS score <9 should be intubated to protect their airway and ensure adequate oxygenation and ventilation. This is usually achieved with a rapid sequence intubation which includes preoxygenation, cricoid pressure and in-line neck stabilisation.

Breathing and ventilation

Oxygenation should be maintained with an SaO_2 ≥95%. Monitor the patient with oximetry and regular arterial blood gases. $PaCO_2$ should be maintained at 35–40 mmHg; routine hyperventilation is not indicated. High inspiratory pressures should be avoided by using low PEEP (5 cm H_2O) and tidal volumes <8 mL/kg.

Circulation

Maintain mean arterial pressure (MAP) ≥80 mmHg (assume that ICP is 20 mmHg when not measured). Aim for a cerebral perfusion pressure (CPP) ≥60 mmHg if ICP is monitored and is raised (>20 mmHg).

$$CPP = MAP - ICP$$

Avoid hypovolaemia, giving volume resuscitation as required with iso/hyperosmolar crystalloid or blood products and avoid albumin [7].

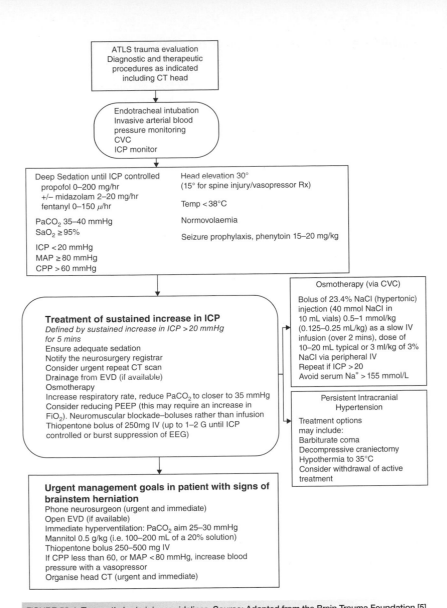

FIGURE 59.4 **Traumatic brain injury guidelines. Source: Adapted from the Brain Trauma Foundation [5].**

Note that cervical spine injury and major extracranial injuries are commonly associated with severe TBI (refer to Chapter 62 Cervical spine injuries).

Disability and Exposure: neurological assessment

Record GCS score and note pupil size and responsiveness. Examine for localising signs.

A CT head scan should be performed as soon as practical and surgical triage should determine if craniotomy is indicated and/or brain monitoring is required (e.g. ICP, JvO_2).

Patients with severe head injury will require management in the ICU.

Seizures

Seizures are common following head injuries and require urgent attention. Patients may require resuscitation – remember the basic principles (ABC) and obtain intravenous access.

Pharmacological management of seizures

Benzodiazepines are first line (and often easily available) choices.

- Lorazepam 0.1 mg/kg (for patient < 50 kg, adult dose 4 mg) administered at rate of 2 mg/min (this is the most effective treatment)
- Midazolam 0.2 mg/kg (consider intranasal or rectal route if there is no IV access, especially in children)
- Diazepam 0.2 mg/kg administered at rate of 5–10 mg/min, also available as rectal suppository
- Propofol 2–5 mg/kg

Note that all of these agents will cause sedation and possibly airway obstruction or apnoea; ongoing airway management is therefore required.

Once stabilised, establish the aetiology of the seizure with blood tests – FBE, U&Es, LFTs, Ca^{2+}, glucose, clotting profile, drug and alcohol screen, and drug levels of antiepileptic medications.

Treat hypoglycaemia if suspected.

Prophylaxis medication for seizures

Phenytoin 15 mg/kg is used for seizure prophylaxis, administered at an infusion rate of 50 mg/min.

Lamotrigine and levetiracetam should only be administered under instruction from a neurologist or neurosurgeon.

Ongoing management

The ongoing management of the head-injured patient requires adherence to the following principles in the trauma centre, operating theatre and ICU.

- Nurse head up 30°
- Set CPP haemodynamic goals

- Maintain ventilation, oxygenation and CO_2 levels
- Set ICP goals
- Maintain temperature
- Control blood sugar
- Maintain appropriate sedation
- Maintain fluid and electrolyte balance
- Administer seizure prophylaxis
- Administer thromboembolism prophylaxis (mechanical, caution with pharmacological)
- Maintain nutritional status

References

1. Jennett B. Assessment of the severity of head injury. *Journal of Neurology, Neurosurgery, and Psychiatry*, 1976;**39**(7):647–655. doi:10.1136/jnnp.39.7.647

2. Teasdale G, Jennett B. Assessment of coma and impaired consciousness. A practical scale. *Lancet*, 1974;**2**(7872):81–84. doi:10.1016/s0140-6736(74)91639-0

3. Stiell IG, Wells GA, Vandemheen K, et al. The Canadian CT Head Rule for patients with minor head injury. *Lancet*, 2001;**357**(9266):1391–1396. doi:10.1016/S0140-6736(00)04561-X

4. NICE. *Head Injury Triage, Assessment, Investigation and Early Management of Head Injury in Children, Young People and Adults*. Clinical Guideline 176. www.nice.org.uk/guidance/cg176

5. Brain Trauma Foundation. *Guidelines for the Management of Severe Traumatic Brain Injury*. www.braintrauma.org

6. Alfred Health. *Trauma ICU Traumatic Brain Injury (TBI) Management Guideline*. Melbourne, Australia: Alfred Health, 2011.

7. SAFE Study Investigators. Saline or albumin for fluid resuscitation in patients with traumatic brain injury. *New England Journal of Medicine*, 2007;**357**(9):874–884. doi:10.1056/NEJMoa067514

Maxillofacial injuries

Joel Symons[1] and Charles Baillieu[2]

[1] The Alfred Hospital and Monash University, Australia
[2] The Alfred Hospital and Southern Health, Australia

Epidemiology

Maxillofacial trauma occurs more often in males (male-to-female ratio, 2:1) and younger patients, and results from interpersonal violence, road trauma, sporting injuries, falls and industrial accidents. Major morbidity can result due to the proximity to the brain and airway; traumatic brain injury occurs in 15–48% of these patients (refer to Chapter 59 Traumatic brain injury) [1]. Associated cervical spine injuries are also common [2] (refer to Chapter 62 Cervical spine injuries), with lower cervical spine injuries occurring with upper mid-face fractures and upper cervical spine injuries occurring more commonly with mandibular fractures. The face has a rich blood supply and facial trauma can result in catastrophic haemorrhage.

Classification of maxillofacial fractures

The facial skeleton consists of a series of vertical (strong) and transverse (weaker) buttresses surrounding the sinuses and covered in paper-thin bone. Its structure acts as a crumple zone, evenly distributing energy to the face and minimising damage to the skull and brain. Anatomical reduction of these buttresses is crucial in re-establishing facial function in maxillofacial trauma [3].

Fractures can be classified as follows (Video 60.1).

Fractures of the lower third

These involve fractures of the mandible, which may be asymmetrical and in two or more places; associated teeth may become loose or avulsed. The temporomandibular joints may be involved which may limit mouth opening. Complex mandibular fractures may result in airway compromise.

Fractures of the middle third

These involve fractures of the maxilla, zygoma and lower half of the naso-orbito-ethmoidal complex and may be classified using the Le Fort classification [4].

Perioperative Medicine for the Junior Clinician, First Edition. Edited by Joel Symons, Paul Myles, Rishi Mehra and Christine Ball.
© 2015 John Wiley & Sons, Ltd. Published 2015 by John Wiley & Sons, Ltd.
Companion website: www.wiley.com/go/perioperativemed

Severe fractures in this area may result in airway compromise.

www.wiley.com/go/perioperativemed

VIDEO 60.1 **Maxillofacial injuries and the Le Fort classification.**

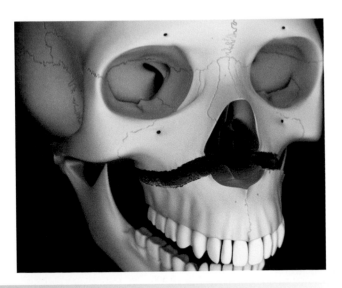

FIGURE 60.1 **Le Fort I fracture.**

A Le Fort I fracture involves the maxilla only (Figure 60.1).

A Le Fort II fracture is through the maxilla and nasal complex and is usually more mobile than a Le Fort I (Figure 60.2). The more serious Le Fort III fracture involves the whole mid-face dissociating from the skull base and facial bones (Figure 60.3).

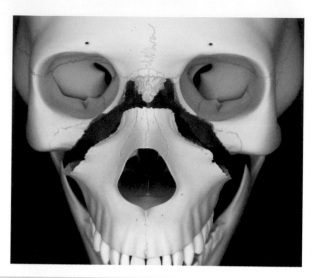

FIGURE 60.2 **Le Fort II fracture.**

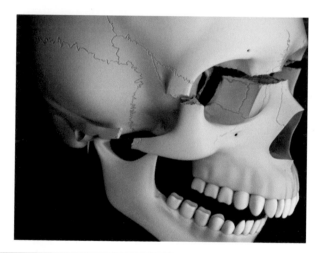

FIGURE 60.3 **Le Fort III fracture.**

In practice, combinations of Le Fort fractures may occur, often with mandibular fractures (Figure 60.4).

Initial assessment

A multidisciplinary approach often requires early involvement of the maxillofacial surgeon, neurosurgeon and ophthalmologist.

In addition to the standardised approach to a trauma patient described in Chapter 58 (Trauma: pretheatre management), particular attention needs to be paid to the following.

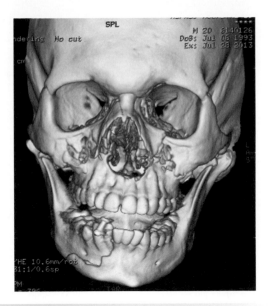

FIGURE 60.4 **Le Fort II and III and right mandibular parasymphyseal fracture.**

History

The mechanism of injury is important because the amount of energy transfer is directly proportional to the resulting tissue damage [4]. Establish whether the patient lost consciousness, has any visual disturbance (photophobia, blurred vision, diplopia, pain, change in vision with eye movement), trouble breathing through their nose or any bloody or clear fluid discharge from their nose or ears, which may indicate a CSF leak. Also enquire about altered hearing, facial numbness, difficulty in opening or closing the mouth, pain on biting down and the presence or absence of normal occlusion.

Examination

This should include:

- *airway assessment*: especially loose teeth, dentures, oropharyngeal bleeding, swelling and tissue displacement
- *bleeding assessment*: life-threatening bleeding may occur from scalp lacerations. Nasal and mandibular fractures and extensive mid-face fractures may also result in extensive bleeding
- *assessment of the eyes and visual pathways*.

Table 60.1 gives a summary of maxillofacial fractures and relevant clinical symptoms and signs.

Management

General management principles for the trauma patient should include particular attention to securing the airway in patients whose airway is at risk, and controlling haemorrhage. An FBE and group and hold should be ordered urgently and appropriate antibiotics administered. The airway should be secured in a

TABLE 60.1 Maxillofacial injuries and relevant clinical symptoms and signs

Fracture	Clinical symptom or sign
Mandibular	Condylar fractures – tender area anterior to the ear meatus, limited mouth opening on one or both sides Teeth malocclusion Painful jaw movement Mobility and crepitus of the mandible adjacent to the fracture Anterior open bite Gingival bleeding and intraoral oedema Paraesthesia or anaesthesia of half of the lower lip, chin, teeth and gingiva (disruption of the inferior alveolar nerve and/or its mental branch in mandibular parasymphyseal, body or angle fractures
Alveolar	Alveolar mobility, loose or avulsed teeth, gingival bleeding
Maxillary	Le Fort I – facial oedema, mobility of the hard palate, maxillary alveolus and teeth Le Fort II – facial oedema, subconjuctival haemorrhage, mobility of the maxilla, telecanthus, epistaxis, CSF rhinorrhoea Le Fort III – massive facial oedema, anterior open bite, epistaxis, CSF rhinorrhoea, movement of all facial bones in relation to the cranial base with manipulation of the teeth and hard palate
Zygomaticomaxillary complex	Depressed malar eminence (flattened cheekbone) Pain on palpating the zygomatic eminence Lateral subconjunctival haemorrhage Step defect along the lateral orbital and infraorbital rims or zygomaticomaxillary buttress Paraesthesia of lateral side of nose and upper lip (impingement of infraorbital nerve) Diplopia on upward gaze (entrapment of inferior rectus muscle) Trismus Intraoral ecchymosis and gingival disruption
Zygomatic arch	Palpable defect and pain over the zygoma Limitation of mandibular movement due to limitation of movement of the mandibular coronoid process
Nasoethmoidal	Telecanthus Epistaxis CSF rhinorrhoea Epiphora (due to blockage of nasolacrimal duct)
Nasal	Displaced nasal bridge or septum (this may be pre-existing) Nasal displacement, crepitus and epistaxis Septal haematoma
Orbital floor	Periorbital oedema, crepitus and ecchymosis/enophthalmos Paraesthesia of lateral side of nose, upper lip and maxillary gingivae (infraorbital nerve damage) Lateral and upward gaze dysfunction (entrapment of medial and inferior rectus muscles) Diplopia on upward gaze (entrapment of inferior rectus muscle)
Frontal bone	Crepitus of the supraorbital rims Paraesthesia of the supraorbital and supratrochlear nerves Frontal lacerations, contusions or haematoma Facial pain Visible depression of the forehead CSF rhinorrhoea (in one-third of patients)

CSF, cerebrospinal fluid.

manner that allows safe transport of the patient to scanning, theatre or the ward. All foreign material, such as tooth fragments, dental appliances and debris, should be cleaned from the airway. Emergency department control of bleeding may require temporary nasopharyngeal or oropharyngeal packing or obturation with inflatable compression devices such as Foley catheters. Manual reduction of fractures may reduce bleeding but should only be attempted by experienced trained clinicians. The availability of plates and screws for open reduction of fractures has removed the need for previously used craniofacial splints and frames; persistent bleeding from postnasal or mid-face fractures will often cease after definitive reduction and internal fixation in the operating theatre. Uncontrollable bleeding from facial fractures that cannot be tamponaded by packing are best managed by early selective embolisation in an angiography suite. Emergency surgical control of the external carotid artery or transmaxillary ligation of the maxillary artery is often not helpful in controlling bleeding.

After stabilisation of the patient in the emergency room, early CT scanning is mandated using a high-resolution, fast acquisition scanner which allows rapid assessment of the bony structures, soft tissues and blood vessels. The images can be reprocessed into whatever views are required and the 3D computer rendering of the external facial skeleton is extremely helpful in management planning with all clinicians involved in the patient's care. Conventional maxillary orthopantomograms or plain skull X-rays have little role in the trauma setting.

All patients with more than insignificant facial injuries need to be assessed by a maxillofacial reconstructive surgeon; plastic and reconstructive surgeons may be required where the maxillofacial surgeons do not have soft tissue reconstruction training. Significant dental trauma also mandates early referral to a dental service. Neurosurgeons, ENT surgeons and ophthalmologists may also be required.

In a major trauma hospital a dedicated craniomaxillofacial trauma service should be involved upon arrival or immediately a craniomaxillofacial injury is identified. Surgical input into airway management, and assessment and planning of craniofacial reconstruction should occur in the emergency department (ED).

Surgical reconstruction of the face is best carried out within 24 hours, but these complex patients may have other significant injuries that take precedence and timing for all surgeries requires a team approach. Delayed reconstruction of the facial skeleton is acceptable, but beyond three to four weeks strong healing may necessitate osteotomies to mobilise and reduce the fractures. Limited toilet procedures and wound closures are performed in the ED or ICU to prevent infective complications whilst waiting for theatre.

Preoperative management on the ward

Airway assessment, as described in Chapter 14 (Airway assessment and planning), is crucial, with particular attention to nasal patency and the presence of trismus. This may occur for mechanical reasons such as mandibular condyle fractures but is usually due to pain and disappears on induction of anaesthesia.

Appropriate blood investigations should be ordered and antibiotics and strict analgesia administered.

Postoperative management

This includes attention to:

* analgesia (refer to Chapter 93 Acute pain). Surgeons will usually perform nerve blocks and local anaesthetic infiltration of the surgical site intraoperatively. Mandibular fractures are usually more painful postoperatively than mid-face ones and this should be accounted for in the analgesic regime
* antibiotic prophylaxis
* postoperative oedema. Steroids (e.g. dexamethasone) should be administered. Postoperative oedema usually worsens in the first 48 hours after injury, especially in Le Fort II and III fractures
* throat packs are often inserted intraoperatively. Despite strict hospital guidelines for their insertion and removal, maintain a high index of suspicion for a retained throat pack in a patient who presents with difficulty breathing postoperatively [5]
* PONV prophylaxis (refer to Chapter 79 Postoperative nausea and vomiting). Most intermaxillary fixation with plates and screws and elastic bands leaves patients with a functional jaw postoperatively. Wiring a patient's mandible and maxilla together is uncommon today but requires wire cutters to be urgently available should the patient experience PONV.

References

1. Jeroukhimov I, Cockburn M, Cohn S. Facial trauma: overview of trauma care. In: Thaller SR, editor. *Facial Trauma*. New York: Marcel Dekker, 2004, p. 11.

2. Lewis VL Jr, Manson PN, Morgan RF, Cerullo LJ, Meyer PR Jr. Facial injuries associated with cervical fractures: recognition, patterns, and management. *Journal of Trauma*, 1985;**25**(1):90–93. doi:10.1016/0030-4220(70)90331-2

3. Perry M. Maxillofacial trauma – developments, innovations and controversies. *Injury*, 2009;**40**(12):1252–1259. doi:10.1016/j.injury.2008.12.015

4. Morosan M, Parbhoo A, Curry N. Anaesthesia and common oral and maxillo-facial emergencies. *Continuing Education in Anaesthesia, Critical Care and Pain*, 2012;**12**(5):257–262. doi:10.1093/bjaceaccp/mks031

5. National Patient Safety Agency. *Reducing the Risk of Retained Throat Packs after Surgery*. www.nrls.npsa.nhs.uk/resources/?entryid45=59853

61 Spinal injuries (excluding cervical spine)

Susan Liew

The Alfred Hospital and Monash University, Australia

Thoracolumbar spine anatomy

The ribcage makes the thoracic spine inherently more stable than the lumbar spine and also makes the C7/T1 and T12/L1 junctions more prone to injury with violent flexion-extension forces. The thoracic spinal cord is more vulnerable to injury because the mid-thoracic area is a watershed area of blood supply, the cord itself takes up a larger proportion of the spinal canal, and it is tethered by the dentate ligaments.

The spinal cord ends at L1. Conus (L1 cord) injuries and cauda equina (nerve roots) injuries can affect bowel and bladder function. Nerve root injuries in the thoracic spine cause only sensory dysfunction.

Patterns of injuries

The spine is best thought of in columns (Figure 61.1) as described by Denis [1], and indications for surgery are guided by the Thoracolumbar Injury Classification and Severity Score (TLICS) [2]. The most common injuries are to the vertebral body. One-column (anterior) injuries (Figure 61.2) are stable and include endplate fractures or crush fractures, generally only requiring symptomatic treatment. Burst fractures (Figure 61.3) can range from being stable (two columns – anterior and middle) with no neurology to very unstable (all three columns) with complete cord neurology (Video 61.1). Figure 61.4 shows an algorithm for surgical decision making and Figure 61.5 shows the TLICS scoring tables.

Fracture-dislocations (Figure 61.6) are a less common three-column injury with primary disruption of the facet joints. Other three-column injuries include Chance fractures (Figure 61.7), 'carrot-stick' fractures seen in the stiff spine of ankylosing spondylitis (Figure 61.8), and purely ligamentous flexion-distraction injuries (Figure 61.9).

Perioperative Medicine for the Junior Clinician, First Edition. Edited by Joel Symons, Paul Myles, Rishi Mehra and Christine Ball.
© 2015 John Wiley & Sons, Ltd. Published 2015 by John Wiley & Sons, Ltd.
Companion website: www.wiley.com/go/perioperativemed

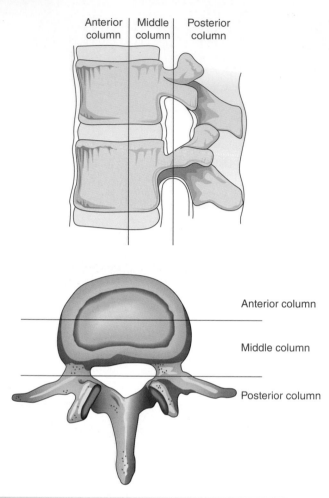

Anterior column | Middle column | Posterior column

Anterior column

Middle column

Posterior column

FIGURE 61.1 **Columns of the vertebral body in sagittal and axial planes.**

Surgical indications for spinal fixation

Most patients with 'complete' spinal cord injuries remain completely paraplegic so the aim of surgery is to achieve bony stability and prevent further injury. Surgery usually does not need to be done urgently in the middle of the night.

> Urgent (immediate) surgery is indicated with progressive cord neurology or occasionally incomplete neurology where decompression (and stabilisation) is performed to stop further progression and optimise neurological recovery.

For injuries without neurology or just nerve root involvement, surgery can be done as soon as practical – ideally on the next available daytime operating list.

(a)   (b)

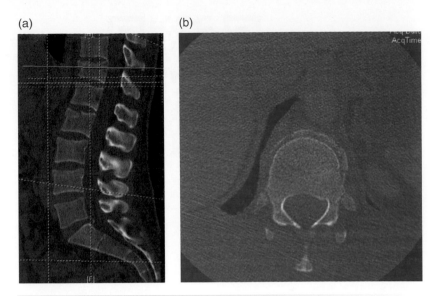

FIGURE 61.2 **Anterior column injury.** (a) Sagittal CT. (b) Axial CT.

(a)   (b)

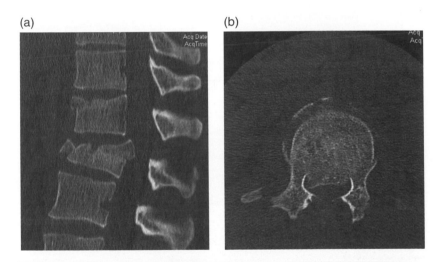

FIGURE 61.3 **Burst fracture.** (a) Sagittal CT. (b) Axial CT.

For some surgeons, it is paramount to determine whether the injury is predominantly caused by an axial force (e.g. burst fracture) or a flexion force (e.g. facet fracture-dislocation) as this determines their surgical approach. The pros and cons of anterior versus posterior surgery for burst fractures are still widely debated, but fracture dislocations must be approached from posterior first to enable reduction of the facets. Regardless, instrumentation spans above and below the unstable level, and usually with the addition of a bone graft. If bone grafting/fusion is not performed, the instrumentation is removed at approximately nine months post surgery.

www.wiley.com/go/perioperativemed

VIDEO 61.1 **Thoracolumbar spinal injuries.**

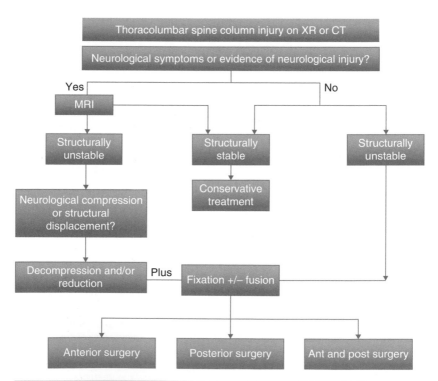

FIGURE 61.4 **Algorithm for surgical decision making.** CT, computed tomography; MRI, magnetic resonance imaging; XR, X-ray.

Injury morphology	
Type	Points
Compression	1
Compression burst	2
Translation rotation	3
Distraction	4

TLICS
*ThoracoLumbar Injury
Classification & Severity score*

Integrity of post ligamentous complex	
Involvement	Points
Intact	0
Indeterminate	2
Injured	3

Injury severity score	
Score	Suggested treatment
3 or less	Conservative
4	Conservative or surgical
5 or more	Surgical

Neurological status	
Involvement	Points
Intact	0
Nerve root	2
Spinal cord injury (complete)	2
Spinal cord injury (incomplete)	3
Cauda equina	3

FIGURE 61.5 **TLICS tables. Source: Vaccaro et al. [2]. Reproduced with permission from Wolters Kluwer Health.**

(a)

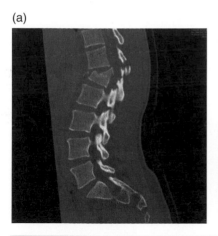

(b)

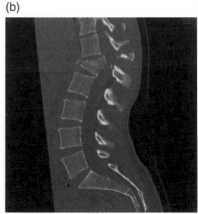

FIGURE 61.6 **Fracture-dislocation. (a) Sagittal CT through the plane of the right facet. (b) Sagittal CT through the plane of the spinous process.**

The physiological response to injury

The physiology of injury and pain is well known, but special consideration must be given to the following.

Spinal cord injury (SCI)

Spinal cord injury causes spinal shock which will manifest as hypotension and bradycardia. It can mask shock from blood loss or be misread as hypovolaemia, so other injuries need to be actively excluded. In thoracic spine injuries, a haemothorax

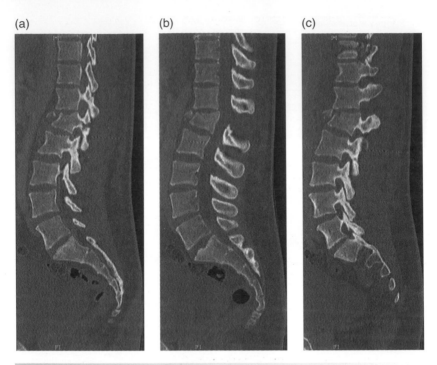

FIGURE 61.7 Chance fracture. (a) Sagittal CT through the plane of the right pedicle. (b) Sagittal CT through the plane of the spinous process. (c) Sagittal CT through the plane of the left pedicle.

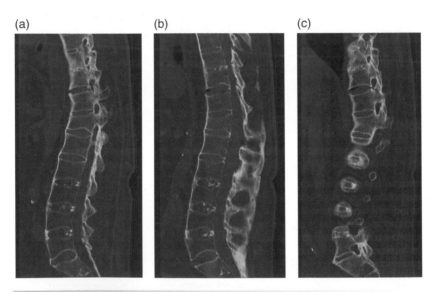

FIGURE 61.8 Carrot-stick fracture. (a) Sagittal CT through the plane of the right facet. (b) Sagittal CT through the plane of the spinous process. (c) Sagittal CT through the plane of the left facet.

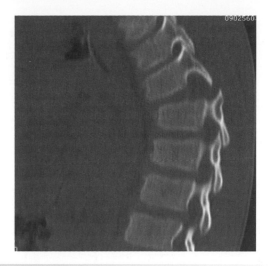

FIGURE 61.9 **Ligamentous injury lateral X-ray.**

or haemopneumothorax may be associated with the spine injury without primary chest injury. High thoracic cord injuries can have a profound effect on respiratory function, so tidal volumes need to be monitored. High-dose steroids are no longer given to SCI patients [3]. Venous thromboembolism prophylaxis, pressure care, and bowel and bladder regimens should be started as soon as possible. Spinal shock can last up to three weeks [4].

Polytrauma

In polytrauma, the physiological response to injury is magnified. Life-threatening conditions are treated first even in the presence of SCI. With severe polytrauma, it may be some days before the patient is 'fit' for surgery. Other factors needing to be taken into account include being able to lie prone (e.g. compromised if there are facial injuries), tolerate moderately long (average two to three hours) surgery, and receive blood transfusion (e.g. Jehovah's witness patient).

The elderly patient or patients with multiple co-morbidities

Ageing and/or the presence of multiple co-morbidities lessens physiological reserve and patients can decompensate and/or decondition rapidly. Optimisation for surgery can be a fine balance between the respiratory (e.g. risk of pneumonia in bed) and cardiac (e.g. risk of MI/arrhythmias with surgery) systems and/or managing the fluid balance, especially after resuscitation in polytrauma. Many patients are also receiving some form of anticoagulation for cardiovascular reasons – get advice and refer early!

Waiting for surgery

The injured spine needs to be protected from further displacement by nursing the patient with spinal precautions, i.e. maintaining neutral position. If a patient is not fit, the risk of surgery is too high or the patient is going to have a prolonged period of 'rest in bed', then the spinal injury can be treated conservatively. Confinement to bed, however, comes with its own unique set of risks, such as pneumonia, pressure

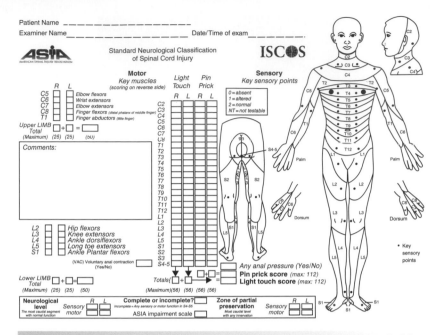

FIGURE 61.10 ASIA Standard Neurological Assessment of Spinal Cord Injury. www.asia-spinalinjury.org/elearning/ISNCSCI_Exam_Sheet_r4.pdf

areas and thromboembolism, which need to be weighed against the risks of surgery, such as the anaesthesia, infection or causing more injury to a traumatised cord.

Documentation of any neurological injury should be done accurately via the ASIA chart (Figure. 61.10).

> Documentation of informed consent means you have discussed with the patient the natural history, treatment options and outcomes, and risks – if you don't know them, don't do it!

References

1. Denis F. Spinal instability as defined by the three-column spine concept in acute spinal trauma. *Clinical Orthopaedics and Related Research*, 1984;**189**:65–76. doi:10.1097/00003086-198410000-00008

2. Vaccaro AR, Lehman RA Jr, Hurlbert RJ, et al. A new classification of thoracolumbar injuries: the importance of injury morphology, the integrity of the posterior ligamentous complex, and neurologic status. *Spine*, 2005;**30**(20):2325–2333. doi:10.1097/01.brs.0000182986.43345.cb

3. Consortium for Spinal Cord Medicine. Early acute management in adults with spinal cord injury: a clinical practice guideline for health-care professionals. *Journal of Spinal Cord Medicine*, 2008;**31**(4):403–479. www.ncbi.nlm.nih.gov/pubmed/18959359

4. Hambly PR, Martin B. Anaesthesia for chronic spinal cord lesions. *Anaesthesia*, 1998;**53**(3):273–289. doi:10.1046/j.1365-2044.1998.00337.x

62 Cervical spine injuries

Peter Hwang and Jin Tee

The Alfred Hospital and Monash University, Australia

Epidemiology

- Spinal cord injuries account for approximately 2–13% of total trauma patients with spine injuries [1–3].
- The incidence of cervical spine injury at a Level 1 trauma centre is 29% (Table 62.1) [1].
- Patients with spine trauma have a mortality rate of 5–17%.
- Level 1 trauma centres have significantly lower mortality rates due to implementation of standardised trauma protocols and algorithms in patients with spine injuries.

Risk factors for mortality in trauma patients with spine injuries include:
- age (≥65 years)
- severe polytrauma
- severe traumatic brain injury
- C1/2 dissociation injuries (usually fatal at the scene)
- severe neurological deficit [1].

Anatomy

The adult cervical spinal cord extends from the medulla oblongata to the C7–T1 vertebral level. It is encircled by the spine column, covered by the dura and adjacent to the densely vascular epidural space. Blood supply is provided by one anterior (ventral two-thirds of the cord) and two posterior spinal arteries (the remaining dorsal region), both branches of the vertebral arteries. They enter the foramen transversarium at the C6 level, perforate the dura at C1, and join to form the basilar artery at the anterior part of the pons.

The spinal cord consists of white matter on the periphery, a central H-shaped mass of grey matter and a small central canal containing cerebrospinal fluid. Of its many

Perioperative Medicine for the Junior Clinician, First Edition. Edited by Joel Symons, Paul Myles, Rishi Mehra and Christine Ball.
© 2015 John Wiley & Sons, Ltd. Published 2015 by John Wiley & Sons, Ltd.
Companion website: www.wiley.com/go/perioperativemed

TABLE 62.1 Spine injury characteristics of 965 trauma patients with spine injuries seen at the Alfred Hospital, Melbourne from 1 May 2009 to 1 January 2011

Spine injury characteristics (per segment)	Number (n = 2333)	Incidence (per total spine injuries)
C0–2	189	8.1%
• Occipital condyle	26	1.1%
• C1 burst	35	1.5%
• Odontoid (Type 2)	47	2%
• Odontoid (Types 1 & 3)	17	0.7%
• C2 Hangman's	18	0.8%
• C1/2 dissociation	11	0.5%
• C1/2 misc.	35	1.5%
C3–7	497	21.3%
• DLC only	76	3.3%
• Compression	344	14.7%
• Burst	5	0.2%
• Distraction	28	1.2%
• Translation or rotation	44	1.9%
T1–12	893	38.3%
• DLC only	3	0.1%
• Compression	792	33.9%
• Burst	44	1.9%
• Distraction	42	1.8%
• Translation or rotation	12	0.5%
L1–5	691	29.6%
• DLC only	0	0
• Compression	612	26.2%
• Burst	61	2.6%
• Distraction	15	0.6%
• Translation or rotation	3	0.1%
Sacrococcygeal	63	2.7%

C1/2 misc., miscellaneous fractures affecting the C1/2 lamina, body, lateral mass or spinous process; DLC, discoligamentous complex.

ascending and descending tracts, three are crucial in examination of the cervical spine trauma patient:

• the corticospinal tract (upper and lower limb muscular control)
• the anterolateral spinothalamic tract (pain, temperature, light touch and pressure sensation)
• the posterior columns (fine touch, vibration and position sense).

Pathophysiology

Management of traumatic spinal cord injury recognises a sequence of two events: (i) primary injury, incurred during the initial insult and unlikely to be modified by therapeutic intervention, and (ii) secondary injury, hours to days following the insult, as a result of a cascade of tissue injury, inflammation and cellular dysfunction.

A pathognomonic feature of secondary injury is spinal cord oedema which, if significant, presents clinically as neurological deterioration and on MRI as cord signal change.

> Independent predictors of poor functional outcome and mortality include shock, hypoxaemia, hypercoagulability, the elderly with poor cardiovascular reserve, and patients with multiple co-morbidities [2,3].

Protecting the cervical spine

Cervical spine fracture and spinal cord injury

This requires rapid assessment and prompt planning. Unrestricted movement is potentially disastrous as unrecognised unstable discoligamentous cervical spine injury may cause cervical vertebra dislodgement and corresponding acute spinal cord compression and injury.

Once cleared of spinal injury, the patient no longer requires spinal precautions and is allowed to sit up or ambulate (particularly important for patients with chest or abdominal injuries).

> As a general rule, a patient with a cervical spine injury that is anatomically aligned or minimally displaced can almost always be treated conservatively with a rigid external orthosis (e.g. halothoracic brace, rigid cervical collar or brace incorporating both elements such as the SOMI brace) (Figure 62.1; Video 62.1)

Concept of spinal stability

There have been many classifications and algorithms designed for cervical spine trauma stability assessments. The most relevant, current and complete algorithm is the Subaxial Cervical Spine Injury Classification System or SLIC [4]. It assesses cervical spine mechanical stability and injury morphology, discoligamentous integrity and the patient's neurological status to recommend operative or non-operative treatment options (Table 62.2).

> The majority of high cervical spine injuries without neurological deficits can be safely managed with an external rigid orthosis. Only those injuries that subluxate or displace during erect imaging of the cervical spine or have significant displacement require surgical consideration.

Perioperative management

> Haemodynamic instability, high intracranial pressures from traumatic brain injury or severe coagulopathy must be treated adequately prior to cervical spine reconstruction and/or spinal cord decompression [2,3].

(a) 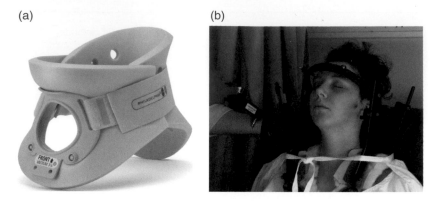 (b)

FIGURE 62.1 (a) Common cervical orthoses include a Philadelphia collar. (b) A halothoracic brace is a method of cervical spine immobilisation.

www.wiley.com/go/perioperativemed

VIDEO 62.1 This video discusses cervical spine injuries and the various methods used to immobilise them.

Suitability for surgery

It may be reasonable to defer definitive spine surgery in critically ill spine trauma patients despite them suffering highly unstable cervical spine injuries with neurological deficits. These patients should be braced in the interim, with either a rigid collar or sitting to 30°, or be immobilised with a halothoracic brace.

Patient positioning

Anterior cervical spine fixation – the patient is positioned supine on the operating table, head slightly lordosed, with a small roll under the lower neck or upper shoulders. Gardner Well tongs (Figure 62.2) or other traction devices may be used to provide traction to the injured cervical segment for fracture reduction if required.

TABLE 62.2 **Subaxial Cervical Spine Injury Classification System (SLIC)**

	Points
Morphology	
No abnormality	0
Compression	1
Burst	+1 = 2
Distraction (e.g. facet perch, hyperextension)	3
Rotation/translation (e.g. facet dislocation, unstable teardrop or advanced stage flexion compression injury)	4
Disco-ligamentous complex (DLC)	
Intact	0
Indeterminate (e.g. isolated interspinous widening, MRI signal change only)	1
Disrupted (e.g. widening of disc space, facet perch or dislocation)	2
Neurological status	
Intact	0
Root injury	1
Complete cord injury	2
Incomplete cord injury	3
Continuous cord compression in setting of neuro deficit (Neuro modifier)	+1

*≤3 = Conservative, 4 = Either method, ≥5 = Operative
Source: Vaccaro et al. [4]. Reproduced with permission of Wolters Kluwer Health.

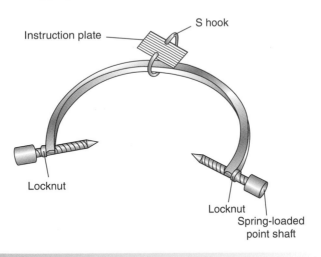

FIGURE 62.2 **Gardner Well tongs.**

For posterior cervical spine fixation, the patient is positioned prone on a surgical pillow, head held with a head clamp.

In both cases, the position of the head and cervical spine is determined intraoperatively using an image intensifier.

Respiratory system

Securing the airway is complex and important. Cervical traction or halo braces present a physical obstacle to airway access.

Commonly used adjunctive intubation techniques include awake fibreoptic intubation enabling simultaneous neurological examination, and indirect video laryngoscopy, with or without manual inline stabilisation. A reinforced tracheal tube is also essential to prevent kinking during patient positioning and perioperatively, during surgical retraction. This should be changed to a regular tube at surgical conclusion if the patient is going to the ICU.

Immediate postoperative period

> Immediate postoperative tracheal extubation may be contraindicated if extensive, prolonged surgery has occurred (due to peritracheal soft tissue oedema, recurrent laryngeal nerve injury, prone positioning and haemodynamic instability).

Neurogenic shock

> Neurogenic shock can be a potentially devastating complication, leading to multiorgan failure and death if not promptly recognised and treated.

Neurogenic shock is due to autonomic disruption from spinal cord injury, usually above the T4 level, and leads to sympathetic dysfunction, decreased systemic vascular resistance, and hypotension and bradycardia from unopposed vagal activity. Treatment includes both fluid loading and vasopressor support as it can be difficult to rule out concurrent or haemorrhagic shock perioperatively.

Haemodynamic goals for a spinal cord-injured patient include maintaining a mean arterial pressure of 85–90 mmHg and avoiding systolic blood pressure less than 90 mmHg in the first week [5].

References

1. Tee JW, Chan CH, Fitzgerald MC, Liew SM, Rosenfeld JV. Epidemiological trends of spine trauma: an Australian level 1 trauma centre study. *Global Spine Journal*, 2013;**3**(2):75–84. doi:10.1055/s-0033-1337124

2. Tee J, Chan C, Fitzgerald M, Liew S, Rosenfeld J. Early predictors of functional disability following spine trauma: a Level 1 trauma center study. *Spine*, 2013;**38**(12):999–1007. doi:10.1097/BRS.0b013e31828432a3

3. Tee JW, Chan PC, Gruen RL, et al. Early predictors of mortality after spine trauma: a level 1 Australian trauma center study. *Spine*, 2013;**38**(2):169–177. doi: 10.1097/BRS.0b013e3182634cbf

4. Vaccaro AR, Hulbert J, Patel AA, et al. The subaxial cervical spine injury classification system. *Spine*, 2007;**32**(21):2365–2374.

5. Ryken TC, Hurlbert RJ, Hadley MN, et al. The acute cardiopulmonary management of patients with cervical spinal cord injuries. *Neurosurgery*, 2013;**72**(Suppl 2):84–92. doi:10.1227/NEU.0b013e318276ee16

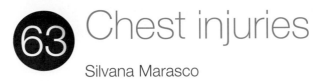

63 Chest injuries

Silvana Marasco

The Alfred Hospital and Monash University, Australia

Major chest injuries are associated with a mortality rate of approximately 10% and account for over 25% of all trauma deaths.

Trauma reception

Initial triage assesses the patient's mechanism of injury, apparent injuries, haemodynamic and respiratory stability. Wide-bore intravenous access and arterial monitoring are essential. In patients with respiratory distress, the airway should be secured by tracheal intubation. The initial survey assesses for breath sounds and considers tension pneumothorax (absent breath sounds, deviated trachea away from the affected side and haemodynamic instability) (Figure 63.1). If a pneumothorax is suspected, a small-bore intercostal catheter (ICC) should be inserted into the second intercostal space in the mid-clavicular line.

Chest X-ray and CT scans (where the patient is sufficiently stable) provide invaluable information.

There should be a low threshold for inserting ICCs bilaterally [1]. ICC bleeding of more than 1500 mL initially and more than 250 mL/hr ongoing are indications for surgical exploration.

Any penetrating injury within the 'cardiac box' (area between the nipples, below the clavicles and above the costal margin) should be treated with a high degree of suspicion. An unstable patient with penetrating injury in this area warrants an immediate thoracotomy. A stable patient should be assessed with a FAST or TTE (refer to Chapter 58 Trauma: pretheatre management and Chapter 64 Abdominal injuries). Any pericardial collection warrants exploration.

Emergency department thoracotomy

This management strategy is best reserved for patients with penetrating injury and witnessed signs of life at the scene (with short scene and transport time) or on arrival in the ED. There is little place for ED thoracotomy in blunt chest injury due to dismal survival rates; this should be limited to those patients arriving with signs of life and arresting in the ED [2]. ED thoracotomy is performed through the left fourth intercostal space, extending from the sternum as far laterally as required [3]. The aim of ED thoracotomy is to relieve life-threatening conditions such as pericardial tamponade, control intrathoracic haemorrhage or massive air leak, provide temporising repair to cardiac injuries and perform internal cardiac massage if required.

Perioperative Medicine for the Junior Clinician, First Edition. Edited by Joel Symons, Paul Myles, Rishi Mehra and Christine Ball.
© 2015 John Wiley & Sons, Ltd. Published 2015 by John Wiley & Sons, Ltd.
Companion website: www.wiley.com/go/perioperativemed

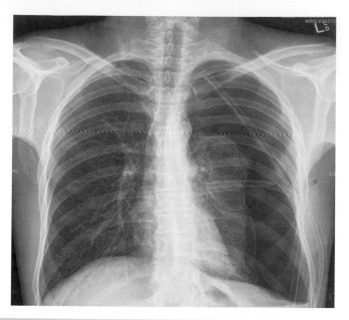

FIGURE 63.1 **Left pneumothorax with failure of lung re-expansion despite two intercostal catheters.**

Postoperative management of ICCs

Intercostal catheters are kept at 20 cm H_2O suction (Figure 63.2). Presence of a swing in the water chamber indicates that the tube is in the pleural space, and loss of swing indicates that either the tube is blocked or the pleural space is adhesed. An air leak is demonstrated by bubbling in the underwater seal (Video 63.1). Ongoing air leaks must always be checked for system leaks (dressing not airtight, tubing connector loose). If an ICC blocks and there is evidence of ongoing air leak (worsening pneumothorax or respiratory status, surgical emphysema), then a second ICC should be placed. Once an air leak appears to resolve, the ICC should be clamped for 4–6 hours and a chest X-ray taken to ensure no occult air leak is continuing. If there is no evidence of ongoing air leak, then the ICC can be removed.

Intercostal catheters placed for haemothorax can be removed once drainage losses are no more than 20 mL/hr for six hours. Any retained collection confers a risk of empyema or trapped lung, and should be referred to the cardiothoracic unit for consideration of thoracoscopic drainage (Figure 63.3). Further ICC placement is rarely helpful in retained haemothorax which is usually organised thrombus.

Specific injuries

Airway and lungs

Intrathoracic tracheobronchial injuries are rare and typically occur close to the carina (a relatively fixed point). Mortality is high due to difficulty with ventilation and oxygenation. Most lung injuries can be managed conservatively with ICC drainage. Massive air leak (interfering with ventilation), prolonged air leak (continuing more than five days) or repeated blockage of ICCs are all indications for operative intervention.

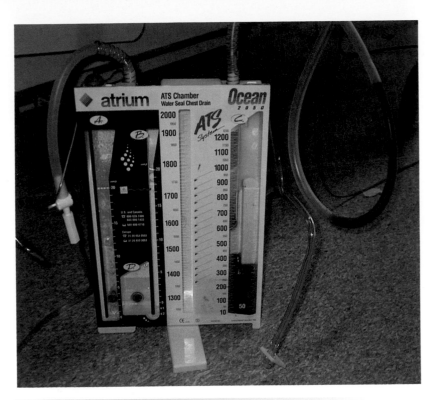

FIGURE 63.2 Underwater seal chest drain.

www.wiley.com/go/perioperativemed

VIDEO 63.1 An intercostal catheter collection system consists of three separate chambers which allow removal of air and fluid and provision of negative pressure to the pleural space.

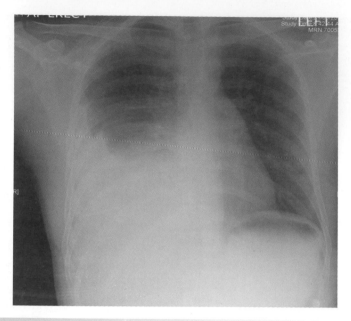

FIGURE 63.3 **Right haemothorax.**

The vast majority of lung injuries can be repaired. Rarely, lobectomy or pneumonectomy is required for uncontrollable air leak or bleeding. However, emergency pneumonectomy is associated with very poor survival rates (0–50%) [4]. Pulmonary contusion is present in approximately 30% of blunt chest trauma and is a risk factor for acute respiratory distress syndrome, pneumonia and prolonged ventilation. Management is supportive, aiming to keep the lungs dry, with ventilation strategies aimed at minimising barotrauma.

Cardiac injury

Penetrating cardiac injuries require immediate operative intervention. Temporising measures in ED thoracotomy can include using a Foley catheter to tamponade any chamber breach or placing a clamp across a torn atrial appendage. Blunt cardiac trauma has been associated with tricuspid valve disruption which can be surgically repaired once the patient has been stabilised.

Major vascular injury

Generally, the patient will only reach the hospital alive with such an injury if it has self-tamponaded or is contained. Aortic transection occurs as the result of sudden deceleration causing a tear at a relatively 'fixed' point of the aorta (where the descending aorta gives rise to the left subclavian artery). This injury can be treated with endovascular stenting. Other vascular injuries can be directly sutured, bypassed or ligated, depending on their nature and position.

Chest wall and diaphragm

Chest wall injuries are the main cause of bleeding after thoracic trauma. Rib fractures occur frequently (Figure 63.4). Fracture of the first rib or scapula indicates a significant force and is invariably associated with other injuries. Flail chest is a condition of paradoxical chest wall movement due to three or more ribs fractured in more than one place creating a floating segment of chest wall (Video 63.2). Often associated with pulmonary contusion, flail chest is a risk for respiratory failure and will often require invasive ventilator support. There is increasing evidence to support operative management of these patients with rib fixation [5].

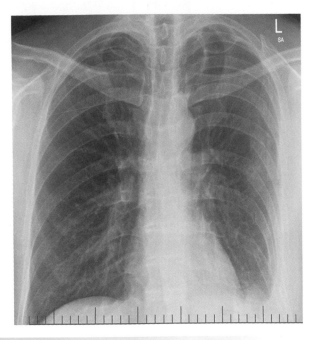

FIGURE 63.4 **Multiple left posterior rib fractures.**

www.wiley.com/go/perioperativemed

VIDEO 63.2 **A video demonstrating a flail chest injury with free-floating flail segment.**

Diaphragmatic injuries are notoriously difficult to identify on standard imaging modalities unless there is obvious herniation of abdominal contents into the chest. Thoracoscopy is the gold standard screening tool if there is a high degree of suspicion. Diaphragmatic injuries can be corrected by either a thoracic or abdominal approach, the choice often being dictated by other injuries.

References

1. Fitzgerald M, Mackenzie CF, Marasco S, Hoyle R, Kossmann T. Pleural decompression and drainage during trauma reception and resuscitation. *Injury*, 2008;**39**(1):9–20. doi:10.1016/j.injury.2007.07.021

2. Bastos R, Baisden CE, Harker L, Calhoon JH. Penetrating thoracic trauma. *Seminars in Thoracic and Cardiovascular Surgery*, 2008;**20**(1):19–25. doi:10.1053/j.semtcvs.2008.01.003

3. Hunt PA, Greaves I, Owens WA. Emergency thoracotomy in thoracic trauma – a review. *Injury*, 2006;**37**(1):1–19. doi:10.1016/j.injury.2005.02.014

4. Martin MJ, McDonald JM, Mullenix PS, Steele SR, Demetriades D. Operative management and outcomes of traumatic lung resection. *Journal of the American College of Surgeons*, 2006;**203**(3):336–344. doi:10.1016/j.jamcollsurg.2006.05.009

5. Marasco SF, Davies AR, Cooper J, et al. Prospective randomized controlled trial of operative rib fixation in traumatic flail chest. *Journal of the American College of Surgeons*, 2013;**216**(5):924–932. doi:10.1016/j.jamcollsurg.2012.12.024

Abdominal injuries

Katherine Martin

The Alfred Hospital, Australia

The trauma patient presents clinicians with the challenge of identifying all life-threatening and potentially disabling injuries in a timely fashion, and then prioritising the procedures and management required. Many of these injuries lie within the abdomen.

Epidemiology

Trauma is the leading cause of death in Australians between the ages of 1 and 44. Overall, it is the third leading cause of death, behind malignancy and cardiovascular disease. Injury accounts for nearly 10% of all deaths globally, with an age-standardised rate of 74.3 per 100,000 [1]. Haemorrhage is the most common cause of preventable death in trauma [2].

The majority of trauma in Australia and New Zealand occurs via blunt mechanisms. In the 12 months from July 2012 until June 2013, the Alfred Hospital in Melbourne, Victoria, admitted 1293 severely injured trauma and burn patients. Of these, 96% were injured as a result of blunt mechanism. Almost 500 of these severely injured patients sustained a significant abdominal injury, and 174 required laparotomy.

General perioperative considerations

Abdominal trauma

Injuries to the abdomen can involve many of the body's systems (Figure 64.1).

Trauma reception and resuscitation

Trauma reception and resuscitation are the co-ordinated, systematic approach to the assessment and treatment of the trauma patient. The advanced trauma life support (ATLS) programme is widely regarded as the gold standard in the early management of trauma victims. The systematic attention to airway, breathing and circulation, with assessment and simultaneous treatment of immediately life-threatening injuries, can be applied to trauma patients regardless of mechanism, age or gender (refer to Chapter 58 Trauma: pretheatre management) [3].

Perioperative Medicine for the Junior Clinician, First Edition. Edited by Joel Symons, Paul Myles, Rishi Mehra and Christine Ball.
© 2015 John Wiley & Sons, Ltd. Published 2015 by John Wiley & Sons, Ltd.
Companion website: www.wiley.com/go/perioperativemed

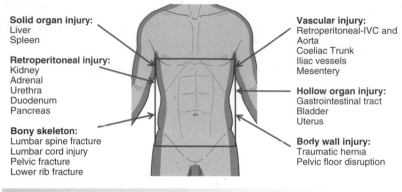

Solid organ injury:
Liver
Spleen

Retroperitoneal injury:
Kidney
Adrenal
Urethra
Duodenum
Pancreas

Bony skeleton:
Lumbar spine fracture
Lumbar cord injury
Pelvic fracture
Lower rib fracture

Vascular injury:
Retroperitoneal-IVC and
Aorta
Coeliac Trunk
Iliac vessels
Mesentery

Hollow organ injury:
Gastrointestinal tract
Bladder
Uterus

Body wall injury:
Traumatic hernia
Pelvic floor disruption

FIGURE 64.1 Injuries of the abdomen.

Preoperative assessment

The preoperative assessment of the trauma patient ideally begins with the involvement of the anaesthetist in the resuscitation room. Specific attention should be paid to the following aspects of initial assessment, in the patient with abdominal trauma.

- *Airway:* Patients will often have a full stomach, and are at risk of vomiting and aspiration. Suspicion of lumbar spine injury may prevent the patient from sitting up.
- *Breathing:* Intra-abdominal injury resulting in splinting of the diaphragm, and associated chest injury including rib fractures, haemothorax, pneumothorax, pulmonary contusions and diaphragm rupture can result in impaired mechanical ventilation and gas exchange. Hypovolaemia results in tachypnoea. Both chest injury and hypovolaemia result in increased work of breathing, and therefore increased CO_2 production. Early intubation and mechanical ventilation should be considered in these patients.
- *Circulation*: The abdomen is the most common source of blood loss in hypotensive trauma patients. Bleeding may be intraperitoneal or extraperitoneal, and is often from multiple sources. Clinical examination of the abdomen is only reliable if positive findings such as seatbelt bruising, distension or peritonism are present. FAST is commonly used in the assessment of the hypotensive patient (refer to Chapter 58 Trauma: pretheatre management). The identification of free intraperitoneal fluid in a hypotensive patient indicates bleeding until proven otherwise. Pelvic fractures seen on plain radiograph also indicate a potential source of blood loss. Resuscitation should focus on restoring blood volume using blood products in preference to crystalloid.

Adjuncts to the primary survey include ECG, urinary catheter (and examination of the urine for haematuria), venous bloods for FBE, U&E, clotting profile and cross-match. Women of child-bearing age should have a serum beta-human chorionic gonadotrophin (HCG) performed.

The secondary survey involves a thorough head-to-toe examination of the patient. This is then followed by specific investigations. CT scan with arterial phase intravenous contrast, from the eighth thoracic vertebra to beyond the pubic symphysis, is the investigation of choice in patients with evidence of abdominal injury [4]. Patients who have sustained an injury which makes clinical examination of

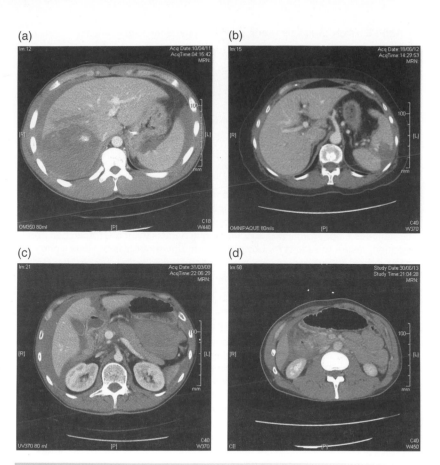

FIGURE 64.2 **Abdominal injuries seen on CT scan.** (a) Hepatic laceration with evidence of arterial bleeding. (b) Splenic laceration with evidence of arterial bleeding. (c) Hepatic injury with associated pancreatic laceration and large-volume haemoperitoneum. (d) Periduodenal haematoma and free gas suggestive of duodenal injury.

the abdomen difficult (for example, traumatic brain injury) also benefit from CT to exclude most intra-abdominal injuries. Figure 64.2 depicts examples of intra-abdominal injuries seen on CT scan. It should be noted that patients who remain hypotensive despite resuscitation, or only transiently respond to resuscitation, are generally not safe to scan in most institutions.

If the anaesthetist has not been involved in the initial assessment, they should endeavour to receive a verbal handover at the bedside from the physician who has been the team leader thus far. A useful acronym used by prehospital and in-hospital personnel is **MIST**:

- **M**echanism and time of injury
- **I**njuries found or suspected
- **S**ymptoms and signs
- **T**reatment initiated.

The **AMPLE** history is another useful acronym commonly used in trauma:

* **A**llergies
* **M**edications
* **P**ast Illness/**P**regnancy
* **L**ast Meal
* **E**vents/**E**nvironment related to injury.

Prior to any surgical procedure being undertaken for abdominal trauma, a thorough assessment of the trunk should be performed, with particular attention to the following.

Ventilation

High-energy blunt abdominal trauma is commonly associated with chest injury. Pneumothoraces may not be seen on supine or erect CXR and patients ideally should have a CT scan of the trunk. If not, reassessment via palpation (feeling for subcutaneous emphysema) and auscultation is necessary. If a CT scan has been performed, review to assess for obvious pneumothorax or less obvious signs such as subcutaneous gas, particularly if associated with rib fractures. If a CT scan has not been performed, and rib fractures are present or there has been a clinical suspicion for pneumothorax, then a repeated CXR in the erect position should be taken.

Assessment of circulation and volume of blood loss

The abdomen is a common source of bleeding in hypovolaemic trauma patients; it may contain 3–5 L in a 70 kg male. Tachypnoea, tachycardia, hypotension or a narrowed pulse pressure, peripheral pallor and clamminess all indicate intravascular hypovolaemia. The preoperative assessment must include taking note of the following.

* *Fluid resuscitation*: fluid given during the resuscitation (both en route to hospital and on arrival), and the response to this treatment should be noted. A massive transfusion may still be in progress on transfer of the patient to theatre.
* *Core body temperature*: hypothermia is associated with coagulopathy and increased mortality. Every effort should be made to rewarm cold patients and maintain body heat.
* *Arterial blood gas analysis*: base deficit is a marker of tissue perfusion. A base deficit >8 indicates significant tissue hypoperfusion, and is an important predictor of the need for operative intervention for bleeding [5].
* *Evidence of adequate end-organ perfusion*: urine output and conscious state.
* Timing of most recent venous blood analysis should be noted. FBE, U&E and clotting profile should be repeated regularly while active resuscitation is ongoing and definitive control of bleeding is yet to be achieved.

Thoracolumbar spine assessment

Thoracolumbar spine assessment (refer to Chapter 61 Spinal injuries) requires a complete radiological assessment. This may be via CT scan or plain radiographs. Where possible, the thoracolumbar spine should be assessed prior to operative intervention in order to facilitate patient positioning during the procedure, and on extubation.

Conclusion

Major trauma is common. Medical professionals involved in the management of these patients need a sound understanding of the principles of the initial assessment, in order to quickly identify life-threatening intra-abdominal injury.

Patients requiring surgical intervention for abdominal injury are often bleeding and require urgent transfer to theatre. Surgical and anaesthetic staff work together to resuscitate the patient and achieve definitive control of bleeding, thus minimising preventable morbidity and mortality.

References

1. Lozano R, Naghavi M, Foreman K, et al. Global and regional mortality from 235 causes of death for 20 age groups in 1990 and 2010: a systematic analysis for the Global Burden of Disease Study 2010. *Lancet*, 2012;**380**(9859):2095–2128. doi:10.1016/S0140-6736(12)61728-0

2. Kauvar DS, Lefering R, Wade CE. Impact of hemorrhage on trauma outcome: an overview of epidemiology, clinical presentations, and therapeutic considerations. *Journal of Trauma*, 2006;**60**(6 Suppl):S3–11. doi:10.1097/01.ta.0000199961.02677.19

3. American College of Surgeons. *Advanced Trauma Life Support (ATLS)*, 9th edn. Chicago, IL: American College of Surgeons, 2012.

4. Hoff WS, Holevar M, Nagy KK, et al. Practice management guidelines for the evaluation of blunt abdominal trauma: the East Practice Management Guidelines Work Group. *Journal of Trauma*, 2002;**53**(3):602–615. doi:10.1097/01.TA.0000025413.43206.97

5. Ordonez CA, Badiel M, Pino LF, et al. Damage control resuscitation: early decision strategies in abdominal gunshot wounds using an easy 'ABCD' mnemonic. *Journal of Trauma and Acute Care Surgery*, 2012;**73**(5):1074–1078. doi:10.1097/TA.0b013e31826fc780

65 Burns

Jamie Smart

The Alfred Hospital, Australia

Burn injury is a common form of trauma. Carelessness, inattention, alcohol, drugs and pre-existing medical problems are all significant contributors. Total body surface area (TBSA) burned (>40%), increasing age (>60 years) and inhalation injury are the three major risk factors for mortality [1].

Pathophysiology

Burns cause local injury and the release of inflammatory mediators. Effective resuscitation can limit the size of the local injury.

If the tissue damage is of significant size (>10–15%), circulating mediators of inflammation are released, triggering a systemic inflammatory response. Clinical features include (normal) tissue oedema, tachycardia and tachypnoea, fever and leucocytosis (Figure 65.1).

Burn shock

'Burn shock' describes a state of poor tissue and organ perfusion following major burn injury, with decreased intravascular volume, increased systemic vascular resistance and reduced cardiac output [2].

Circulating inflammatory mediators disrupt the integrity of the microcirculation in all tissues. Proteins move out of the intravascular space, decreasing intravascular colloid osmotic pressure and allowing an outpouring of fluids into the interstitial space [3]. This leads to decreased tissue perfusion and ultimately multiorgan failure.

Effective resuscitation restores capillary integrity to near normal and reduces morbidity and mortality. The Parkland Formula remains the gold standard for fluid resuscitation. It is inexpensive and effective. No other formula improves outcome (Table 65.1). Subsequent fluid administration should be based on endpoints of resuscitation, with urinary output the most easily monitored. The Parkland Formula recommends the use of a balanced salt, crystalloid (Hartmann's) solution.

Over-resuscitation: fluid creep

'Fluid creep' refers to the use of volumes beyond recognised protocols leading to worsening oedema and increased complications. Lung injury, compartment syndromes and death have been associated with over-resuscitation [4]. Colloids,

Perioperative Medicine for the Junior Clinician, First Edition. Edited by Joel Symons, Paul Myles, Rishi Mehra and Christine Ball.
© 2015 John Wiley & Sons, Ltd. Published 2015 by John Wiley & Sons, Ltd.
Companion website: www.wiley.com/go/perioperativemed

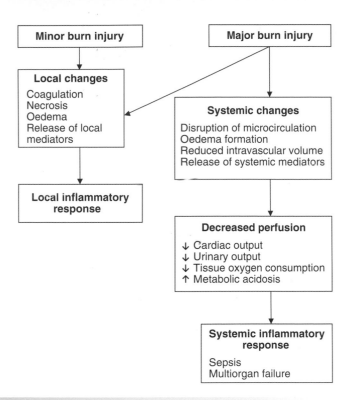

FIGURE 65.1 **The pathophysiology of burn injury.**

hypertonic saline and albumin have all been used to decrease the administered volume of fluid, but as there is no evidence of improved outcome, it is difficult to justify their use in the acute setting.

Inhalation injury

Inhalation injury is a predictor of morbidity and mortality and is classified according to the site of damage.

- *Upper airway injury*: superheated air or steam damages airway mucosa, leading to early airway oedema and rapid, life-threatening obstruction.
- *Lower respiratory tract injury*: relates to the direct effects of the toxic products of combustion. Chemicals dissolve in the mucosa causing membrane damage, ulceration, necrosis and oedema.
- *Systemic intoxication*: carbon monoxide combines readily with haemoglobin. The resulting compound, carboxyhaemoglobin, significantly reduces the oxygen-carrying capacity of blood. Suspect this in patients caught in fires in enclosed spaces (Table 65.2). Co-oximetry is the investigation of choice. Treatment of carbon monoxide poisoning is 100% oxygen, decreasing the half-life of carboxyhaemoglobin from 240 min to 40 min. There is no evidence that hyperbaric oxygen provides a significantly better outcome.
- *Systemic inflammatory response*: the lungs can also be affected by systemic inflammation with loss of endothelial integrity and oedema formation.

TABLE 65.1 The Parkland Formula

	Age Formula
Adults	3–4 mL crystalloid/kg body weight/%TBSA burn (e.g. Hartmann's solution)
Children	3–4 mL crystalloid/kg body weight/%TBSA burn (e.g. Hartmann's solution) plus maintenance (5% glucose +/– 20 mmol KCl in 0.45% saline) Maintenance: 100 mL/kg up to 10 kg plus 50 mL/kg from 10–20 kg plus 20 mL/kg for each kg over 20 kg

Volume calculated is an estimate of fluid requirements in the first 24 hours. Half of volume should be administered in the first 8 hours, from the time of injury.

TABLE 65.2 Signs and symptoms of carbon monoxide poisoning

COHb%	Symptoms
0–15	None
15–20	Headache, confusion
20–40	Nausea and vomiting, disorientation
40–60	Hallucinations, fits, coma
>60	Death

COHb, carboxyhaemoglobin.

Hypermetabolism

The inflammatory response to major burn injury drives a hypermetabolic state which develops in proportion to the size of the burn. Metabolic rate increases to 1.5 times normal but is greatly influenced by ambient temperature. Keeping patients at a thermoneutral temperature (28–32°) minimises the increase in metabolic rate. Feeding should be commenced early to match nutritional needs.

Coagulation

Both the thrombotic and fibrinolytic systems become activated. In the acute phase, clotting factors decrease due to consumption and haemodilution [5]. Later a thrombogenic state develops, making thromboprophylaxis essential.

Infection and sepsis

Immune suppression causes an increased risk of infection. Any infection should be investigated and treated promptly, with antibiotic therapy directed by the results of microbial cultures [6].

Pharmacology

Pharmacokinetics alter significantly in burn injury. Drug clearance, total body water and plasma proteins levels are all affected. Drug administration must be tailored to the individual patient.

The muscle relaxant suxamethonium should not be used after 48 hours due to the risk of an exaggerated, potentially fatal flux of potassium following depolarisation of extrajunctional skeletal muscle acetylcholine receptors.

Initial evaluation and resuscitation

History

A comprehensive history is vital and should be directed to burn factors and patient factors.

A – Airway

The airway should be reviewed and the cervical spine controlled. Assess for airway burns, as obstruction from oedema may be rapid (Box 65.1). If there is any doubt or concern, intubate early. Impending airway obstruction is best managed by an anaesthetist with skilled assistance (refer to Chapter 14 Airway assessment and planning).

B – Breathing

Administer 100% oxygen. Observe the breathing pattern and provide ventilatory assistance if necessary. Circumferential chest burns may severely compromise breathing, in which case early escharotomy is indicated.

C – Circulation

Control any obvious haemorrhage and assess for potential blood loss. Insert two large-bore cannulae through intact skin. Commence fluid resuscitation as per the Parkland Formula.

D – Disability/Neurological Status

The common causes for decreased consciousness include head injury, carbon monoxide, alcohol, drugs, epilepsy, hypoxaemia and shock.

E – Exposure

Assess the depth and size of the burn. Burn depth can be classified as superficial or partial (confined to epidermis and dermis) or full thickness (destruction of dermis).

BOX 65.1 Factors associated with airway burn

Facial involvement
Singed nasal hairs
Hoarse voice
Productive cough
Carbonaceous sputum
Stridor
Obstructive respiratory pattern

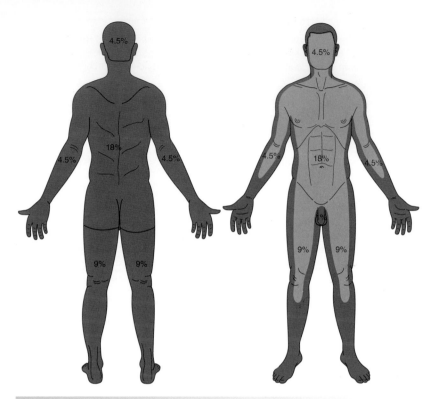

FIGURE 65.2 **The rule of 9s for assessing burn size.**

Size of the burn (%TBSA) is commonly assessed using the 'rule of 9s' (Figure 65.2).

Other considerations include a secondary survey, analgesia, early surgery and transfer to a burns centre (Box 65.2).

Preoperative preparation

Preoperative assessment of the burns patient should take particular note of:

- preoperative condition, cardiorespiratory status and temperature
- extent of injury and proposed surgery
- airway issues
- vascular access
- availability of blood products
- fasting guidelines
- communication with ICU, surgeons and theatre.

Initial excision and biological closure

Surgical management involves early excision and grafting, with the aim of eliminating all burned tissue. The benefits of this approach include decreased rates of sepsis, less overall blood loss, fewer respiratory complications and decreased mortality.

Pain management

Good pain management reduces the incidence of complications such as chronic pain, anxiety, depression and post-traumatic stress disorder (refer to Chapter 93 Acute pain, Chapter 94 Neuropathic pain and Chapter 95 The chronic pain patient).

Effective pain management requires a multimodal approach, targeted at the different types of pain experienced by the patient:

* background pain – a constant nociceptive pain
* breakthrough pain
* procedural pain – dressing changes, baths and mobilisation
* neuropathic pain.

References

1. Ryan CM, Schoenfeld DA, Thorpe WP, Sheridan RL, Cassem EH, Tompkins RG. Objective estimates of the probability of death from burn injuries. *New England Journal of Medicine*,1998;**338**(6):362–366. doi:10.1056/Nejm199802053380604

2. Latenser BA. Critical care of the burn patient: the first 48 hours. *Critical Care Medicine*, 2008;**37**(10):2819–2826.

3. Demling RH. The burn edema process: current concepts. *Journal of Burn Care and Rehabilitation*, 2005;**26**(3):207–227.

4. Rex S. Burn injuries. *Current Opinion in Critical Care*, 2012;**18**(6):671–676. doi:10.1097/Mcc.0b013e328359fd6e

5. Lavrentieva A. Replacement of specific coagulation factors in patients with burn: a review. *Burns*, 2013;**39**(4):543–548. doi:10.1016/j.burns.2012.12.009

6. MacLennan N, Heimbach DM, Cullen BF. Anesthesia for major thermal injury. *Anesthesiology*, 1998;**89**(3):749–770. doi:10.1097/00000542-199809000-00027

65

66 Bleeding disorders

Paul Coughlan

Eastern Health and Monash University, Australia

Recognised haemostatic disorders that increase the perioperative risk of bleeding include the following.

- Coagulation factor deficiencies
  - Von Willebrand disease (vWD)
  - Haemophilia A (factor VIII deficiency)
  - Haemophilia B (factor IX deficiency)
  - Rare clotting factor deficiencies
- Thrombocytopenia and platelet function defects
- Acquired clotting factor deficiencies
  - Liver failure
  - Disseminated intravascular coagulation
  - Acquired factor VIII inhibitor
- Connective tissue disorders
- Therapeutic anticoagulation/antiplatelet medication

Pathophysiology

Normal haemostasis is activated by disruption of the endothelial lining of blood vessels. Conceptually, this process is divided into primary haemostasis and coagulation but in reality they act co-operatively (Figure 66.1; Video 66.1).

Primary haemostasis (platelet activation and recruitment)

Tissue damage leads to binding and activation of von Willebrand factor (vWF) which binds platelet surface receptors, leading to adhesion. Additional platelet binding results in a haemostatic platelet plug.

Von Willebrand factor is synthesised in endothelial cells and secreted into the blood and subendothelial matrix. A significant amount of vWF is retained in Weibel-Palade bodies and can be released either by stress/trauma or by therapeutically administering desmopressin (DDAVP).

Perioperative Medicine for the Junior Clinician, First Edition. Edited by Joel Symons, Paul Myles, Rishi Mehra and Christine Ball.
© 2015 John Wiley & Sons, Ltd. Published 2015 by John Wiley & Sons, Ltd.
Companion website: www.wiley.com/go/perioperativemed

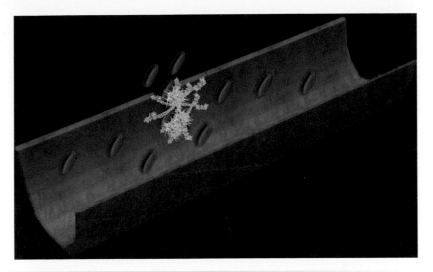

FIGURE 66.1 The concurrent processes of primary haemostasis and the coagulation cascade. The result is a process that reduces and eventually stops blood loss. In this figure, activated platelets and thrombin act together to form a plug.

www.wiley.com/go/perioperativemed

VIDEO 66.1 Coagulation is divided into two processes: primary haemostasis and the coagulation cascade. Whilst conceptually separate, both of these processes occur in parallel. The result is a thrombin mesh to stem bleeding.

Coagulation

Tissue injury exposes tissue factor (TF) which, together with activated factor VII, activates factor X. Factor Xa cleaves and activates prothrombin, forming thrombin and activating a feedback loop with co-factors V and VIII, and factors IX and XI. Further thrombin production generates fibrin from fibrinogen, leading to a haemostatic clot.

Where thrombin production is decreased, such as in haemophilia, not only is clot formation delayed but the quality and stability are poor, leading to a high risk of delayed rebleeding.

Physical factors are also important in haemostasis, including vessel wall spasm and physical compression by tamponade, which explains why patients with connective tissue disorders are at increased risk of post-traumatic bleeding (e.g. corticosteroids, Ehlers–Danlos).

Coagulation and platelet activation have limited capacity to stop bleeding from larger vessels. It is therefore absolutely critical in patients with bleeding disorders that careful surgical technique is employed and tissue disruption is kept to a minimum. The simplest operation with least surgical trauma by the most skilful surgeon will give the best haemostatic outcome.

Principles of management of the patient with a known bleeding disorder

Establish a precise diagnosis of the bleeding disorder. Take a clinical history of the patient's individual and family bleeding problems. Re-establish normal haemostasis preoperatively. Continue treatment until the risk of surgical bleeding has passed.

Von Willebrand disease [1] (Table 66.1)

Patients with vWD usually have a history of bleeding together with abnormal vWF levels. Patients with known Type II or III disease should be managed in conjunction with a haematologist (preferably the regional haemophilia centre). Patients with Type I vWD should have had a trial DDAVP infusion demonstrating an appropriate haemostatic response. DDAVP is a derivative of ADH. It stimulates the release of vWF from endothelial storage bodies and effects last several hours.

Minor procedures may be managed with perioperative oral tranexamic acid.

For other surgery with low bleeding risk, treat with tranexamic acid 1 g orally three times daily (commencing preoperatively) for 72 hours post procedure, together with a pre-procedure dose of DDAVP (30 mcg/kg by slow IV infusion). Patients having major surgery usually require further doses of DDVAP or vWF infusions and should be co-managed with a haematologist. Repeated doses of DDAVP can cause clinically significant hyponatraemia and appropriate monitoring is required.

Haemophilia

Haemophilia (A or B) is an X-linked inherited deficiency of either factor VIII or factor IX. Rarely, female carriers may have a mild bleeding disorder.

Haemophilia patients having surgery should be managed in a regional haemophilia centre [2]. All patients with moderate (<5% factor level) or severe (<1%) disease should have a treatment plan in place for management of spontaneous bleeds or surgical procedures.

Occasionally patients with mild haemophilia (factor level >5%) will be identified incidentally preoperatively because they have a prolonged APTT or, possibly, a mild bleeding history. These patients require careful assessment by a haematologist.

TABLE 66.1 Von Willebrand disease

	Type I	Type II	Type III
	Mild/moderate deficiency of vWF	Functional abnormality of vWF	Severe deficiency of vWF
Clinical spectrum	Mild. May be asymptomatic. Post-traumatic bleeding	Variable	Severe bleeding disorder. Similar to haemophilia
Frequency	Common	Uncommon	Rare
Inheritance	Autosomal dominant	Variable	Recessive
Screening tests	APTT – normal or mildly prolonged PFA-100 usually abnormal	APTT, PFA-100 variably abnormal	APTT, PFA-100 markedly abnormal
Further testing	vWF antigen, vWF activity Factor VIII level	vWF antigen, vWF activity Factor VIII level Multimer analysis	vWF antigen, vWF activity Factor VIII level Molecular studies
Perioperative treatment options	Tranexamic acid DDAVP vWF concentrate (not usually required)	Tranexamic acid DDAVP (contraindicated in Type IIB) vWF concentrate	vWF concentrate

APTT, activated partial thrombin time; DDAP, desmopressin; vWF, von Willebrand factor.

The routine use of clotting factor concentrates should be avoided as it can lead to inhibitor formation, thereby transforming patients into a severe phenotype.

Thrombocytopenia

In general, a platelet count $>100 \times 10^9$/L is safe for major surgery and $>50 \times 10^9$/L is adequate for minor procedures.

For elective procedures where platelet counts fall below these threshold levels, careful assessment is required (Box 66.1). Underlying problems such as liver disease (especially hepatitis C), portal hypertension, drug side effects, lymphoproliferative disorders, consumptive coagulopathy, primary bone marrow disease and inherited thrombocytopenias need to be considered. In the absence of an obvious underlying disease, undiagnosed idiopathic thrombocytopenic purpura (ITP) is likely and a short course of prednisolone (e.g. 0.5–1.0 mg/kg for 7–10 days) preoperatively may well correct the thrombocytopenia. High-dose IV immunoglobulin (1 g/kg) may also be appropriate if a response is required in a shorter time. For urgent surgery, platelet transfusion immediately preoperatively may be appropriate with further transfusions intraoperatively and/or post procedure as required.

Assessment of a patient for risk of perioperative bleeding

This is a common clinical scenario: a patient has a past history of perioperative bleeding. Are they at risk of perioperative bleeding in future?

Factors to consider include the following.

- What was the nature of the previous bleeding event?
- What was the surgical procedure?
- Was red cell transfusion required at the time?
- Has the patient had other surgical procedures and if so, what was the outcome (e.g. appendicectomy, cholecystectomy, dental extractions, circumcision)?
- In female patients, are periods abnormally heavy?
- Has bleeding or bruising after trauma been appropriate, e.g. minor trauma with major bruising?
- Has the patient ever had unprovoked (or minimally provoked) joint or muscle bleeding?
- Does the patient experience bleeding on a day-to-day basis with minor trauma?
- Is there a well-established family history of bleeding?
- Consider targeted testing [3] (Box 66.2).

Normal INR, APTT and platelet count do not in themselves reliably exclude a bleeding disorder. Moderate reductions in clotting factor levels do not necessarily cause abnormalities in routine coagulation tests. Variations in local laboratory reagents and assay methods will cause differing sensitivity to clotting factor deficiencies. The most useful predictor of perioperative bleeding is previous recurrent postoperative bleeding, unexpected need for transfusion or remedial surgical intervention.

References

1. Rodeghiero F, Castaman G, Tosetto A. How I treat von Willebrand disease. *Blood*, 2009;**114**(6):1158–1165. doi:10.1182/Blood-2009-01-153296

2. Australian Haemophilia Centre Directors' Organisation. *Guideline for the Management of Patients with Haemophilia Undergoing Surgical Procedures.* www.ahcdo.org.au/

3. Perry DJ, Todd T. *A Practical Guide to Laboratory Haemostasis.* www.practical-haemostasis.com

Human immunodeficiency virus infection

Anna Pierce

The Alfred Hospital, Australia

For people living with the human immunodeficiency virus (HIV), effective antiretroviral therapy (ART) has resulted in a reduction in mortality and increased life expectancy [1]. As a result, the HIV-infected population is ageing with an increasing number of co-morbidities, increasing the likelihood of requiring surgical interventions for both HIV-related and non-HIV-related conditions.

Human immunodeficiency virus infection itself is not a significant independent risk factor for major surgical procedures [2]. There are now many studies that demonstrate similar postoperative mortality in HIV-negative and HIV-infected patients [3]. Some studies have reported increased complications, particularly pneumonia, in patients with HIV, and others have shown poorer outcomes in those with lower CD4 cell counts [3]. More recently, a Canadian group reviewed patients undergoing surgical procedures in an attempt to identify factors that predict short-term postoperative mortality in patients with HIV [4]. They found that a diagnosis of acquired immune deficiency syndrome (AIDS) prior to surgery was not a risk factor for 30-day postoperative mortality; however, emergency hospital admission was a strong predictor of postoperative mortality. Other predictors included prior surgery, older age, CD4 cell count <200 cells/mL, Haemoglobin (Hb) <120 g/L or white cell count (WCC) >11 g/L within 90 days of surgery.

Preoperative assessment

In general, the preoperative assessment of the HIV-infected patient is similar to that for any other patient. Particular attention should be paid to co-morbidities that may present, some of which are more prevalent in HIV-infected patients.

Cardiovascular disease

There is an increased rate of coronary artery disease in HIV-infected patients and it is now an important cause of death. A number of factors contribute to this increased risk, including HIV infection itself, traditional cardiovascular risk factors and ART.

Perioperative Medicine for the Junior Clinician, First Edition. Edited by Joel Symons, Paul Myles, Rishi Mehra and Christine Ball.
© 2015 John Wiley & Sons, Ltd. Published 2015 by John Wiley & Sons, Ltd.
Companion website: www.wiley.com/go/perioperativemed

Liver disease

Patients with HIV may have hepatic dysfunction. This may be due to adverse effects from ART or co-existing liver disease. Patients may be co-infected with hepatitis B or hepatitis C and may be at risk of bleeding due to coagulopathy or thrombocytopenia.

Renal dysfunction

There is an increased prevalence of renal dysfunction in HIV-infected patients. This may be related to HIV itself or other causes, including ART, in particular tenofovir. Renal function should be assessed preoperatively as reduced renal function may affect the dosing of anaesthetic or other medications. In addition, if renal function deteriorates after surgery, the dosing of ART may also need to be altered.

Chronic pulmonary disease

Human immunodeficiency virus infection is associated with an increased risk of pulmonary disease. A large proportion of HIV-infected patients are smokers, and the risk of bacterial pneumonia is also increased. There is also an increased risk of postoperative pneumonia [3].

Diabetes

The prevalence of diabetes and insulin resistance is increased [5].

Thrombocytopenia

This is particularly important to assess in those with advanced liver disease, but may also be immune mediated (ITP) associated with HIV.

Neutropenia

Neutropenia may be associated with advanced immunosuppression, but may also be drug related, e.g. Bactrim or AZT.

Routine baseline assessment should include FBE, U&E, LFT, glucose and clotting profile.

In addition, HIV disease status should be assessed by history of opportunistic infections or other HIV-related complications, plus recent CD4 cell count and HIV viral load. CD4 cell count is used to assess degree of immune suppression and need for prophylaxis against opportunistic infections. As noted above, some studies have shown poorer outcomes in those with low CD4 cell counts, and one study showed improved outcomes when the viral load was suppressed below 30,000 copies/mL [3].

Perioperative management

During the preoperative period, antiretroviral therapy should be continued. If it is necessary to cease oral medications, all antiretroviral drugs should be discontinued to minimise the risk of development of drug resistance. It is particularly preferable not to cease ARTs in patients co-infected with hepatitis B virus (HBV) as ceasing the ART that also has activity against HBV may result in a flare of hepatitis.

The patient's HIV physician should be notified about the procedure and be made aware of their admission to hospital.

One of the major considerations in the HIV-infected patient presenting for surgery is the potential for drug interactions. ART are classified into four main classes.

* Reverse transcriptase inhibitors (of which there are two types: nucleoside/nucleotide reverse transcriptase inhibitors [NRTIs] and non-nucleoside reverse transcriptase inhibitors [NNRTIs])
* Protease inhibitors (PIs)
* Entry inhibitors
* Integrase inhibitors

A summary of these antiretrovirals may be found in Table 67.1.

Protease inhibitors and NNRTIs are metabolised via the cytochrome P450 system and have significant interactions with many other agents. In particular, the use of protease inhibitors and the benzodiazepines midazolam and triazolam is contraindicated. It is essential to assess for any potential drug interactions before

TABLE 67.1 Summary of the different types of ART drugs currently available

Drug class	Available drugs
Nucleoside reverse transcriptase inhibitor (NRTI)	Zidovudine (AZT) Lamivudine (3TC)* Abacavir Kivexa (abacavir/lamivudine) Trizivir (abacavir/lamivudine/zidovudine) Didanosine (DDI) Emtricitabine (FTC)* Tenofovir* Truvada (tenofovir/emtricitabine)
Non-nucleoside reverse transcriptase inhibitor (NNRTI)	Nevirapine Evavirenz Etravirine Rilpivirine
Protease inhibitor (PI)	Indinavir Saquinavir Lopinavir/ritonavir Fosamprenavir Atazanavir Tipranavir Darunavir Ritonavir
Entry inhibitor	Enfuvertide (T20) Maraviroc
Integrase inhibitor	Raltegravir Elvitegravir Dolutegravir
Combined agent	Atripla (tenofovir/emtricitabine/efavirenz) Eviplera (tenofovir/emtricitabine/rilpivirine)

*These drugs also have activity against hepatitis B.

new drugs are administered. Fortunately, there are no significant interactions with inhalational general anaesthetic agents.

Some useful online resources for ARTs include the following.

- University of Liverpool drug interactions site, available at www.hiv-drug interactions.org. An app for smart phones is also available
- *HIV Drug-Drug Interactions*, available at www.hivguidelines.org/clinical-guidelines/adults/hiv-drug-drug-interactions
- Department of Health and Human Services *Guidelines for the Use of Antiretroviral Agents in HIV-1 Infected Adults and Adolescents*, available at www.aidsinfo.nih.gov
- Johns Hopkins Poc-IT Center, available at www.hopkins-hivguide.org
- PDR Network, available at www.pdr.net
- Epocrates medical software, available at www.epocrates.com.

References

1. Antiretroviral Therapy Cohort Collaboration. Life expectancy of individuals on combination antiretroviral therapy in high-income countries: a collaborative analysis of 14 cohort studies. *Lancet*, 2008;**372**(9635):293–299. doi:10.1016/S0140-6736(08)61113-7

2. Harris HW, Schecter WP. Surgical risk assessment and management in patients with HIV disease. *Gastroenterology Clinics of North America*, 1997;**26**(2):377–391. doi:10.1016/s0889-8553(05)70300-9

3. Horberg MA, Hurley LB, Klein DB, et al. Surgical outcomes in human immunodeficiency virus-infected patients in the era of highly active antiretroviral therapy. *Archives of Surgery*, 2006;**141**(12):1238–1245. doi:10.1001/archsurg.141.12.1238

4. Wiseman SM, Forrest JI, Chan JE, et al. Factors predictive of 30-day postoperative mortality in HIV/AIDS patients in the era of highly active antiretroviral therapy. *Annals of Surgery*, 2012;**256**(1):170–176. doi:10.1097/SLA.0b013e318255896b

5. Stanley TL, Grinspoon SK. Body composition and metabolic changes in HIV-infected patients. *Journal of Infectious Diseases*, 2012;**205**(Suppl 3):S383–390. doi:10.1093/infdis/jis205

68 Exposure to blood-borne viruses

Anna Pierce

The Alfred Hospital, Australia

Occupational exposures to blood and body fluids occur frequently in healthcare workers (HCWs), putting them at risk of infection with blood-borne viruses such as human immunodeficiency virus (HIV), hepatitis B virus (HBV) and hepatitis C virus (HCV). As well as the possibility of infection and chronic illness, the HCW must also deal with the emotional and psychological stress of the exposure, and the potential long-term employment implications of viral infection.

Exposures that may put a HCW at risk of infection with blood-borne viruses include percutaneous injury (needlestick or cut with a sharp object) or contact of mucous membrane or non-intact skin (e.g. exposed skin that is chapped, abraded or has dermatitis) with blood, tissue or other body fluids that are potentially infectious [1].

Potentially infectious body fluids include blood, any body fluids containing visible blood, cerebrospinal fluid, synovial fluid, pleural fluid, peritoneal fluid, pericardial fluid and amniotic fluid. Semen and vaginal fluids have not been implicated in occupational transmission of HIV, HBV or HCV. Faeces, nasal secretions, saliva, sputum, sweat, tears, urine and vomitus are not considered potentially infectious unless they contain blood. The risk for transmission of HBV, HCV and HIV infection from these fluids and materials is extremely low [1].

Risk of infection after needlestick injury or other exposure

The risk of transmission varies between the different viruses, the immune status of the HCW (particularly for HBV), the nature of the injury received and the availability and use of postexposure prophylaxis (PEP) [2].

Human immunodeficiency virus

The average transmission risk is estimated to be 0.3% (95% CI 0.2–0.5%) [3] for percutaneous exposure to HIV-infected blood and 0.09% (95% CI 0.0006–0.5%) for mucous membrane exposure. Several factors have been identified as being

Perioperative Medicine for the Junior Clinician, First Edition. Edited by Joel Symons, Paul Myles, Rishi Mehra and Christine Ball.
© 2015 John Wiley & Sons, Ltd. Published 2015 by John Wiley & Sons, Ltd.
Companion website: www.wiley.com/go/perioperativemed

associated with increased transmission risk, including visible contamination of the device with blood, a procedure that involves a needle being placed directly into a vein or artery and a deep injury. In addition, the risk is also increased if the source has terminal illness. This probably reflects a higher HIV viral load in the source.

Hepatitis B virus

The risk of transmission of HBV is variable and is related to the titre of source HBV DNA. This correlates with the hepatitis B e-antigen (HBeAg) status of the source with the transmission risk ranging from 2% (source HBeAg negative) to 40% (source HBeAg positive) [4]. All HCWs should be vaccinated against HBV and postvaccination serology should be performed. HCWs are protected from infection if they have protective levels of hepatitis B surface antibody (HBsAb).

Hepatitis C virus

The average incidence of anti-HCV seroconversion after accidental percutaneous exposure from an HCV-positive source is 1.8% (range 0–7%) [5].

Management of a needlestick injury or other exposure to blood-borne viruses

All hospitals and healthcare organisations should have clear guidelines for the management of exposures to blood-borne viruses. This includes protocols for reporting of incidents, availability of experts for consultation (infectious diseases physicians, staff health physicians), mechanisms for timely source and HCW testing, and prescription of PEP if required. Outpatient follow-up of the HCW afterwards is also required.

First aid

Sites of needlestick injury and other skin sites should be washed with soap and water and an occlusive dressing applied. *Do not squeeze the site*. Mucous membranes should be rinsed with water immediately.

Report the incident immediately.

Evaluation of the exposure and the source

Any exposure that puts a HCW at potential risk of infection should be followed up. The most important thing to determine is the HIV, HBV and HCV status of the source, if this is not already known. The source patient should be informed that an exposure has occurred, and they should have serological testing for HIV, HBV and HCV.

Testing of the source should be done with appropriate counselling and consent as per applicable local laws [1].

The exposed HCW should also have blood taken for baseline serological testing for HBsAb, HIV and HCV. If the exposed HCW has protective HBsAb (≥ 10 IU/L), the source's results are all negative and there are no known risk factors for blood-borne viruses, no further follow-up is required.

Management and follow-up (Table 68.1)

Hepatitis B

When the source is negative for HBsAg and the exposed HCW is negative for HBsAb (< 10 IU/L) and does not have documented evidence of previously being vaccinated with a course of hepatitis B vaccination and/or antibodies > 10 IU/L, the HCW should be vaccinated.

If the source is positive for HBsAg and the exposed HCW has no documented evidence of being fully vaccinated or has been vaccinated but no documentation of ever having protective antibodies, hepatitis B immunoglobulin should be administered and vaccination initiated.

Human immunodeficiency virus

If the source is positive for HIV antibodies, an infectious diseases clinician should be contacted immediately to discuss the need for PEP. PEP should be initiated as soon as possible following exposure, preferably within two hours. If the source cannot be tested in a timely manner and is at high risk for HIV infection, PEP should be initiated and can be ceased if the source subsequently tests negative.

TABLE 68.1 Recommended follow-up schedule for healthcare workers

Source	Four weeks	Six weeks	Three months	Six months
Hep C positive		Hep C PCR Hep C Ab	Hep C Ab	Hep C Ab
HIV positive		HIV Ag/Ab	HIV Ag/Ab	
Unknown		Hep C Ab HIV Ag/Ab	Hep C Ab HIV Ag/Ab	Hep C Ab
Hep BsAg positive with recipient non-responder to vaccine	Second dose of HepB IgG (should have had first dose at time of exposure)		Hep B sAg	
High risk for Hep C* with negative serology at time of exposure		Hep C Ab	Hep C Ab	Hep C Ab
High risk for HIV* with negative serology at time of exposure		Hep C Ab HIV Ag/Ab	Hep C Ab HIV Ag/Ab	
Low risk with negative serology at time of exposure		Nil	Nil	Nil

*Definition of 'at risk' for:
HIV: men who have sex with men (MSM) with unprotected sex within the 6 weeks prior to the incident
Hep C: current intravenous drug user (IVDU) and/or MSM with unprotected sex within the 6 weeks prior to the incident.

Hepatitis C

If the source is positive for hepatitis C antibodies, further testing and follow-up are required. A test for hepatitis C RNA should be performed on the source blood to determine if the source has chronic hepatitis C infection. There is no PEP available for hepatitis C; HCWs exposed to an HCV-infected source should be followed up closely and referred for early treatment if seroconversion occurs.

References

1. US Public Health Service. Updated US Public Health Service guidelines for the management of occupational exposures to HBV, HCV, and HIV and recommendations for postexposure prophylaxis. *MMWR Recommendations and Reports*, 2001;**50**(RR-11):1–52.

2. National Institute for Occupational Safety and Health (NIOSH). *Preventing Needlestick Injuries in Health Care Settings.* Publication No. 2000-108. Cincinnati, OH: National Institute for Occupational Safety and Health, 1999. www.cdc.gov/niosh/docs/2000-108/pdfs/2000-108.pdf

3. Kuhar DT, Henderson DK, Struble KA, et al. Updated US Public Health Service guidelines for the management of occupational exposures to human immunodeficiency virus and recommendations for postexposure prophylaxis. *Infection Control and Hospital Epidemiology*, 2013;**34**(9):875–892. doi:0.1086/672271

4. Gerberding JL. Management of occupational exposures to blood-borne viruses. *New England Journal of Medicine*, 1995;**332**(7):444–451. doi:10.1056/NEJM199502163320707

5. Alter MJ. The epidemiology of acute and chronic hepatitis C. *Clinics in Liver Disease*, 1997;**1**(3):559–568. doi:10.1016/s1089-3261(05)70321-4

69 The patient with psychiatric illness

Steven Ellen[1] and James Olver[2]

[1] The Alfred Hospital and Monash University, Australia
[2] The University of Melbourne, Australia

Psychiatric disorders are common; about one in five people suffers a psychiatric disorder in any given year. In a hospital setting they are even more common; the added stress of being sick, the fear associated with being in hospital, and the physiological changes to the brain that accompany illness and treatments all exaggerate mental illness. It is important to recognise patients who have mental illness, to know when and how urgently to act and whether to seek specialist assistance. Psychiatric issues are often overlooked in the perioperative period but their recognition and treatment should be a minimum standard of care.

The three most typical psychiatric scenarios in the perioperative period are:

- pre-existing psychiatric conditions that impact on surgical care, e.g. a patient with schizophrenia awaiting an operation who needs medications adjusted or special care with communication
- psychiatric conditions which lead to surgical care, e.g. a suicide attempt which leads to an admission to a trauma unit
- surgical patients who develop a mental health complication, e.g. depression or delirium, after major surgery.

A psychiatric assessment in these circumstances should begin with a history and some basic questions such as:

- How do you feel you are coping?
- How long have you been feeling like this?
- How bad is it?
- Do you ever feel like giving up or are you suicidal?
- What help have you sought so far?
- Is there anything we can help with whilst you are in hospital?

Simple open questions work best, preferably in a calm environment. The clinical pressures presented by the perioperative environment often lead to rushed consultations where patients are less likely to be forthcoming. However, when time is short, a brief screen can still be done and the consultation can be completed later, often by other professionals. Nurses, social workers, psychologists and psychiatrists are all skilled in following up brief screens, and non-urgent problems can be referred to the family doctor.

Perioperative Medicine for the Junior Clinician, First Edition. Edited by Joel Symons, Paul Myles, Rishi Mehra and Christine Ball.
© 2015 John Wiley & Sons, Ltd. Published 2015 by John Wiley & Sons, Ltd.
Companion website: www.wiley.com/go/perioperativemed

Assessing the urgency of the situation is critical, particularly how quickly a review is needed and whether any increase in nursing observation level is required. If the patient has self-harmed, is agitated or aggressive, this will be crucial. Also, medications often need to be adjusted for surgery but some cannot be stopped suddenly – especially clozapine, lithium and benzodiazepines.

Finally, assess whether the patient requires specialist referral. Nearly all hospitals have access to allied health workers who are well versed in psychological assessment. Larger services will also have a 'consultation-liaison' (CL) psychiatry service. CL psychiatry, also known as psychological medicine or psychosomatic medicine, is the subspecialty of psychiatry that addresses mental health in medical settings. Basic advice (like medication changes) can sometimes be handled over the phone; more complex problems require formal assessment. All suicide attempts and any new diagnosis of a major mental disorder require formal assessment, and many other problems will benefit from psychiatric input – especially behaviour management (either in delirium or with personality problems), consent issues, psychological adjustment to illness or treatment, and unusual diagnostic dilemmas.

Common problems [1]

Delirium

Delirium in the postoperative period is very common and often missed, especially when presenting symptoms are those of depression (hypoactive delirium) and hallucinations or delusions (hyperactive delirium). It is important to note that delirium is characterised by a fluctuation of the conscious state so a normal assessment at one point does not exclude it. Overnight nursing notes are useful as delirium is often worse at night. Corroborative history can be sought from family and carers; they will be invaluable in reporting critical changes in delirium such as change of personality and behaviour over a period of days and alterations in memory, orientation and attention. Always do a cognitive test for any odd or atypical behaviour. The most popular is the Folstein Mini-Mental State Examination [2].

Depression [3]

Depression is a common cause of failure to adequately rehabilitate after surgery, leading to prolonged hospital stay and increased risks of postsurgical complications. Patients cannot concentrate, lack motivation and often have trouble explaining their mood. There are a number of screening tools available but simple enquiry about depressed mood and associated features such as feelings of guilt, failure, burden and hopelessness might uncover a problem that slows recovery and delays discharge if not recognised. Note that biological symptoms of depression such as sleep and appetite disturbance are non-specific in medically ill patients. Specific questions relating to thoughts of death and suicide should always be asked.

Psychiatric medications

Psychiatric medications often take years to be stabilised. In major psychiatric disorders, do not cease or change doses without checking why the drug was prescribed and liaising with the treating clinician. The risks need to be balanced and appreciated.

Self-harm

Self-harm always needs to be assessed. Do not dismiss it as a simple cry for help. Consider whether extra nursing observations are needed whilst awaiting a formal assessment.

Drug and alcohol problems

Drug and alcohol problems are common and often missed. Withdrawal for most begins within about 24 hours, which is often the postoperative period. Withdrawal symptoms can easily be mistaken for postoperative complications. Always check with the patient and if in doubt, institute appropriate withdrawal regimens. Alcohol and benzodiazepine withdrawals are easy to treat but can be life-threatening if missed. The simplest treatment is the tapered use of a long-acting benzodiazepine that is dosed according to the withdrawal symptoms measured on the alcohol withdrawal scale.

Schizophrenia and bipolar disorder

Patients with chronic psychiatric conditions such as schizophrenia and bipolar disorder can sometimes appear lacking in comprehension and may be mistaken for being intellectually impaired. This is usually not the case; it is far more likely to simply be an issue of communication style. It should not be assumed that these patients cannot consent and or that they do not need explanations. The surgery should be explained simply yet carefully, checking that they understand, and with an understanding of their communication style.

It is important to note that capacity and consent are specific for limited situations and are not generalisable. For example, a patient with schizophrenia may not be able to consent to psychiatric treatment but may have good understanding of their medical and surgical problems.

Advice should always be sought if there is any concern about the patient's competence to consent to a procedure.

References

1. Selzer R, Ellen S. *Psych-Lite: Psychiatry That's Easy to Read*. New York: McGraw-Hill, 2010.
2. Folstein MF, Folstein SE, McHugh PR. 'Mini-mental state'. A practical method for grading the cognitive state of patients for the clinician. *Journal of Psychiatric Research*, 1975;**12**(3):189–198.
3. Olver JS, Hopwood MJ. Depression and physical illness. *Medical Journal of Australia*, 2012;**1**(Suppl 4):9–12. doi:10.5694/Mjao12.10597

70 Obstetric patients having non-obstetric surgery

Maggie Wong

The Royal Women's Hospital and Monash University, Australia

Between 0.75% and 2% of pregnant women undergo non-obstetric surgery during pregnancy. The most common indications are intra-abdominal sepsis, trauma and malignancy. Appendicectomy is the most commonly performed procedure, with cholecystectomy ranking second.

Management goals

Refer to Table 70.1.

Physiological considerations

Discussion of the physiological changes of pregnancy can be found in standard texts; some major changes are mentioned below (Table 70.2).

The physiological changes of pregnancy are related to the hormonal effects (predominantly progesterone and oestrogen), the mechanical effects of the gravid uterus, which becomes an abdominal organ after 20 weeks gestation, the increased metabolic demand of the developing fetus and the dilated, low-resistance placental circulation, functionally resembling that of a shunt.

Pharmacological considerations [1]

There are significant pregnancy-related pharmacokinetic changes, namely increased volume of distribution, altered plasma protein binding, (physiological) hypoalbuminaemia, increased alpha-1 glycoprotein and altered drug clearance.

Pregnant patients will naturally have concerns about the effect of surgery and anaesthesia on the unborn child. To date, no anaesthetic agent has been clearly shown to be harmful to the human fetus, and women should be reassured prior to

Perioperative Medicine for the Junior Clinician, First Edition. Edited by Joel Symons, Paul Myles, Rishi Mehra and Christine Ball.
© 2015 John Wiley & Sons, Ltd. Published 2015 by John Wiley & Sons, Ltd.
Companion website: www.wiley.com/go/perioperativemed

TABLE 70.1 Maternal and fetal goals

Maternal goals	Fetal goals
Maintain physiological homeostasis	Maintain uteroplacental perfusion to minimise fetal asphyxia
	Minimise unnecessary drug exposure
	Minimise the risk of preterm labour and fetal loss

TABLE 70.2 Physiological considerations during pregnancy

Organ system	Changes	Consequences	Management
Respiratory	Mucosal oedema and tissue friability in upper airway	Increased risk of difficult laryngoscopy and intubation	Be prepared for a difficult airway – have the necessary equipment and assistance
	Reduced FRC and increased V/Q mismatch	Accelerated hypoxaemia during periods of apnoea	Adequate preoxygenation to minimise desaturation
	Progesterone-mediated increase in alveolar minute ventilation	More rapid onset of inhalation induction	
	Mechanical ventilation – hypocapnia	Uteroplacental vaso-constriction, left maternal oxyhaemoglobin dissociation curve shift, reducing oxygen delivery to fetus	Avoid hyperventilation
	Mechanical ventilation, CO_2 pneumoperitonem – hypercapnia	Limits gradient for CO_2 transfer to maternal blood leading to fetal acidosis	Increase ventilation to maintain normocapnia
Cardiovascular	Heart tilted anteriorly and leftward	ST/T wave changes, left axis deviation on ECG	Beware of misinterpreted ischaemic changes
	Greater increase in plasma volume than red cell mass	Physiological anaemia of pregnancy	
	Aortocaval compression (from second trimester)	Supine hypotensive syndrome	Lateral uterine tilt to maintain venous return and cardiac output
	Uteroplacental circulation: • low resistance system • perfusion mainly pressure dependent • not autoregulated	Maternal hypotension will lead to reduced uteroplacental flow	Maintain maternal blood pressure, alpha-adrenergic agonists being agents of choice
	Epidural veins engorgement (collateral venous return from lower extremities)	Compressed lumbar epidural/ intrathecal space, more extensive local anaesthetic spread	Reduced neuraxial local anaesthetic dosage
Gastrointestinal	Stomach displaced by gravid uterus Decreased lower oeso-phageal sphincter tone	Increased risk of reflux and aspiration	Combination antacid-antihistamine-2 (effervescent ranitidine) prophylaxis, rapid sequence induction
Haematological	Hypercoagulable state	Increased risk of thromboembolic complications	Thromboembolism prophylaxis

undergoing anaesthesia during pregnancy. When used in clinically relevant doses and concentrations, there is no proof of teratogenicity in humans of [2]:

- volatile agents
- barbiturates, ketamine, benzodiazepines
- opioids
- local anaesthetics
- muscle relaxants (these polar molecules do not cross the placenta in significant amounts).

While there is no specific recommendation on anaesthetic techniques, regional anaesthesia should be employed whenever possible to avoid complications of general anaesthesia in the pregnant population.

Specific anaesthetic medications that have been studied for teratogenic effects

With scavenging systems in place, studies have failed to show an association between nitrous oxide exposure and fetal loss and birth defects. The association between benzodiazepine (diazepam) use and craniofacial deformities (cleft palate, with or without cleft lip) has been refuted. Animal studies suggest anaesthetic agents influence early brain development by altering its anatomical organisation and causing functional consequences in the form of learning and memory deficit [3]. It is unclear whether results from animal studies can be extrapolated to the fetal brain.

Adverse fetal outcomes

These include premature labour, prematurity and fetal loss. Pregnancy outcomes following non-obstetric surgery are summarised in Table 70.3 [4].

Appendicitis with peritonitis is associated with a higher rate of adverse fetal outcome [4] and when compared with the non-pregnant population, appendiceal perforation is much more common in pregnant patients [5].

The laparoscopic approach is the preferred route to treat intra-abdominal pathology because of documented maternal benefits, i.e. reduced postoperative pain, faster recovery, shorter length of hospital stay, smaller incidence of thromboembolic events

TABLE 70.3 **Pregnancy outcomes following non-obstetric surgery [4]**

Event	Incidence
Maternal death	0.06%
Miscarriage	5.8% – all trimesters 10.5% – first trimester
Premature labour	3.5%
Fetal loss	2.5%
Prematurity	8.2%
Major birth defects (non-obstetric surgery in first trimester)	3.9% (1–3% in general population)

and lower rate of postoperative ileus [5]. However, concerns for fetal well-being during laparoscopic surgery include direct uterine and/or fetal trauma, fetal acidosis from carbon dioxide absorption and decreased uteroplacental blood flow from reduced maternal cardiac output secondary to raised intra-abdominal pressure.

Perioperative fetal monitoring and obstetric management

Antepartum fetal assessment should be performed to decrease the risk of intrauterine demise. Non-stress testing (NST), based on the coupling of palpable fetal movements and fetal heart rate (FHR) acceleration, generally forms the initial assessment tool. FHR variability and accelerations are observed in response to fetal movement [6]. Continuous FHR monitoring is feasible from 18 weeks gestation, and FHR variability can be monitored from 25 to 27 weeks gestation. Most term fetuses have many of these accelerations in a 20–30-minute period of recording, indicating the absence of acidosis. Premature, growth restricted and medicated or anaesthetised fetuses exhibit reduced fetal movement-FHR acceleration couplings. Less mature fetuses have smaller accelerations, but they should still demonstrate some degree of acceleration with palpated fetal movement. A non-reactive/abnormal NST, a sensitive marker for worsening hypoxaemia or acidosis, signifies a compromised fetus.

FHR measured by an external doppler ultrasound transducer together with the simultaneous documentation of uterine activity by an external tocodynamometer monitor comprises the cardiotocogram (CTG). Uterine activity seen on the CTG may indicate the onset of preterm labour. An obstetrician should be consulted on the appropriateness and interpretation of fetal monitoring and its management.

The American College of Obstetricians and Gynecologists Committee Opinion on Non-obstetric Surgery During Pregnancy [7] makes the following recommendations.

- A multidisciplinary team approach is important to optimise maternal and fetal safety.
- A pregnant woman should never be denied indicated surgery, regardless of trimester.
- Elective surgery should be postponed until after delivery.
- If possible, non-urgent surgery should be performed in the second trimester to minimise the risk of spontaneous abortion and premature labour.
- Surgery should be performed at an institution with obstetric and neonatal services.
- The decision to use fetal monitoring should be individualised.
  - If the fetus is considered *previable*, it is generally sufficient to confirm the fetal heart rate by doppler before and after surgery.
  - If the fetus is considered *viable*, as a minimum, CTG should be performed before and after surgery to assess fetal well-being and the absence of uterine activity.
  - Intraoperative fetal monitoring may be appropriate if the fetus is viable, monitoring is feasible, and caesarean delivery is possible during the planned surgery.

References

1. Gaiser R. Physiologic changes of pregnancy. In: Chestnut DH, Polley LS, Tsen LC, Wong CA, editors. *Chestnut's Obstetric Anesthesia: Principles and Practice*, 4th edn. Philadelphia, PA: Mosby Elsevier, 2009. doi:10.1016/b978-0-323-05541-3.00002-8

2. Van de Velde M. Nonobstetric surgery during pregnancy. In: Chestnut DH, Polley LS, Tsen LC, Wong CA, editors. *Chestnut's Obstetric Anesthesia: Principles and Practice*, 4th edn. Philadelphia, PA: Mosby Elsevier, 2009. doi:10.1016/b978-0-323-05541-3.00017-x

3. Palanisamy A. Maternal anesthesia and fetal neurodevelopment. *International Journal of Obstetric Anesthesia*, 2012;**21**(2):152–162. doi:10.1016/j.ijoa.2012.01.005

4. Cohen-Kerem R, Railton C, Oren D, Lishner M, Koren G. Pregnancy outcome following non-obstetric surgical intervention. *American Journal of Surgery*, 2005;**190**(3):467–473. doi:10.1016/j.amjsurg.2005.03.033

5. Bakker OJ. Systematic review and meta-analysis of safety of laparoscopic versus open appendicectomy for suspected appendicitis in pregnancy. *British Journal of Surgery*, 2012; **99**: 1470–1478. doi:10.1002/bjs.8890

6. Moaveni DM, Birnbach DJ, Ranasinghe JS, Yasin SY. Fetal assessment for anesthesiologists: are you evaluating the other patient? *Anesthesia and Analgesia*, 2013;**116**(6):1278–1292. doi:10.1213/ANE.0b013e31828d33c5

7. American College of Obstetricians and Gynecologists Committee on Obstetric Practice. ACOG Committee Opinion No. 474: Nonobstetric surgery during pregnancy. *Obstetrics and Gynecology*, 2011;**117**(2 part 1):420–421.

71 The elderly patient

Yana Sunderland

Northern Health, Australia

Surgical outcomes in the elderly

The elderly are increasingly represented amongst elective surgical patients, due to the ageing population and improved health status, as well as developments in surgical and medical expertise. Studies have shown that older patients have higher rates of postoperative complications and mortality [1,2].

This increased complication rate is mainly due to medical, rather than surgical complications. The elderly have increased frequency of common postoperative complications, as well as geriatric syndromes, such as delirium and falls. They are also at risk of deteriorating function, which can have a major impact on their quality of life, and may result in the need to move to institutional care [3].

Age and co-morbidity are both associated with increased risk of complications. Functional impairment (inability to perform activities of daily living independently), which is common in older patients, also increases adverse outcomes, including mortality [1–3].

Approach to the assessment of elderly patients

There is still no well-established approach to estimating perioperative risk in elderly patients. Traditional operative assessment tools such as the American Society of Anesthesiologists (ASA) physical classification system have some correlation with outcomes. However, more comprehensive scoring systems that include functional and co-morbidity scores, as well as markers of frailty such as falls and cognitive impairment, may better predict outcomes [3].

More recently, the Comprehensive Geriatric Assessment (CGA) has been used in preoperative assessment. The CGA is widely used in geriatric assessment and management of elderly medical patients. It involves multidimensional assessment that takes medical, functional, psychological and social factors into consideration. The CGA has shown improved outcomes in some surgical groups, such as orthopaedic patients undergoing elective arthroplasty [4]. It can be modified to suit a particular population, including surgical patients,

Perioperative Medicine for the Junior Clinician, First Edition. Edited by Joel Symons, Paul Myles, Rishi Mehra and Christine Ball.
© 2015 John Wiley & Sons, Ltd. Published 2015 by John Wiley & Sons, Ltd.
Companion website: www.wiley.com/go/perioperativemed

but should include key parameters such as a measure of cognition and function as well as medical co-morbidity.

Some of the key factors to be considered when assessing elderly patients are highlighted below.

Impact of the surgical condition

The impact of the surgical condition on the patient's health and quality of life is important in all patients, but may have a greater impact in the elderly. Common examples include poorly controlled pain in orthopaedic patients waiting for arthroplasty, leading to deconditioning. Similarly, inadequate iron replacement in iron-deficient patients waiting for colorectal surgery may increase the risk of postoperative transfusion.

Specific screening systems review

Cardiorespiratory system

Questions regarding shortness of breath and exercise tolerance are important, as symptoms of undiagnosed cardiovascular or respiratory disease may go unrecognised or be attributed to the ageing process by the patient. Similarly, ability to test exercise capacity may be limited due to mobility issues such as arthritis, so ischaemia or cardiac failure may be masked.

'Geriatric Giants'

The 'Geriatric Giants' are a group of syndromes found predominantly in the elderly. The importance of these syndromes is that they may mask underlying conditions and are markers of frailty and poorer postoperative outcomes.

Falls
Ask about falls in the last 12 months and review the circumstances. Look for undiagnosed cardiac (arrhythmias, valvular lesions) and neurological disease, cognitive or functional impairment. All patients who have had falls are at increased risk in the postoperative period.

Cognition
Patients with cognitive impairment have a higher risk of complications including delirium, falls and mortality. Common tools used for screening include the Abbreviated Mental Test (AMT), which is a 10-question screening test, and Folstein's Mini-Mental State Examination (MMSE), a 30-question test used in screening and assessment of dementia (refer to Chapter 69 The patient with psychiatric illness and Chapter 90 Postoperative delirium and postoperative cognitive dysfunction).

Continence
Patients with pre-existing continence issues are at increased risk of urinary retention, failing 'trials of void' and urinary tract infections. Continence issues can also lead to increased risk of other complications postoperatively, such as falls and delirium.

Medication review

The preoperative assessment is a good opportunity to review indications for all medications and cease any that are no longer required.

Limit NSAID use in the postoperative period as they increase the risk of stress ulcers and renal impairment. There are no clear guidelines pertaining to patients on multiple antihypertensive medications, though postoperative hypotension is very common in older surgical patients. Benzodiazepines may cause delirium, drowsiness and falls, so should be avoided postoperatively. However, patients on high chronic doses should be weaned gradually, to avoid a withdrawal syndrome.

Functional impairment and social history

Functional impairment is common and increases the risk of postoperative complications. Examples of screening tools include the Modified Barthel Index and the Katz Index of Independence of Daily Living.

Patients with functional impairment may benefit from preoperative intervention such as prescription of a gait aid, home modification or a preoperative exercise programme. Early postoperative allied health assessment for these patients is essential.

A social history detailing supports and living circumstances will aid in predicting the need for inpatient rehabilitation or support services.

Patient expectations and goals of care

Discussing the patient's goals and expectations regarding their surgery and recovery is important. Elderly patients may have unrealistic expectations regarding the benefits of surgery. They may attribute poor health from other conditions to their surgical condition. A more realistic expectation regarding benefits will help when making decisions to proceed.

When considering surgical risk in elderly patients, it is important to remember that deterioration of function and cognition can occur (refer to Chapter 90 Postoperative delirium and postoperative cognitive dysfunction). Most elderly patients consider cognitive and functional outcomes to be more important than mortality when considering an acceptable burden of treatment [5].

The preoperative period is a good time to ask if a patient has participated in advance care planning (refer to Chapter 20 Medical futility and end-of-life care). This is the process of considering future medical intervention and end-of-life care; it may involve appointment of a proxy in case the patient is unable to make medical decisions in the future. This process can help to clarify the patient's goals of treatment and help guide decision making with regard to intervention, if the surgical course is complicated.

References

1. Polanczyk CA, Marcantonio E, Goldman L, et al. Impact of age on perioperative complications and length of stay in patients undergoing noncardiac surgery. *Annals of Internal Medicine*, 2001;**134**(8):637–643. doi:10.7326/0003-4819-134-8-200104170-00008
2. Turrentine FE, Wang H, Simpson VB, Jones RS. Surgical risk factors, morbidity, and mortality in elderly patients. *Journal of the American College of Surgeons*, 2006;**203**(6):865–877. doi:10.1016/j.jamcollsurg.2006.08.026

3. Robinson TN, Eiseman B, Wallace JI, et al. Redefining geriatric preoperative assessment using frailty, disability and co-morbidity. *Annals of Surgery*, 2009;**250**(3):449–455. doi:10.1097/SLA.0b013e3181b45598

4. Harari D, Hopper A, Dhesi J, Babic-Illman G, Lockwood L, Martin F. Proactive care of older people undergoing surgery ('POPS'): designing, embedding, evaluating and funding a comprehensive geriatric assessment service for older elective surgical patients. *Age and Ageing*, 2007;**36**(2):190–196. doi:10.1093/ageing/afl163

5. Fried TR, Bradley EH, Towle VR, Allore H. Understanding the treatment preferences of seriously ill patients. *New England Journal of Medicine*, 2002;**346**(14):1061–1066. doi:10.1056/NEJMsa012528

Allergies and anaphylaxis

Helen Kolawole

Frankston Hospital and Monash University, Australia

Allergic reactions and anaphylaxis are infrequent but potentially life-threatening. During anaesthesia, they may occur immediately on induction when cardiovascular and respiratory physiology is often deranged. They may be resistant to prompt treatment and pose a challenge in identifying the cause of the reaction as many possible allergens are presented to perioperative patients.

The incidence of anaphylactic reactions in patients undergoing general anaesthesia is in the order of 1:3000 to 1:20,000 [1]. The mortality is 3–9% from severe reactions with 2% having significant residual brain damage [2].

In 10% of cases, only one defining sign is present, e.g. cardiac arrest or hypotension; 30% of patients have no cutaneous signs and this is more likely where there is significant hypotension.

The time between exposure to an IV agent and the reaction is usually 5–10 minutes, but it can be within seconds.

The pathological mechanism in most cases of perioperative anaphylaxis is allergic anaphylaxis, i.e. IgE mediated.

Management of anaphylaxis under anaesthesia [3]

The principles of management are termination of mast cell degranulation and interruption of the mediator-related cycle, modulation of vascular and bronchial smooth muscle tone, and replacement of intravascular volume.

Adrenaline

Adrenaline is pivotal in the management of anaphylaxis because it produces vasoconstriction and suppresses bronchoconstriction, increases cardiac output, and reduces mucosal oedema and mediator release.

Perioperative Medicine for the Junior Clinician, First Edition. Edited by Joel Symons, Paul Myles, Rishi Mehra and Christine Ball.
© 2015 John Wiley & Sons, Ltd. Published 2015 by John Wiley & Sons, Ltd.
Companion website: www.wiley.com/go/perioperativemed

There are also risks in administering adrenaline either from inadvertent overdose or increased patient sensitivity to adrenaline, e.g. extremes of age and patients with coronary artery disease. The management of anaphylaxis requires careful titration of adrenaline with continuous monitoring of physiological responses.

Fluid resuscitation

With anaphylaxis, 35–75% of the blood volume may extravasate in 10–15 minutes. Multiple fluid boluses of 20 mL/kg may be required.

Steroids

There is no evidence that steroids improve outcome in anaphylaxis [4]. They may be useful in cases where there is a protracted reaction or a biphasic response.

Antihistamines

Antihistamines do not have a role in the acute phase of anaphylaxis crisis management.

Follow-up of suspected perioperative allergic reactions

Investigation of anaphylaxis consists of three components:

1. careful information gathering to ensure all possible drugs/products are considered to reduce the incidence of false-negative assessments
2. measurement of products of mast cell degranulation, i.e. tryptase
3. skin testing for the relevant drugs/substances.

Tryptase

Alpha-tryptase is a protease enzyme that is stored in granules in mast cells and basophils. It is also elevated in systemic mastocytosis.

The peak tryptase level occurs 30 minutes to two hours after onset of reaction; its half-life is 90 minutes. Following death, the circulation stops and tryptase is no longer cleared.

False-negative tests occur where the anaphylaxis mechanism involves basophils, as tryptase levels are lower than in mast cells. False-positive tests can occur in cases of extreme stress such as trauma, myocardial infarction and hypoxia.

Skin testing

Skin testing is the current gold standard for investigating IgE-mediated allergic reactions that occur under anaesthesia [5]. Skin testing is the most useful for neuromuscular blocking drugs (NMBD), latex, beta-lactam antibiotics and chlorhexidine. It is also the only way of determining cross-reactivity between different NMBDs when one has induced anaphylaxis.

Skin testing is undertaken four to six weeks after the event to ensure mast cell recovery has occurred, reducing the risk of false-negative testing. Unfortunately, skin testing may not identify a cause in up to 50% of cases.

Management of anaphylaxis is summarised in Box 72.1.

Specific triggers of perioperative anaphylaxis

Neuromuscular blocking drugs

These account for 50–70% of perioperative anaphylaxis. Anaphylaxis occurs in 1:6500 with life-threatening reactions occurring in 1:10,000 [6]. There is a female preponderance 1:2.5–4 [4]. Only 15–30% of patients have previously been exposed to a NMBD. Suxamethonium appears to have the highest incidence.

Latex

Latex accounts for 5–22% of perioperative anaphylaxis. The most likely causative agents are latex surgical or examination gloves, latex balloons, e.g. catheters, and latex condoms, e.g. some ultrasound probe covers.

Antibiotics

Antibiotics account for 15–20% of perioperative anaphylaxis. Penicillins and cephalosporins (beta-lactam antibiotics) cause 70% of these reactions; the next most common is vancomycin. The most serious reactions occur in individuals with no history of allergy.

Colloids

These account for 4–9% of perioperative reactions. Reactions are severe in 20% of patients and typically occur 20 minutes after starting infusion.

Chlorhexidine

There are reports of anaphylaxis to chlorhexidine-impregnated central venous catheters (CVC), urethral gels, implanted surgical mesh, mouthwash, skin preparations and vaginal administration of chlorhexidine. It is likely that this will be an increasing problem in the perioperative period because chlorhexidine has become so ubiquitous. There have been numerous unpublished and published cases where a second reaction to chlorhexidine has been inadvertently triggered.

Dyes

Isosulfan blue and patent blue cause anaphylaxis with extensive cross-reactivity. The incidence is 0.15–2%, occurring up to 30 minutes after injection.

Local anaesthetics

These are responsible for less than 0.6% of anaphylaxis cases. Immunologically mediated reactions are unusual. Reactions are usually vasovagal, related to IV adrenaline, anxiety and local anaesthetic toxic complications.

Induction agents

Propofol anaphylaxis occurs in 1:60,000. Propofol contains additives such as soybean oil, glycerol and egg lecithin. Egg lecithin is purified from egg yolk. Propofol is likely to be safe in the majority of egg-allergic children who do *not* have a history of egg anaphylaxis. Anaphylaxis to barbiturates, ketamine and benzodiazepines is extremely rare.

Opioids

Anaphylaxis is rare but minor histamine reactions are not uncommon. Reactions consist mainly of non-specific mast cell activation, particularly skin mast cells.

Conclusion

Perioperative anaphylaxis is likely to remain an unpredictable cause of morbidity and mortality. The only method available to reduce the incidence is to decrease inadvertent reactions. All patients must be questioned preoperatively about previous adverse reactions in the perioperative period and if patients have unexplained reactions, this should prompt further investigation.

References

1. Mertes PM, Tajima K, Regnier-Kimmoun MA, et al. Perioperative anaphylaxis. *Medical Clinics of North America*, 2010;**94**(4):761–789, xi. doi:10.1016/j.mcna.2010.04.002

2. Mertes PM, Malinovsky JM, Jouffroy L, et al. Reducing the risk of anaphylaxis during anesthesia: 2011 updated guidelines for clinical practice. *Journal of Investigational Allergology and Clinical Immunology*, 2011;**21**(6):442–453. www.ncbi.nlm.nih.gov/pubmed/21995177

3. Australian and New Zealand Anaesthetic Allergy Group. Anaphylaxis Management Guidelines. www.anzaag.com/Mgmt%20Resources.aspx

4. Choo KJ, Simons E, Sheikh A. Glucocorticoids for the treatment of anaphylaxis: Cochrane systematic review. *Allergy*, 2010;**65**(10):1205–1211. doi:10.1111/j.1398-9995.2010.02424.x

5. Ebo DG, Fisher MM, Hagendorens MM, Bridts CH, Stevens WJ. Anaphylaxis during anaesthesia: diagnostic approach. *Allergy*, 2007;**62**(5):471–487. doi:10.1111/j.1398-s.2007.01347.x

6. Dewachter P, Mouton-Faivre C. What investigation after an anaphylactic reaction during anaesthesia? *Current Opinion in Anesthesiology*, 2008;**21**(3):363–368. doi:10.1097/Aco.0b013e3282ff85e1

73 Obesity

Jennifer Carden

Victorian Anaesthetic Group, Australia

As the prevalence of obesity increases worldwide, more obese surgical patients will require anaesthesia and perioperative care, with increased risk of postoperative morbidity and mortality.

Definitions

Overweight/obesity is defined as abnormal or excessive fat accumulation that may impair health [1].

Clinically, obesity in adults is usually defined and classified in terms of Body Mass Index (BMI).

$$BMI = weight\ in\ kilograms/height\ in\ metres^2\ (kg/m^2)$$

A range of factors, including the nature of the diet, ethnic group, genetic predisposition and activity level, affect the incidence of obesity co-morbidities.

Clinically, the BMI does not take into account whether the weight is fat or muscle nor the distribution of body fat. Central obesity most particularly predisposes patients to many of the co-morbidities associated with excess body fat (Table 73.1). Measurements such as waist circumference and waist-to-hip ratio may be more useful when considering risk.

Epidemiology

In 2011–12, over 60% of Australian adults were overweight or obese [2]. Obesity is the fifth leading risk for global deaths [1].

In the surgical patient population, obese patients are more highly represented because of the higher risk of surgical disease. The co-existing cardiac, respiratory and diabetic complications, as well as mobilisation issues, add to the perioperative problems (Box 73.1).

Perioperative Medicine for the Junior Clinician, First Edition. Edited by Joel Symons, Paul Myles, Rishi Mehra and Christine Ball.
© 2015 John Wiley & Sons, Ltd. Published 2015 by John Wiley & Sons, Ltd.
Companion website: www.wiley.com/go/perioperativemed

TABLE 73.1 Classification of adults according to Body Mass Index (BMI)[a]

Classification	BMI	Risk of co-morbidities
Underweight	< 18.50	Low (but risk of other clinical problems increased)
Normal	18.50–24.99	Average
Overweight:	≥ 25.00	
Preobese	25.00–29.99	Increased
Obese class I	30.00–34.99	Moderate
Obese class II	35.00–39.99	Severe
Obese class III	≥ 40.00	Very severe

[a] These BMI values are age-independent and the same for both sexes. However, BMI may not correspond to the same degree of fatness in different populations due, in part, to differences in body proportions. The table shows a simplistic relationship between BMI of the diet, ethnic group and activity level. The risks associated with increasing BMI are continuous and graded and begin at a BM above 25. The interpretation of BMI gradings in relation to risk may differ for different populations. Both BMI and a measure of fat distribution (waist circumference or waist: hip ration (WHR)) are important in calculating the risk of obesity co-morbidity/ies. Source: World Health Organization [6]. Reproduced with permission from WHO.

BOX 73.1 Co-morbidities associated with obesity

Cardiovascular

Hypertension
Ischaemia
Heart failure
Cardiomyopathy
Arrhythmias (atrial fibrillation)
Right heart failure
Pulmonary hypertension

Vascular

Peripheral vascular disease
Venous insufficiency/ulcers
Deep vein thrombosis and thromboembolism

Respiratory

Sleep apnoea
Hypoventilation syndrome
Asthma

Metabolic

Diabetes
Insulin resistance
Metabolic syndrome
Dyslipidaemia

Gynaecological

Infertility and menstrual problems
Incontinence – urinary/faecal
Obstetric complications

Musculoskeletal

Osteoarthritis
Gout
Low back pain
Immobility
Accident proneness (fractures)

Psychosocial

Depression
Anxiety
Phobias

Cancer

Breast
Colorectal
Prostate
Endometrial

Skin

Infections
Intertrigo
Poor wound healing

Gastrointestinal

Gastro-oesophageal reflux
Non-alcoholic steatohepatitis
Gallstones
Hiatus hernia

73

Pathophysiological changes in obesity

Metabolic

Secretion of hormones and inflammatory bioactive peptides (adipocytokines) by excessive central abdominal visceral fat causes many of the adverse effects on the cardiovascular and metabolic system (metabolic syndrome) [3].

Cardiovascular system

An increase in basal metabolic rate, cardiac output (stroke volume), total blood volume and myocardial work may result in cardiomyopathy, cardiac failure and arrhythmias.

Respiratory physiology

These patients have an increase in O_2 consumption, CO_2 production, minute ventilation and work of breathing. They have a higher incidence of atelectasis and ventilation perfusion mismatch with a reduced functional residual capacity (hence reduced oxygen reserve) and sleep-disordered breathing. They are at higher risk of hypoxia, apnoea and respiratory failure.

Gastrointestinal

Hiatus hernia, increased intra-abdominal pressure and non-alcoholic steatohepatitis (NASH)/cirrhosis are common. There is a higher risk of gastric acid regurgitation and aspiration during general anaesthesia.

Increased total body fat results in reduced mobility, increased metabolic rate, fat infiltration, compression of the airway and reduced mobility of joints. There is a higher risk of difficult bag mask ventilation [4] and difficult intubation [5].

Preoperative management

Organisational

The hospital should provide an environment that is safe for patients and staff. Theatres and wards should have appropriate lifting devices, chairs, beds and operating tables with the correct weight-loading capacity.

The social prejudice and associated low self-esteem, depression and social phobias may lead to a reluctance to seek medical attention. Patients may have had past negative experiences with healthcare professionals. Patients should be treated with compassion and understanding.

Preoperative medical assessment

Assessment should focus on optimising patient co-morbidities. Investigations should be guided by clinical judgement and will depend on the degree of obesity, the patient's medical history and the nature of the surgery. A lower threshold for investigating cardiac and respiratory risks is advisable, especially for major surgery.

The patient should be counselled to aim for a preoperative achievable weight loss strategy (e.g. 5% of total body weight), as this may reduce the incidence of complications. Use the preoperative phase to provide information about future weight loss as well as the usual preoperative consent process outlining risks.

Diabetes
Perioperative hyperglycaemia is associated with poor outcome (refer to Chapter 26 Diabetes medication and Chapter 49 Diabetes mellitus).

Obstructive sleep apnoea
Patients with a history of OSA (snoring, witnessed apnoeas, daytime sleepiness) should have polysomnography (sleep studies) and institution of early positive airway pressure treatment, if time permits, before surgery. If the OSA is not well controlled, a higher level of postoperative monitoring (ICU/HDU) may be required (refer to Chapter 40 Obstructive sleep apnoea).

Airway assessment
Careful airway assessment is important (refer to Chapter 14 Airway assessment and planning).

Intraoperative management

General anaesthesia may present problems with managing the patient's airway and achieving adequate ventilation.

Regional techniques and IV access might be more difficult due to subcutaneous fat limiting access; ultrasound may be useful in both cases. Occasionally, central venous access may be required and should be considered preoperatively if the patient requires longer-term IV access.

Blood pressure measurement may be difficult on the obese arm; a wide cuff or an arterial line may be required.

Obese patients are particularly at risk of nerve injuries during surgery so careful positioning on the operating table is necessary.

Pharmacology

Alterations in the way anaesthetic and other perioperative drugs are handled may be due to:

- an increase in lean body mass (higher dosing required)
- an increase in total body fat (lipid-soluble drugs have prolonged elimination)
- an increase in metabolic rate, cardiac output and glomerular filtration rate (drugs excreted in the kidneys have a shorter half-life)
- end-organ damage (liver, cardiac, renal impairment) may reduce clearance.

Airway issues

The anaesthetist should anticipate airway difficulty and plan for safe management of the airway (e.g. videolaryngoscopy or fibreoptic intubation), and consider preoperative prophylaxis to reduce gastric pH. Good positioning and adequate preoxygenation increase the time available for securing the airway. An increased risk of gastric acid aspiration sometimes mandates a rapid sequence induction, giving consideration to the anticipated difficulty of intubation. Note that cricoid pressure may reduce the risk of aspiration but if not properly applied, may increase difficulty of tracheal intubation.

Adequate ventilation is best guided by the principles of protective lung ventilation, including PEEP and recruitment manoeuvres, and perhaps administration of higher oxygen concentration. The Trendelenburg or sitting position will improve oxygenation. Tidal volume should be calculated on ideal body weight rather than total body weight to limit risk of barotrauma.

Postoperative management

Postoperative nausea and vomiting is common, so combination antiemetic prophylaxis is recommended (refer to Chapter 79 Postoperative nausea and vomiting).

Multimodal analgesia and regional techniques (opioid sparing) will reduce PONV and risk of respiratory depression.

Prophylaxis against deep venous thrombosis and pulmonary embolism is imperative in this high-risk group (refer to Chapter 24 Thromboprophylaxis).

Respiratory complications

- Administer supplemental oxygen postoperatively.
- Monitor oxygen saturation.
- Use CPAP (OSA).
- Consider the need for high-acuity care (HDU and ICU) for respiratory monitoring and support in high-risk patients recovering from major surgery.

References

1. World Health Organisation (WHO). *Obesity and Overweight*. Fact sheet no. 311. www.who.int/mediacentre/factsheets/fs311/en/

2. Australian Bureau of Statistics. *4338.0 - Profiles of Health*. Canberra, Australia: Australian Bureau of Statistics, 2013.

3. Grundy SM, Brewer HB Jr, Cleeman JI, et al. Definition of metabolic syndrome: report of the National Heart, Lung, and Blood Institute/American Heart Association conference on scientific issues related to definition. *Circulation*, 2004;**109**(3):433–438. doi:10.1161/01. CIR.0000111245.75752.C6

4. Langeron O, Masso E, Huraux C, et al. Prediction of difficult mask ventilation. *Anesthesiology*, 2000;**92**(5):1229–1236. www.ncbi.nlm.nih.gov/pubmed/10781266

5. Brodsky JB, Lemmens HJ, Brock-Utne JG, Vierra M, Saidman LJ. Morbid obesity and tracheal intubation. *Anesthesia and Analgesia*, 2002;**94**(3):732–736. www.ncbi.nlm.nih.gov/pubmed/11867407

6. World Health Organisation (WHO). *Obesity: Preventing and Managing the Global Epidemic*. Report of a WHO Consultation. WHO Technical Report Series 894. Geneva: World Health Organization, 2000.

Goal-directed therapy

Andrew Toner[1] and Mark Hamilton[2]

[1] St George's Hospital, United Kingdom
[2] St George's Hospital and Medical School, United Kingdom

Good cardiovascular performance in the perioperative period is associated with optimal surgical recovery. When tissue blood flow and oxygen delivery are compromised, there is an increased incidence of organ dysfunction and postoperative complications. Preventive treatments focused on augmenting haemodynamics can be standardised using goal-directed therapy (GDT). Such an approach has demonstrated efficacy over conventional care in some, but not all randomised trials [1].

Definition

Goal-directed therapy is defined as the titration of IV fluids, with or without vasoactive agents, to achieve a physiological goal that is dynamically measured by invasive blood pressure monitoring or non-invasive methods such as oesophageal doppler.

The problem

In health, the cardiovascular system ensures there is adequate blood flow, oxygen delivery and waste product removal to meet the metabolic needs of the organs and tissues of the body. A common measurement of such cardiovascular performance is global oxygen delivery calculated by the following equation:

$$Oxygen\ delivery = heart\ rate \times stroke\ volume \times Hb \times SaO_2 \times constant$$

In surgical patients, many perioperative factors have the potential to impair tissue perfusion, by negatively impacting on the components of oxygen delivery (Table 74.1).

Routine management

Surgical patients will routinely receive maintenance IV fluids, oxygen supplementation, chest physiotherapy and blood transfusions to keep haemoglobin levels above locally defined thresholds (commonly 8–10 g/dL). Further quantities of

Perioperative Medicine for the Junior Clinician, First Edition. Edited by Joel Symons, Paul Myles, Rishi Mehra and Christine Ball.
© 2015 John Wiley & Sons, Ltd. Published 2015 by John Wiley & Sons, Ltd.
Companion website: www.wiley.com/go/perioperativemed

TABLE 74.1 Perioperative factors that reduce oxygen delivery

	Decreased heart rate	Decreased stroke volume	Decreased haemoglobin	Decreased SaO_2
Fasting		X		
Anaesthetic/ analgesic drugs	X	X		
Blood loss		X	X	
Fluid shifts		X		
Inflammation		X		X
Pain				X
Immobilisation				X

www.wiley.com/go/perioperativemed

VIDEO 74.1 Goal-directed therapy may assist in optimising fluid therapy during the perioperative period.

IV fluids are often prescribed by perioperative physicians, in order to support haemodynamic performance. The amount and timing of fluid are influenced by measured losses, conventional indicators of poor global perfusion (e.g. oliguria) and personal preferences – all of which can be unreliable. Fluid practice is thus highly variable and non-standardised. If cardiac performance remains inadequate despite these measures, the clinical manifestations will be detected relatively late in the postoperative course, e.g. acute kidney injury (AKI). At this point, advanced monitoring and haemodynamic support can be instituted reactively in an attempt to rescue the patient, but may not be successful.

Goal-directed therapy (Video 74.1)

Elective use of advanced haemodynamic monitoring in a critical care facility enables proactive cardiovascular support before organ dysfunction develops – this is the basis of GDT. In phase 1, stroke volume is optimised by titrating IV fluid boluses to effect, e.g. 250 mL crystalloid solution. If a fluid bolus leads to an increase in cardiac preload and a subsequent rise in stroke volume greater than 10%, it is repeated until further fluid administration has a negligible impact on stroke volume (the presumed top of the Frank–Starling curve is reached) (Figure 74.1, Figure 74.2).

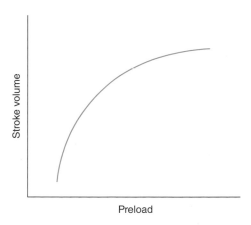

FIGURE 74.1 **Frank–Starling curve.**

(a)

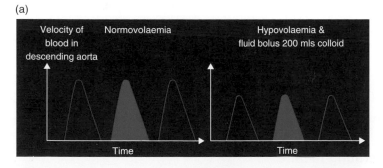

(b)

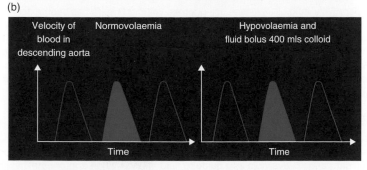

FIGURE 74.2 **(a)** Typical oesophageal doppler velocity profile. The left shows normovolaemia, the right shows hypovolaemia with an initial bolus of fluid. **(b)** Further oesophageal doppler velocity profiles. A subsequent bolus of additional fluid shows a return to normovolaemia.

In phase 2, inotropes can be used to further augment stroke volume and heart rate, so that the selected goals are reached. Commonly, the goal is a global oxygen delivery value of 600 mL/min/m^2, a threshold targeted in patient populations exhibiting superior surgical recovery. Alternatively, goals can be tailored to the individual patient. For example, mixed venous oxygen saturation reflects the balance between oxygen delivery and oxygen consumption in a given subject, and has been successfully utilised to guide GDT [2].

Risk–benefit balance

The potential benefits of GDT are three-fold. First, pre-emptive cardiovascular support reduces the sequelae of tissue hypoxia. Second, fluid optimisation attenuates the sympathetic drive associated with hypovolaemia and hypoperfusion, and may reduce cardiac work. Third, the consequences of excessive fluids and tissue oedema are avoided.

Like all interventions in medicine, fluids and inotropes can be harmful as well as beneficial. Inotropes in particular, increase cardiac work for the benefit of the other vital organs. Patients with established cardiovascular disease will be most vulnerable to rising cardiac demands. To mitigate this risk, GDT safety limits can be used to stop or cap inotropic support in the presence of tachycardia, ischaemic ECG changes or chest pain.

Overall, the role of GDT is to provide standardised haemodynamic support for a finite period (up to eight postoperative hours), in order to counteract the physiological disturbances associated with surgery. When delivered in this way, improvements in hospital morbidity have been demonstrated. Prolonged administration of GDT guided by pulmonary artery catheters has not demonstrated a mortality benefit in high-risk surgical patients, and may be harmful in mixed groups of critically ill patients.

Clinical applications

The principles of GDT can be applied in various clinical settings beyond critical care facilities.

Operating theatre

Intraoperatively, fluid optimisation using stroke volume targets has been extensively investigated. A number of early trials reported improved surgical recovery compared with standard fluid care but as many aspects of surgical practice have changed in the intervening years (e.g. shorter fasting protocols, avoidance of bowel preparation, laparoscopic surgery), the current relevance of these findings has been questioned. Indeed, the most recent studies of goal-directed fluid therapy showed no benefit overall [3,4].

Surgical ward

Fluid optimisation can be achieved in surgical ward patients by utilising appropriate goals as a substitute for stroke volume monitoring. For example, central venous oxygen saturation is available as a guide to fluid titration when appropriate invasive lines are *in situ*. Surrogate markers of cardiac output can also be used as a basis for fluid optimisation, e.g. urine output, capillary refill, lactate, acid–base balance. The key application of GDT principles in this setting is to give small, rapid fluid boluses and measure the response against a predetermined parameter. If patients exhibit signs of global hypoperfusion despite fluid optimisation, then escalation to critical care is warranted.

Emergency department

The benefits of GDT in patients presenting to emergency departments with severe sepsis gained widespread recognition with the publication of a landmark paper by Rivers et al. [5]. Several international, multicentre trials are under way in an attempt to reproduce these results, with a recent trial failing to demonstrate a benefit [6].

References

1. Hamilton MA, Cecconi M, Rhodes A. A systematic review and meta-analysis on the use of preemptive hemodynamic intervention to improve postoperative outcomes in moderate and high-risk surgical patients. *Anesthesia and Analgesia*, 2011;**112**(6):1392–1402. doi:10.1213/ANE.0b013e3181eeaae5

2. Donati A, Loggi S, Preiser JC, et al. Goal-directed intraoperative therapy reduces morbidity and length of hospital stay in high-risk surgical patients. *Chest*, 2007;**132**(6):1817–1824. doi:10.1378/chest.07-0621

3. Challand C, Struthers R, Sneyd JR, et al. Randomized controlled trial of intraoperative goal-directed fluid therapy in aerobically fit and unfit patients having major colorectal surgery. *British Journal of Anaesthesia*, 2012;**108**(1):53–62. doi:10.1093/bja/aer273

4. Srinivasa S, Taylor MH, Singh PP, Yu TC, Soop M, Hill AG. Randomized clinical trial of goal-directed fluid therapy within an enhanced recovery protocol for elective colectomy. *British Journal of Surgery*, 2013;**100**(1):66–74. doi:10.1002/bjs.8940

5. Rivers E, Nguyen B, Havstad S, et al. Early goal-directed therapy in the treatment of severe sepsis and septic shock. *New England Journal of Medicine*, 2001;**345**(19):1368–1377. doi:10.1056/NEJMoa010307

6. Pro CI, Yealy DM, Kellum JA, et al. A randomized trial of protocol-based care for early septic shock. *New England Journal of Medicine*, 2014;**370**(18):1683–1693. doi:10.1056/NEJMoa1401602

74

75 Fluids and electrolytes

David Story

The University of Melbourne, Australia

Intravenous fluids are a cornerstone of perioperative care. Intraoperative fluid therapy is dealt with by anaesthetists but junior doctors often prescribe preoperative and later postoperative fluids. Appropriate choice and administration of IV fluids can reduce organ failure, while incorrect dosing can cause, or worsen, organ injury. Vulnerable patients with diminished physiological reserve are at greatest risk [1]. Because fluid therapy can have these important clinical effects on body fluid volumes and fluid chemistry, fluids must be prescribed with the same care as any other drug [1,2].

One way to consider fluid therapy is with the mnemonic TROL.

- T – Type
- R – Rate
- O – Outcome
- L – Limits

An example is Hartmann's solution (Type) at 2 mL/kg/hr (Rate) to maintain systolic blood pressure > 100 mmHg (Outcome) and the central venous pressure < 10 mmHg (Limit).

Type

Intravenous fluids can be broadly divided into three types: crystalloids, colloids and blood products. Crystalloids are central to fluid therapy. Colloid use is controversial and the need for blood products should be reassessed during any fluid therapy. There is no ideal IV fluid [1].

Crystalloids versus colloids

Crystalloids (Table 75.1) are solutions that leave a crystal residue if all the water is evaporated. In solution, they have small ions that easily cross membranes. Colloids have larger molecules (colloid) made from protein (albumin and gelatin) or starch and usually have a crystalloid carrier similar to saline or Plasmalyte (Table 75.1). While colloids have the theoretical advantage of better plasma retention, there is little clinical evidence for outcome advantage with colloids

Perioperative Medicine for the Junior Clinician, First Edition. Edited by Joel Symons, Paul Myles, Rishi Mehra and Christine Ball.
© 2015 John Wiley & Sons, Ltd. Published 2015 by John Wiley & Sons, Ltd.
Companion website: www.wiley.com/go/perioperativemed

TABLE 75.1 **Concentration of ions in commonly used IV fluids**

Strong Ion	Hartmann's	5% Dextrose	Plasmalyte	Normal saline
Sodium, mmol/L	129	0	140	154
Chloride, mmol/L	109	0	98	154
Potassium, mmol/L	5	0	5	0
Calcium, mmol/L	2	0	0	0
Magnesium, mmol/L	0	0	3	0
Acetate, mmol/L	0	0	27	0
Gluconate, mmol/L	0	0	23	0
Lactate, mmol/L	29	0	0	0
Glucose, mmol/L	0	278	0	0

compared with crystalloids and some evidence of harm [3]. For patients with isolated brain injury, there is good evidence that 0.9% saline is superior to 4% albumin [1]. Further, the starch colloids may cause harm in patients with sepsis or at risk of renal dysfunction, both of which are common in many hospital patients [1,3].

There are a few widely used perioperative IV fluids, with the most common and least physiological being 0.9% saline (Table 75.1), often called 'normal' saline [4]. There is increasing evidence that saline is associated with worse outcome in many surgical patients, particularly acute kidney injury [1]. Hartmann's (Table 75.1) is a more physiological solution widely used by anaesthetists and very similar to Ringer's lactate [2] used in the United States. Another more balanced salt fluid is Plasmalyte (Table 75.1) which, unlike Hartmann's, does not have calcium, an added feature for those who worry about compatibility of blood products with Hartmann's solution (an over-rated issue).

Rate

The IV fluid administration rate will depend on the indication [2,5]. A patient who is hypovolaemic and hypotensive requires fluid resuscitation, often with boluses of 20 mL/kg of crystalloid given as quickly as possible. Steps must be taken to treat underlying fluid loss, particularly haemorrhage. For adults, the maintenance fluid rate is about 1.5 mL/kg/hr or 30–40 mL/kg/day [5]. Aggressive but not emergency volume resuscitation is typically about 10 mL/kg/hr.

Outcome

The outcome or endpoint of fluid therapy is usually a haemodynamic outcome, blood pressure and/or heart rate, but also includes end-organ changes such as increased urine output [1]. These may or may not be valid indices of fluid status.

Limits

Preoperative patients needing emergency surgery for bleeding or arterial rupture may benefit from blood pressure constraints (hypotensive resuscitation) [4]. Otherwise, limits will usually be based on measures of filling ranging from clinical and less accurate, such as CVP, to technical but more precise measures, such as left ventricular end-diastolic volume (LVEDV) estimates from TTE. Because of autoregulation, organ perfusion plateaus once an adequate blood pressure is reached and excess fluid is associated with worse outcome [1].

Electrolytes

The electrolyte content of a fluid (see Table 75.1) and subsequent tonicity will affect the distribution of the fluid through body water and the effect on electrolytes, particularly in the extracellular fluid, including plasma [1,5].

A rough, bedside description of body water is that 60% of body weight is water. Of that water, two-thirds (Figure 75.1) is intracellular fluid (ICF), including red blood cells (RBC). One-third is extracellular fluid (ECF), of which one-quarter is intravascular. Therefore, one-twelfth of total body water (5% body weight) is plasma water, the target for initial resuscitation [2]. Because sodium is an extracellular ion, sodium containing fluids such as Hartmann's or 0.9% saline will distribute through the ECF, leaving about a quarter in plasma. In contrast, dextrose (5% dextrose) acts like water because glucose is taken up into cells, and therefore into the intracellular fluid, and the water will follow. Only one-twelfth will remain in plasma, making dextrose a poor resuscitation fluid; additionally, it results in undesirable hyperglycaemia. Dextrose alone is a poor maintenance fluid because of hyponatraemia.

'Normal' 0.9% saline is associated with hyperchloraemic metabolic acidosis. If saline is used to resuscitate a patient with lactic acidaemia, the superimposed hyperchloraemic acidosis will worsen the acidaemia [2]. All IV fluids (Table 75.1) can be associated with electrolyte abnormalities, particularly if large volumes are administered quickly. Saline will also be associated with hypocalcaemia, hypomagnesaemia and, at times, hypokalaemia [5,6].

Like all patient care, while clinical assessment is essential, laboratory testing is an important supplement. Patients who are receiving large volumes of fluids and/or are critically ill should have frequent testing and correction of clinical chemistry [5,6]. Patients on maintenance fluids may need supplemental potassium [5]. It is important to remember that considerable information can be obtained from a venous blood gas sample. Spot urine chemistry combined with urine output can help match fluid therapy with water and electrolyte excretion.

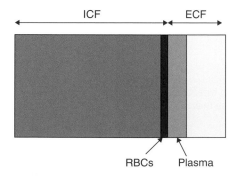

FIGURE 75.1 **Body water distribution. ECF, extracellular fluid; ICF, intracellular fluid; RBC, red blood cell.**

> REMEMBER: If there is bleeding or a patient needs fluid therapy but you are uncertain about the TROL: CALL FOR HELP.

References

1. Myburgh JA, Mythen MG. Resuscitation fluids. *New England Journal of Medicine*, 2013;**369**(13):1243–1251. doi:10.1056/NEJMra1208627

2. Piper GL, Kaplan LJ. Fluid and electrolyte management for the surgical patient. *Surgical Clinics of North America*, 2012;**92**(2):189–205. doi:10.1016/j.suc.2012.01.004

3. Perel P, Roberts I, Ker K. Colloids versus crystalloids for fluid resuscitation in critically ill patients. *Cochrane Database of Systematic Reviews*, 2013;**2**:CD000567. doi:10.1002/14651858. CD000567.pub6

4. Santry HP, Alam HB. Fluid resuscitation: past, present, and the future. *Shock*, 2010;**33**(3): 229–241. doi:10.1097/SHK.0b013e3181c30f0c

5. Knight A. Prescribing intravenous fluids: how to get it right. *British Journal of Hospital Medicine (London)*, 2010;**71**(4):M57–58, M60. doi:10.12968/hmed.2010.71.sup4.47530

6. Hilton AK, Pellegrino VA, Scheinkestel CD. Avoiding common problems associated with intravenous fluid therapy. *Medical Journal of Australia*, 2008;**189**(9):509–513. www.ncbi.nlm.nih.gov/pubmed/18976194

Electrolyte abnormalities

Lloyd Roberts[1] and Carlos Scheinkestel[2]

[1] The Alfred Hospital, Australia
[2] The Alfred Hospital and Monash University, Australia

Abnormalities in K^+ and Na^+ concentrations are among the more common electrolyte disturbances (e.g. hypokalaemia occurs in 0.7% of the population and hypernatraemia in 0.5%). Extremes of serum K^+ and Na^+ and rapid rates of change are associated with morbidity and mortality [1].

Potassium derangements

* Hypokalaemia: serum K^+ <3.5 mmol/L
* Hyperkalaemia: serum K^+ >5.0 mmol/L (>6 mmol/L is potentially dangerous)

Aetiology

Clinically, drugs are the most common cause of hypokalaemia, while >80% of hyperkalaemia is caused by renal impairment, with drugs commonly contributing (Tables 76.1 and 76.2).

Consequences

Symptoms are more likely with more extreme values and rapid rates of change (Table 76.3) [2].

Management

Treat the underlying cause and recheck K^+ level after treatment.

Hypokalaemia

Replace K^+. On average, serum K^+ decreases by 0.3 mmol/L per 100 mmol total body K^+ depletion, but this relationship is highly variable. Oral administration is usually safer than IV but avoid in gastric stasis. Details of oral K^+ supplements can be found in Table 76.4.

Hypokalaemia is usually accompanied by decreased chloride so KCl is the ideal replacement. If the patient has diarrhoea or metabolic acidosis, consider $KHCO_3$ or KCO_3. Administer IV potassium where oral administration is impractical or with severe hypokalaemia – up to 10 mmol in 100 mL volume with saline per hour (ideally as a premade bag). Avoid 5% dextrose which may shift K^+ intracellularly [3]. K^+ is

Perioperative Medicine for the Junior Clinician, First Edition. Edited by Joel Symons, Paul Myles, Rishi Mehra and Christine Ball.
© 2015 John Wiley & Sons, Ltd. Published 2015 by John Wiley & Sons, Ltd.
Companion website: www.wiley.com/go/perioperativemed

TABLE 76.1 Causes of hypokalaemia

	Drug causes	Other causes
↑ Losses (most common cause, via kidney or gastrointestinal tract)	Laxatives, diuretics, fludrocortisone, high-dose glucocorticoids, amphotericin B, aminoglycosides	Diarrhoea, vomiting (mainly kidney losses), glycosuria, diabetic ketoacidosis, volume depletion, primary hyperaldosteronism, hypomagnesaemia
↓ Intake (<25 mmol/day)		Poor oral intake
Intracellular K⁺ shifts	Insulin, salbutamol	↑ pH, stress, delirium tremens, hyperthyroidism
Factitious		Diluted sample

TABLE 76.2 Causes of hyperkalaemia

	Drug causes	Other causes
↓ Excretion	ACE inhibitors/angiotensin receptor blockers, K⁺-sparing diuretics (e.g. spironolactone), cyclosporine, tacrolimus, trimethoprim	Renal insufficiency, mineralocorticoid deficiency (e.g. Addison's disease, usual steroids omitted)
↑ Intake	KCl	Massive blood transfusion
Extracellular K⁺ shifts	Beta-blockers, digoxin toxicity	Insulin deficiency/resistance, uncontrolled diabetes, acidosis, cell lysis (surgery, trauma, rhabdomyolysis)
K⁺ release in arm/ collection tube		Haemolysis during phlebotomy, thrombocytosis, severe leucocytosis, repeated fist clenching with tourniquet on

ACE, angiotensin converting enzyme.

TABLE 76.3 Consequences of potassium derangements

Range (mmol/L)	Clinical and ECG features
<2.0	Ascending paralysis and respiratory arrest possible
<2.5	Rhabdomyolysis possible
2.5–3.0	Constipation, mild weakness
3.0–3.5	Asymptomatic, but ↑ risk of arrhythmias with HF, LVH or cardiac ischaemia (aim for K⁺ >4.0 mmol/L)
3.5–5	Normal range
6.0–7.0	↑ Risk of ECG changes (e.g. peaked T waves) and arrhythmias (especially with rapid rise, acidosis or hypoxia) though sensitivity of ECG for hyperkalaemia is poor
7.0–8.0	Potential ascending paralysis, flattened P waves, long PR interval, widened QRS complex
8.0–9.0	Lost P wave, loss of ST segment leading to a sine wave
>9.0	Ventricular fibrillation and standstill

ECG, electrocardiogram; HF, heart failure; LVH, left ventricular hypertrophy.

TABLE 76.4 **Oral potassium supplements**

	Slow release (e.g. Slow K®, Span K®)	Chlorvescent®
mmol of K+	8 mmol/tablet	14 mmol/tablet
Other ions	8 mmol Cl-/tablet	8 mmol Cl-, also HCO_3^- CO_3^{2-}
Duration of release	3–4 hours	
Presentation	Tablet	Effervescent, salty taste

also available as 20–40 mmol in 1000 mL saline (maximum recommended infusion rate is 20 mmol K+/hr). More rapid or concentrated replacement requires cardiac monitoring in a critical care area and potentially central access.

Consider correcting hypomagnesaemia to assist with correction of hypokalaemia. Since oral magnesium has poor bioavailability, administer IV: $MgSO_4$ or $MgCl_2$, 10 mmol over 1 hour in 100 mL 0.9% saline. Recheck K+ after replacement (with U&E or blood gas), either immediately (if critically low K+) or after initial replacement where K+ losses are ongoing. Check again the next day.

Hyperkalaemia [4]

> Remember, the most common cause of severe hyperkalaemia is iatrogenic from K+ replacement, especially IV.

Treat if K+ >6.5 mmol/L (or 6 mmol/L if unable to exclude an acute rise in K+) and confirm treatment effectiveness with repeat K+ measurements (Table 76.5).

Prevention of hyperkalaemia and hypokalaemia

The normal K+ requirement is ~0.7–1 mmol/kg/day [5]. K+ supplementation is not usually required on the first 1–2 postoperative days unless there is preoperative hypokalaemia. Check serum K+ on day three, or earlier if there are risk factors, for K+ derangement (e.g. renal impairment, maintenance fluids, K+-raising or -lowering drugs, preoperative hypokalaemia).

Sodium derangements [6]

- Hyponatraemia: serum Na+ <135 mmol/L
- Hypernatraemia: serum Na+ >145 mmol/L

Aetiology

Hyponatraemia
The most common cause is hypotonic fluids in patients with high ADH secretion due to the stress response, pain, nausea and vomiting. This persists for 12 hours (minor surgery) to four days (major surgery) postoperatively [7].

TABLE 76.5 **Drug treatment of hyperkalaemia**

Drug	Onset	Duration and notes
If there are ECG changes, administer immediately for cardiac protection (does not lower K⁺)		
10 mL of 10% Ca gluconate/ $CaCl_2$ IV over 2–5 mins (unless digoxin toxicity)	1–3 mins	15–30 mins Ca gluconate is preferred for peripheral IV administration (less irritant to veins)
Rapid-acting agents to transiently shift K⁺ intracellularly		
50 mL of 50% glucose and 10 units Actrapid IV stat	10–20 mins	2–3 hours
Salbutamol 10–20 mg nebulized over 10 mins	20–30 mins	2–3 hours Some patients do not respond to salbutamol [2] Potential small (0.15 mmol/L) initial rise in K⁺
Each of the above two agents ↓ K⁺ by 0.65 mmol/L • combination of both ↓ by 1.2 mmol/L		
$NaHCO_3$ 50 mmol over 5–15 mins (if metabolic acidosis)	Delayed (>60 mins) [2]	Less effective than glucose and insulin and salbutamol
Slower acting agents to remove K⁺ from the body		
Resonium 15–30 g orally or as retention enema	4–6 hours orally, or 1 hour as enema (works in colon)	Maximal effect at 6 hours Caution in constipated patients and avoid combination with sorbitol (risk of bowel necrosis)
Furosemide IV	1 hour	Only effective if adequate renal function
Rapid removal of K⁺ from the body		
Haemodialysis	15–30 mins	Faster with high flux against zero K⁺ dialysate – not CRRT which is too slow
Prevention of recurrence		
Cease K⁺-raising drugs Consider regular diuretics Treat other underlying causes, e.g. fludrocortisone for Addison's disease		

CRRT, continuous renal replacement therapy; ECG, electrocardiogram; IV, intravenous.

Hypernatraemia

The most common cause is water loss from the GI tract (diarrhoea), kidneys (diuretics or diabetes insipidus (DI), e.g. due to lithium therapy (nephrogenic DI), brain injury (central DI)) or skin: fever, burns. Na⁺ gain is usually iatrogenic, e.g. hypertonic saline for burns, trauma or brain injury.

The consequences of both hyponatraemia and hypernatraemia are neurological – lethargy, weakness, nausea, vomiting, headache, irritability, seizures, coma and death. Permanent injury is more likely with acute serum Na⁺ changes to < 125 mmol/L or > 160 mmol/L.

Treatment

Hyponatraemia

Note that hypoglycaemia may present with similar symptoms. Measure blood glucose and send samples for serum glucose, urine and serum Na^+ and osmolality. If there are neurological symptoms (headache, drowsiness or seizures), obtain urgent expert advice.

Profound acute hyponatraemia ($Na^+ < 125$ mmol/L present for <48 hours) with neurology requires rapid elevation of Na^+ (e.g. with 2 mL/kg 3% saline over 20 mins, repeated as required, with frequent rechecking of serum Na^+) to control symptoms, then slower correction – delays may increase the risk of permanent neurological abnormalities or death.

Chronic hyponatraemia requires slow correction – rapid correction risks osmotic demyelination (central pontine myelinolysis).

Always consider other causes for neurological abnormalities, especially if hyponatraemia is less severe (>125 mmol/L).

Asymptomatic hyponatraemia

Chronic mild hyponatraemia, commonly seen in cardiac and liver failure, may be resistant to (and not require) correction. Otherwise, aim to correct slowly (≤ 8 mmol/L/ day rise in Na^+). Cease hypotonic fluids, treat the underlying cause and assess volume status. Euvolaemia or hypervolaemia is suggestive of SIADH which is managed with fluid restriction and avoidance of isotonic and hypotonic fluids. Acute hypovolaemic hyponatraemia often corrects with fluid repletion with isotonic saline.

Hypernatraemia

The rate of correction is proportional to the rate of onset of the hypernatraemia, and the presence and severity of neurological symptoms. It should not exceed 10 mmol/L/day as overly rapid correction risks cerebral oedema and death.

↑ Na^+ due to water loss:

- treat cause, e.g. ddAVP for central DI
- administer hypotonic fluids IV, e.g. 5% dextrose or 4% dextrose in 0.18% NaCl with monitoring of blood sugar levels, especially in those with diabetes
- sterile water IV requires central access.

↑ Na^+ due to Na^+ gain:

- cease hypertonic fluids
- if Na^+ fails to correct, consider diuretics, replacing urinary losses with hypotonic fluids.

Prevention of hyponatraemia and hypernatraemia

Measure serum Na^+ daily in patients receiving maintenance fluids. Use isotonic fluids (e.g. 0.9% NaCl) during the initial (24–96 hours) period of high ADH secretion postoperatively. Avoid hypotonic fluids if Na^+ is low or falling rapidly (>8 mmol/L/day).

References

1. Leung AA, McAlister FA, Rogers SO Jr, Pazo V, Wright A, Bates DW. Preoperative hyponatremia and perioperative complications. *Archives of Internal Medicine*, 2012;**172**(19):1474–1481. doi:10.1001/archinternmed.2012.3992

2. Ahee P, Crowe AV. The management of hyperkalaemia in the emergency department. *Journal of Accident and Emergency Medicine*, 2000;**17**(3):188–191. doi:10.1136/emj.17.3.188

3. Agarwal A, Wingo CS. Treatment of hypokalemia. *New England Journal of Medicine*, 1999;**340**(2):154–155. doi:10.1056/NEJM199901143400220

4. Mahoney BA, Smith WA, Lo DS, Tsoi K, Tonelli M, Clase CM. Emergency interventions for hyperkalaemia. *Cochrane Database of Systematic Reviews*, 2005;**2**:CD003235. doi:10.1002/14651858.CD003235.pub2

5. Rassam SS, Counsell DJ. Perioperative electrolyte and fluid balance. *Continuing Education in Anaesthesia, Critical Care and Pain*, 2005;**5**(5):157–160. doi:10.1093/bjaceaccp/mki042

6. Hilton AK, Pellegrino VA, Scheinkestel CD. Avoiding common problems associated with intravenous fluid therapy. *Medical Journal of Australia*, 2008;**189**(9):509–513. www.ncbi.nlm.nih.gov/pubmed/18976194

7. Gosling P. Salt of the earth or a drop in the ocean? A pathophysiological approach to fluid resuscitation. *Emergency Medicine Journal*, 2003;**20**(4):306–315. doi:10.1136/emj.20.4.306

76

Blood transfusion

Amanda Davis

The Alfred Hospital and Monash University, Australia

Pretransfusion testing

Pretransfusion testing identifies ABO, Rhesus D (RhD) blood type and any red cell alloantibodies developed due to sensitising, e.g. pregnancy or previous transfusion. Cross-match compatible blood prevents acute haemolytic transfusion reactions due to ABO incompatibility or red cell alloantibodies. Care with collecting and labelling blood samples is vital as mislabelling can lead to fatal haemolytic transfusion reactions.

ABO typing

The antigen(s) on the patient's red cells must be consistent with the naturally occurring isohaemagglutinins (anti-A/anti-B) present in the patient's plasma/serum (Table 77.1).

RhD testing

Rhesus D-positive patients can receive RhD-positive or -negative red cells.

RhD-negative patients are at high risk of developing anti-D if exposed to RhD-positive red cells. This must be avoided in women of child-bearing age since anti-D puts a future pregnancy at risk of haemolytic disease of the newborn.

Antibody screen

Red cell alloantibody testing is performed to detect clinically significant red cell alloantibodies to non-ABO red cell antigens, e.g. anti-Kell.

Perioperative Medicine for the Junior Clinician, First Edition. Edited by Joel Symons, Paul Myles, Rishi Mehra and Christine Ball.
© 2015 John Wiley & Sons, Ltd. Published 2015 by John Wiley & Sons, Ltd.
Companion website: www.wiley.com/go/perioperativemed

TABLE 77.1 **ABO blood groups**

Patient ABO group	Red cell antigens	Isohaemagglutinins	Compatible red cell donor
A	A	Anti-B	A,O
B	B	Anti-A	B,O
AB	AB	–	AB,B,A,O
O	–	Anti-A and anti-B	O

TABLE 77.2 **Emergency provision of red cells**

ABO group	Cross-match	Time (mins)	Testing	Risks of incompatibility
Group O red cells*	None	5	None	Red cell alloantibody
ABO group specific	None	15	ABO/Rh type	Red cell alloantibody
	Abbreviated	30	ABO/Rh type Antibody screen Electronic crossmatch	Screen negative – none Screen positive – red cell alloantibody
	Full	30–60	ABO/Rh type Antibody screen Full cross-match	None

RhD-negative units are reserved for women of child-bearing age.

Cross-match: electronic and serological

If the antibody screen is negative and there is no history of red cell alloantibodies, then ABO- and RhD-compatible blood is provided, usually by performing an electronic cross-match. Where the antibody screen is positive or there is a history of red cell alloantibodies, a serological cross-match is performed (Table 77.2). As patients develop antibodies, provision of compatible blood becomes more difficult.

Checking of blood products prior to administration to the patient is vital to ensure that the correct blood product is administered to the correct patient (Figure 77.1; Video 77.1).

Blood components

Information about whole blood components can be obtained at www.transfusion.com.au [1].

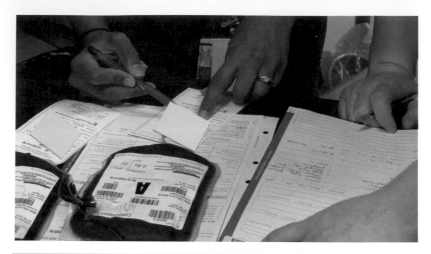

FIGURE 77.1 Checking of blood prior to administration.

www.wiley.com/go/perioperativemed

VIDEO 77.1 Blood transfusion is common in the perioperative period and clinicians must be aware of the risks and benefits for individual patients.

Indications for red cells, platelets, fresh frozen plasma and cryoprecipitate

Haemoglobin should be optimised prior to any elective surgery (refer to Chapter 17 Anaemia) and the Australian National Blood Authority *Patient Blood Management Guidelines*: www.blood.gov.au/pbm-guidelines [2].

Transfusions may be given prophylactically to improve tissue oxygenation using red cells, or prevent bleeding using fresh frozen plasma (FFP), platelets and cryoprecipitate. The 'number' used to trigger transfusion will vary depending on the clinical situation but generally the patient's clinical condition and the presence, source, volume and speed of blood loss are more appropriate parameters to consider.

Minimal evidence exists for the prophylactic use of FFP, cryoprecipitate or platelets prior to procedures. Abnormal coagulation tests do not predict bleeding and FFP fails to correct prothrombin time and bleeding in patients with mild coagulation abnormalities. FFP and cryoprecipitate use in transfusion support has undergone several comprehensive reviews [3,4].

Prophylactic platelet transfusions are mainly relevant to patients with bone marrow failure disorders and severe thrombocytopenia (platelet count < 10 × 10^9/L). They are generally ineffective in conditions of increased platelet destruction, e.g. ITP, immune thrombocytopenic purpura, thrombotic thrombocytopenic purpura, heparin-induced thrombocytopenia, and therefore, in the absence of significant bleeding, would be contraindicated.

Indications for prothrombin complex concentrates

The prothrombin complex concentrate (Prothrombinex) made in Australia contains factors II, IX and X with low levels of factor VII. It is licensed for use in warfarin reversal. In most scenarios it should be used in conjunction with FFP and vitamin K.

Complications of transfusion

If a reaction is suspected, the transfusion should be stopped, vital signs checked, IV access maintained, clerical check of the unit performed (check patient identity and that the unit is tagged and compatible for that patient), supportive care for the patient provided and a transfusion reaction investigation initiated.

Transfusion-transmitted infection has been greatly reduced over recent decades [5–7]. Current infectious and non-infectious risk estimates are available on a publicly accessible website [1]. Some of the more common types of acute transfusion reactions are discussed below. Table 77.3 summarises the acute and delayed transfusion reactions which can occur.

TABLE 77.3 **Transfusion reactions**

	Acute	**Delayed**
Immune	• Haemolytic • Allergic • Febrile non-haemolytic • Transfusion-related acute lung injury	• Post-transfusion purpura • Haemolytic • Transfusion-associated graft versus host disease
Non-immune	• Volume overload • Citrate toxicity • K⁺ toxicity • Bacterial contamination • Hypothermia	• Iron overload • Infectious

Acute haemolytic transfusion reactions

Acute haemolytic transfusion reactions are most often due to ABO incompatibility. Hospitals should develop robust systems to correctly identify patients for sample collection and administration of blood [8].

Transfusion-related acute lung injury

Transfusion-related acute lung injury (TRALI) is associated with transfusion of blood products containing plasma, with features similar to acute lung injury. Previously, TRALI was the leading cause of transfusion-associated mortality. However, the rates have diminished, probably due to the preferential use of male plasma. Treatment is supportive and approximately 80% of patients improve within 48–96 hours [7].

Transfusion-associated circulatory overload

Transfusion-associated circulatory overload (TACO) is common and patients with poor cardiac function and chronic anaemia are at risk. TACO usually manifests within hours of transfusion and is characterised by dyspnoea, orthopnoea, cyanosis, tachycardia, peripheral oedema and hypertension [7]. TACO can be avoided by transfusing slowly, close monitoring and diuretic use as required.

Allergic reactions

Allergic reactions vary from mild to severe. The allergen is usually a plasma protein. Mild reactions include localised urticaria which can be treated with antihistamines and transfusion continued slowly when the reaction resolves. Moderate-to-severe reactions usually involve more generalised rash, respiratory symptoms such as bronchospasm, laryngeal oedema, gastrointestinal symptoms and potentially anaphylactic shock. Acute management includes stopping the transfusion and treating as for anaphylactic or anaphylactoid reactions (refer to Chapter 72 Allergies and anaphylaxis) [7].

Bacterial contamination

Platelets pose the greatest risk of septic transfusion reactions due to bacterial contamination. Reactions are usually associated with fever and chills, vomiting and hypotension and may lead to septic shock, oliguria and disseminated intravascular coagulation (DIC). Management includes ceasing the transfusion, administration of broad-spectrum antibiotics, supportive care and culture of the patient and the unit [7].

Massive transfusion

Transfusion support in the haemorrhaging patient is one aspect of a multidisciplinary approach which includes surgical haemostasis and other local measures. Organisation and communication are crucial.

Where blood loss is rapid, a guide of two red cell units to one unit of FFP can be used to prevent dilutional coagulopathy. Where the fibrinogen is < 1.0 g/L, cryoprecipitate may also be used [2,4,9]. In the absence of administered platelets or increased consumption, for each blood volume of resuscitation the platelet count will fall by about half. The target platelet count in a seriously bleeding patient should be around 50–100 × 10^9/L. The patient should be kept warm and complications such as citrate toxicity monitored and treated. Pharmacological adjuncts to blood components include tranexamic acid and topical therapies. Recombinant VIIa has not proven to be useful and has been associated with adverse events [10].

References

1. ARCBS Transfusion medicine services website: www.transfusion.com.au

2. National Blood Authority Australia. *Patient Blood Management Guidelines*. www.blood.gov.au/pbm-guidelines

3. Stanworth SJ. The evidence-based use of FFP and cryoprecipitate for abnormalities of coagulation tests and clinical coagulopathy. *Hematology ASH Education Program*, 2007:179–186. doi: 10.1182/asheducation-2007.1.179

4. Roback JD, Caldwell S, Carson J, et al. Evidence-based practice guidelines for plasma transfusion. *Transfusion*, 2010;**50**(6):1227–1239. doi:10.1111/j.1537-2995.2010.02632.x

5. www.shotuk.org

6. www.nba.gov.au

7. Popovsky MA. *Transfusion Reactions*, 3rd edn. Bethesda, MD: AABB Press, 2007.

8. Murphy MF, Fraser E, Miles D, et al. How do we monitor hospital transfusion practice using an end-to-end electronic transfusion management system? *Transfusion*, 2012;**52**(12):2502–2512. doi:10.1111/J.1537-2995.2011.03509.X

9. Dzik WH, Blajchman MA, Fergusson D, et al. Clinical review: Canadian National Advisory Committee on Blood and Blood Products – Massive Transfusion Consensus Conference 2011: report of the panel. *Critical Care*, 2011;**15**(6):242. doi:10.1186/Cc10498

10. Yank V, Tuohy CV, Logan AC, et al. Systematic review: benefits and harms of in-hospital use of recombinant factor VIIa for off-label indications. *Annals of Internal Medicine*, 2011;**154**(8):529–540. doi:10.7326/0003-4819-154-8-201104190-00004

78 Organ donation

Steve Philpot[1] and Joshua Ihle[2]

[1] The Alfred Hospital and Monash University, Australia
[2] The Alfred Hospital, Australia

Organ transplantation is a definitive treatment for end-stage organ failures, but is limited by organ availability. Organs can be donated by living donors or after death. Death can be established by neurological criteria (brain death) or circulatory criteria (circulatory death). An important part of end-of-life care is offering families information about organ and tissue donation, and supporting them to make a decision that is right for their loved one and their family. In Australia, where consent for organ donation has been given by the family, they have the right to revoke consent at any time up until transfer to the operating theatre. Where consent has been given by the patient themselves (i.e. on the donor register), the family does not have the right to revoke consent.

No staff members involved in the retrieval of organs or the management of potential recipients should be involved in the management or declaration of death of the potential donor.

There are very few absolute contraindications to organ donation, and medical suitability takes into account co-morbidities and age of the potential donor. Successful organ transplantation relies upon expert management of the potential donor in order to prevent ischaemic damage occurring prior to organ retrieval. These patients are almost always managed in the ICU.

Tissue donation differs from solid organ donation in that tissue (such as heart valves, skin and corneas) is less susceptible to ischaemic damage. Since there is less urgency to retrieve tissue after death, patients who are unable to donate organs may still be eligible to be tissue donors. Because tissue transplantation is rarely life-saving, more stringent selection criteria apply.

Families may wish to view the body of the deceased after the donation retrieval surgery and should be supported to do this. Laws in some countries prevent the provision of information that would allow a transplant recipient to identify their donor.

Donation after brain death (DBD)

Brain death is defined as irreversible cessation of all functions of either the brain or brainstem, depending on the country. There are also region-specific differences in how brain death is determined and the following description is based on Australian and New Zealand guidelines [1]. Patients must have been observed for a period of time to be in an apnoeic, unresponsive coma, to have fixed and dilated pupils, and to have no cough reflex. Either clinical testing or radiological testing confirms the diagnosis [2].

Perioperative Medicine for the Junior Clinician, First Edition. Edited by Joel Symons, Paul Myles, Rishi Mehra and Christine Ball.
© 2015 John Wiley & Sons, Ltd. Published 2015 by John Wiley & Sons, Ltd.
Companion website: www.wiley.com/go/perioperativemed

Clinical testing

The patient must meet all preconditions (Box 78.1) and must be shown to have no brainstem reflexes (Table 78.1). Spinal reflexes (such as deep tendon reflexes, plantar responses and head turning) must be distinguished from cranial nerve

---

BOX 78.1 Preconditions. All preconditions must be met before brain death can be determined by clinical criteria

Injury	Insult to brain consistent with brain death (based upon history or neuroimaging)
Observation	Minimum of 4 hr (24 hr after rewarming when therapeutic hypothermia has been instituted) during which time there is: • unresponsive coma (GCS 3) • non-reactive pupils • absent cough reflex • no spontaneous breathing
Clinical	• Normothermia ($>35°C$) • Normotensive (SBP >90 mmHg, MAP >60 mmHg) • Sedative and paralysing drugs excluded • No severe electrolyte, metabolic or endocrine derangements • Intact neuromuscular function • Ability to assess brainstem (at least one eye and one ear) • Able to perform an apnoea test (no severe hypoxia, no C-spine injury)

GCS, Glasgow Coma Score; MAP, mean arterial pressure; SBP, systolic blood pressure.

TABLE 78.1 **Clinical tests. All brainstem reflexes must be absent in order to determine brain death**

Reflex	Test	Response
Coma	Apply painful stimulus to all four limbs	No response within cranial nerve distribution
Pupillary light: II & III	Shine a bright light into the eyes	Pupils >4 mm size with no pupillary constriction
Corneal: V & VII	Touch the cornea with soft cotton wool	No blinking or withdrawal
Response to pain in trigeminal distribution: V & VII	Apply pain over trigeminal distribution, e.g. supraorbital pressure	No facial or limb movement
Vestibulo-ocular: III, IV, VI & VIII	Inspect external auditory canal for patency, rest head up 30°, inject 50 mL of ice-cold saline	No eye movement for at least 60 seconds
Gag: IX & X	Stimulate the posterior pharyngeal wall	No gag response
Cough: X	Stimulate the tracheo-bronchial wall	No cough response
Presence of apnoea	Cease ventilation, continue oxygenation (supply 2 L/min O_2 via catheter or CPAP only)	No respiratory effort despite $PaCO_2 >60$ mmHg (or >20 mmHg above baseline) and pH <7.30

CPAP, continuous positive airway pressure.

TABLE 78.2 Modalities for radiological brain death determination; not all are approved for this purpose [1,3–6]

Imaging modality	Pros	Cons
Four-vessel angiography (intra-arterial)	Gold standard	Transport of patient Interventional Contrast load
Radionuclide imaging	Technetium 99m (Tc-99m) demonstrates perfusion after crossing blood–brain barrier	Transport of patient
Computed tomography (CT) angiography	Improving CT resolution Good specificity Readily available Non-invasive	Transport of patient Contrast load
Magnetic resonance imaging	Will show other features of raised intracranial pressure	Logistically difficult Slow
Transcranial doppler	Useful screening tool prior to confirmatory study Portable	Insufficiently specific Operator dependent
Electroencephalography	Portable	Affected by confounders Does not detect brainstem activity

reflexes, as only the latter exclude brain death. Seizures (including myoclonus) and true extensor/flexor posturing also exclude brain death. If clinical testing cannot be done (see Box 78.1), or where there is doubt about clinical responses, it is recommended that radiological testing be performed. In some jurisdictions, radiological confirmation is mandated [1].

Radiological testing

Brain death can be diagnosed by demonstrating absent intracranial blood flow. Whilst there are several imaging modalities that might suggest this (Table 78.2), four-vessel angiogram and nuclear medicine perfusion scan are highly sensitive and specific. CT angiography and CT perfusion are also accepted in some countries [3,4]. Transcranial Doppler is not sufficiently specific to confirm brain death.

Managing a brain-dead potential organ donor

Brain-dead potential organ donors are ventilated and have an intact and supported circulation until organ procurement. This requires invasive monitoring and specialised care in the ICU and operating theatre (Table 78.3).

Prior to brain death, a sympathetic surge known as Cushing's response (coning) may be seen, resulting in extreme hypertension and tachycardia or bradycardia. If treated, very short-acting antihypertensives should be used, as the response is short-lived and may be followed by profound hypotension immediately after brainstem death.

Diabetes insipidus is common after brain death. It presents as production of large volumes of dilute urine, hypovolaemia and hypernatraemia, and responds to treatment with synthetic ADH as well as replacement of lost intravascular volume with hypotonic fluid. Deficiency of other pituitary hormones may contribute to cardiovascular instability, and may require specific treatment with steroids and/or thyroid hormone replacement.

TABLE 78.3 **Care of the potential donor: management goals**

System	Targets	Therapies
Monitoring	Safe cardiac and haemodynamic monitoring	Arterial line, central venous line +/– cardiac output monitoring, ECG, temperature, fluid balance
Haemodynamic	MAP >70 mmHg or SBP >100 mmHg Urine output > 1 mL/kg/hr	Inotropes/vasopressors +/– fluid Hormonal therapy (thyroxine, steroids, vasopressin)
Respiratory	Lung protective ventilation Optimum ventilatory mode	Minimal FiO_2 for PaO_2 >60 mmHg Tidal volume 6–8 mL/kg Plateau pressure <30 cmH_2O Head of bed elevated >30° Closed circuit suctioning Lung recruitment manoeuvres
Nutrition	Nutrition for potential liver donors BSL 4–10 mmol/L	Nasogastric feeding preferred Insulin
Metabolic	Normalise electrolytes Na^+ 130–150 mmol/L	K^+, Mg^{2+}, PO_4^- replacement Treat diabetes insipidus Appropriate choice of IV fluid
Temperature	Avoid hypothermia	External warming devices, warm fluids, humidified ventilation, external warming
Haematology	Hb >70 g/dL Correction of coagulopathy	Transfusion as indicated
Microbiology	Infection control	Broad-spectrum antibiotics

BSL, blood sugar level; ECG, electrocardiogram; Hb, haemoglobin; IV, intravenous; MAP, mean arterial pressure; SBP, systolic blood pressure.

Anaesthetic management is aimed at continuing the goals set out in Table 78.3. Neuromuscular blockade is mostly required to suppress the effects of spinal reflexes, but anaesthetic and analgesic agents are not. Vasoactive drugs and intraoperative transfusion may be required. Patients should have blood cross-matched, and have large-bore peripheral venous access in addition to central venous access. Other medications commonly used intraoperatively include heparin, high-dose steroids and prophylactic antibiotics.

Donation after circulatory death (DCD)

In patients who are not brain dead but who are expected to make a poor recovery from acute illness, ongoing organ support may be deemed not in their best interest and subsequently withdrawn. Patients are monitored after withdrawal of cardiorespiratory support (WCRS) with the expectation that they will die shortly afterwards, and death is declared after circulatory arrest. Organ retrieval can occur immediately after death. The suitability of organs for donation depends on the time to death after WCRS (about 90 minutes for lung donation, 60 minutes for kidneys and 30 minutes for heart and liver). Transplant recipient outcomes are similar following DCD and DBD.

In some circumstances, DCD may also be considered where unexpected and irreversible cardiac arrest occurs, or after circulatory arrest in a brain-dead person awaiting organ retrieval.

Managing a potential DCD donor

Unlike after brain death, potential DCD donors are alive during the organ donation assessment period, and their comfort and dignity must take priority. Goals of management are as for brain-dead donors (see Table 78.3). Next-of-kin support should be sought for any treatment related to organ donation. The endocrine and physiological consequences of brainstem death are not seen.

WCRS may occur in the operating theatre or in the ICU. If death occurs within the required timeframes, the patient is moved to the operating room, otherwise the patient's palliative care is continued and organ donation does not proceed. If lungs are to be procured, the patient's trachea is reintubated after death to prevent aspiration. Gentle insufflation of the lungs may prevent progressive atelectasis, but ventilation is avoided.

References

1. Australian and New Zealand Intensive Care Society. *The ANZICS Statement on Death and Organ Donation* (Edition 3.1). Melbourne: ANZICS, 2010.

2. Dupas B, Gayet-Delacroix M, Villers D, Antonioli D, Veccherini MF, Soulillou JP. Diagnosis of brain death using two-phase spiral CT. *American Journal of Neuroradiology*, 1998;**19**(4):641–647.

3. Frampas E, Videcoq M, de Kerviler E, et al. CT angiography for brain death diagnosis. *American Journal of Neuroradiology*, 2009;**30**(8):1566–1570. doi:10.3174/ajnr.A1614

4. Gutierrez LG, Rovira A, Portela LA, Leite C, Lucato LT. CT and MR in non-neonatal hypoxic-ischemic encephalopathy: radiological findings with pathophysiological correlations. *Neuroradiology*, 2010;**52**(11):949–976. doi:10.1007/s00234-010-0728-z

5. Gardiner D, Shemie S, Manara A, Opdam H. International perspective on the diagnosis of death. *British Journal of Anaesthesia*, 2012;**108**(Suppl 1):i14–28. doi:10.1093/bja/aer397

6. McKeown DW, Bonser RS, Kellum JA. Management of the heartbeating brain-dead organ donor. *British Journal of Anaesthesia*, 2012;**108**(Suppl 1):i96–107. doi:10.1093/bja/aer351

Part VI
Early postoperative care

79 Postoperative nausea and vomiting

Joel Symons

The Alfred Hospital and Monash University, Australia

Postoperative nausea and vomiting (PONV) refers to any nausea, dry retching or vomiting that occurs during the first 24–48 hours after surgery.

Epidemiology and risk factors

Postoperative nausea and vomiting occurs in 20–30% of all surgical patients after general anaesthesia [1] and up to 70–80% of high–risk surgical patients [2–4].

Table 79.1 summarises the various patient, anaesthesia and surgical risk factors associated with PONV. These risk factors are important as they determine the type and number of antiemetics that will be required for PONV prophylaxis and treatment.

Pathophysiology and mechanism of action

The following brain structures dispersed throughout the medulla oblongata in the brainstem are involved in PONV.

- The 'vomiting centre'
  - An ill-defined area located in the lateral reticular formation of the brainstem
  - It is a 'central pattern generator' that initiates a sequence of neuronal activities throughout the medulla, resulting in vomiting [5]
- The chemoreceptor trigger zone (CRTZ)
  - Situated in the area postrema in the caudal end of the fourth ventricle
  - Outside the blood–brain barrier
  - Inputs to the 'vomiting centre'
  - Has neuronal projections to the nucleus tractus solitarius
  - Receives inputs from vagal afferents in the GI tract, emetogenic toxins, drugs (e.g. opioids and volatile anaesthetics) and metabolites which circulate in the blood and CSF
- The nucleus tractus solitarius (NTS)
  - Situated in the area postrema and lower pons

Perioperative Medicine for the Junior Clinician, First Edition. Edited by Joel Symons, Paul Myles, Rishi Mehra and Christine Ball.
© 2015 John Wiley & Sons, Ltd. Published 2015 by John Wiley & Sons, Ltd.
Companion website: www.wiley.com/go/perioperativemed

	Patient related	Anaesthesia related	Surgery related
Well-established risk factors	Female gender (especially premenopausal, age 15–50 years) Non-smokers Previous PONV History of motion sickness Age (increased in children >3 years compared to younger, but a decrease with age in adults)	Volatile anaesthesia Nitrous oxide Intra- and postoperative opioid use (dose dependent) Duration of anaesthesia (increased exposure to emetogenic agents)	
Less well-established risk factors (weak evidence)	History of migraine Preoperative anxiety	General anaesthesia Neostigmine	Strabismus surgery (especially in the paediatric population – independent risk factor) Gynaecological surgery Ophthalmological surgery Otological surgery Thyroid surgery Cosmetic surgery
Factors that have been proven to be unrelated	Body Mass Index Menstrual cycle phase	Supplemental oxygen Short-acting opioid use (e.g. remifentanil) Absence of gastric tube decompression	

- Inputs to the 'vomiting centre'
- Receives vagal and sympathetic input from the GI tract and glossopharyngeal nerve and vagal input from the oropharynx, limbic and vestibular systems
- Triggers vomiting by stimulating various brainstem nuclei

Numerous neurotransmitter pathways are involved in the nausea and vomiting response, and it is these that are targeted by antiemetic drugs. The receptors and antiemetic drugs acting on these pathways are shown in Figure 79.1 and Video 79.1.

Scoring systems

As alluded to in Table 79.1, PONV scoring systems are important for two reasons. Firstly, as the number of risk factors increases, so does the incidence of PONV. Secondly, the scoring systems guide PONV prophylaxis. In 70% of patients, PONV risk can be correctly classified using the scoring systems in Tables 79.2 and 79.3. These scoring systems are best used pre- and intraoperatively.

Postoperative nausea and vomiting prophylaxis

Postoperative nausea and vomiting prophylaxis can be effectively achieved by following the five simple steps in Figure 79.2.

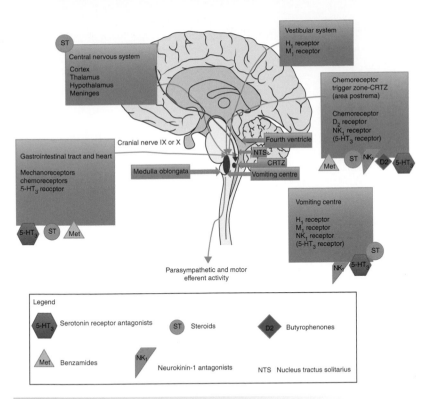

FIGURE 79.1 **Pathophysiology of vomiting and mechanism of action of antiemetics.**

www.wiley.com/go/perioperativemed

VIDEO 79.1 **Pathophysiology of vomiting and mechanism of action of antiemetics.**

TABLE 79.2 **An adult PONV scoring system [3]**

Risk factors for PONV	Number of risk factors	Incidence of PONV (%)
	0	10
Female gender	1	20
History of motion sickness and/or previous PONV	2	40
Non-smoking status	3	60
Postoperative opioid use	4	80

TABLE 79.3 **A paediatric PONV scoring system: Postoperative Vomiting in Children (POVOC) score (for use in children) [10]**

Independent risk factors for PONV	Number of risk factors	Incidence of PONV (%)
	0	9
Duration of surgery >/= 30 min	1	10
Age >/= 3 years	2	30
Strabismus surgery	3	55
History of postoperative vomiting in the child or PONV in his/her relatives	4	70

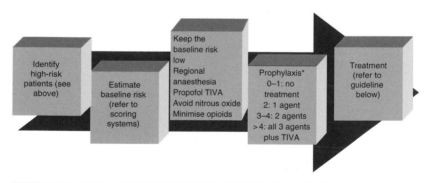

FIGURE 79.2 **The five steps to managing PONV.**

Management of established PONV

The management of established PONV is outlined in Figure 79.3. It commences with a brief exclusion of reversible factors such as hypotension and mechanical obstruction. Further management will depend on whether prophylaxis was or was not administered in theatre.

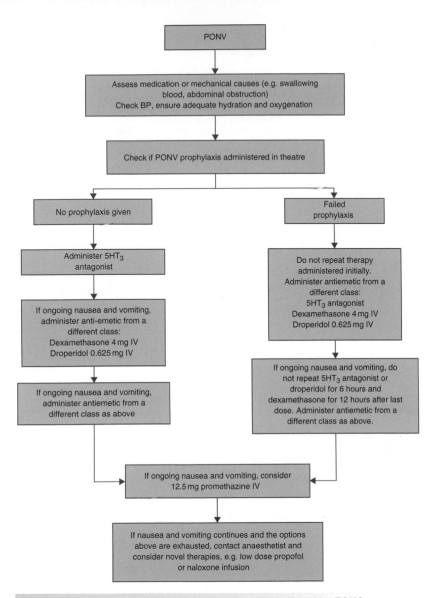

FIGURE 79.3 **Flow diagram for managing postoperative nausea and vomiting (PONV).**

Antiemetic therapy in adults [6–9]

Antiemetic therapy is aimed at blocking receptors involved in the PONV mechanism. One antiemetic usually acts on a number of different receptors, but not on all receptors. It is for this reason that although first-line therapy is usually effective and sufficient, a second or third antiemetic may also be required.

First-line therapy

Table 79.4 outlines the first-line drugs used in antiemetic therapy.

TABLE 79.4 First-line antiemetic agents

Class/ generic names	Dose (adult), timing and mode of administration	Side effects
Serotonin antagonists	**End of surgery**	
Ondansetron	4–8 mg IV/oral/sublingual	Headache, dizziness, constipation, diarrhoea, elevated liver enzymes
Granisetron	0.35–1.5 mg IV/oral	
Tropisetron	2 mg IV	
Dolasetron	12.5 mg IV/oral	
Palonasetron	0.075 mg IV	
Steroids	**Induction of anaesthesia**	
Dexamethasone	4–8 mg IV	Flushing, perineal itching
Butyrophenones	**End of surgery**	
Droperidol	0.625–1.25 mg IV	QTc prolongation, sedation, extrapyramidal side effects
Haloperidol	1 mg IV	

IV, intravenous.

TABLE 79.5 Second-line antiemetic agents

Class/generic names	Dose (adult), timing and mode of administration	Side effects
Cholinergic antagonists	**Night before/day of surgery**	
Scopolamine	1 mg transdermal	Visual disturbances, dry mouth, dizziness
Phenothiazines	**Induction of anaesthesia**	
Promethazine	6.25–25 mg IV	Sedation, restlessness, diarrhoea, agitation, CNS depression, hypotension, extrapyramidal, SVT, neuroleptic syndrome
Prochlorperazine	5–10 mg IV/IM	
Benzamides	**Induction of anaesthesia**	
Metoclopramide	25–50 mg IV	Oculogyric crisis
Antihistamines	**Induction of anaesthesia**	
Dimenhydrinate	1 mg/kg IV	Sedation, dry mouth, blurred vision, urinary retention
Propofol		
Propofol infusion	0.1–0.2 mcg/mL total IV anaesthetic	Hypotension, drowsiness

Class/generic names	Dose (adult), timing and mode of administration	Side effects
Neurokinin-1 antagonists	Preoperatively	
Aprepitant	40 mg oral	Asthenia, diarrhoea, dizziness, hiccups
Opioid antagonists		
Naloxone	0.25 mcg/kg/hr IVI	
Vasopressors		
Ephedrine	0.5 mg/kg IM	
Non-pharmacological		
Acupuncture	P6 acupuncture point	

CNS, central nervous system; IM, intramuscular; IV, intravenous; IVI, intravenous infusion; SVT, supraventricular tachycardia.

Second-line therapy

Second-line therapy can be considered when first-line therapy fails. The patient and clinical situation will determine selection of medication, e.g. use antihistamines where sedation is desirable, use propofol if the patient is in a monitored environment (only under direct supervision of an anaesthetist). These agents are outlined in Table 79.5.

References

1. Dolin SJ, Cashman JN, Bland JM. Effectiveness of acute postoperative pain management:1. Evidence from published data. *British Journal of Anaesthesia*, 2002;**89**:409–423.

2. Tramer MR. A rational approach to the control of postoperative nausea and vomiting: evidence from systematic reviews. Part I. Efficacy and harm of antiemetic interventions, and methodological issues. *Acta Anaesthesiologica Scandinavica*, 2001;**45**:4–13.

3. Apfel CC, Laara E, Koivuranta M, Greim CA, Roewer N. A simplified risk score for predicting postoperative nausea and vomiting: conclusions from cross-validations between two centers. *Anesthesiology*, 1999;**91**(3):693–700. doi:10.1097/00000542-199909000-00022

4. Apfel CC, Korttila K, Abdalla M, et al. A factorial trial of six interventions for the prevention of postoperative nausea and vomiting. *New England Journal of Medicine*, 2004;**350**(24): 2441–2451. doi:10.1056/NEJMoa032196

5. Hornby PJ. Central neurocircuitry associated with emesis. *American Journal of Medicine*, 2001;**111**(Suppl 8A):106S–112S. doi:10.1016/s0002-9343(01)00849-x

6. Gan TJ, Meyer TA, Apfel CC, et al. Society for Ambulatory Anesthesia guidelines for the management of postoperative nausea and vomiting. *Anesthesia and Analgesia*, 2007;**105**(6):1615–1628. doi:10.1213/01.ane.0000295230.55439.f4

7. Pierre S. Nausea and vomiting after surgery. *Continuing Education in Anaesthesia, Critical Care and Pain*, 2013;**13**(1):28–32.

8. Le TP, Gan TJ. Update on the management of postoperative nausea and vomiting and postdischarge nausea and vomiting in ambulatory surgery. *Anesthesiology Clinics*, 2010;**28**(2):225–249.

9. Gan TJ, Diemunsch P, Habib AS, et al. Consensus guidelines for the management of postoperative nausea and vomiting. *Anesthesia and Analgesia*, 2014;**118**(1):85–113. doi:10.1213/ANE.0000000000000002

10. Eberhart LH, Geldner G, Kranke P, et al. The development and validation of a risk score to predict the probability of postoperative vomiting in pediatric patients. *Anesthesia and Analgesia*, 2004;**99**(6):1630–1637. doi:10.1213/01.ANE.0000135639.57715.6C

80 Postoperative fluid therapy

Dashiell Gantner

The Alfred Hospital and Monash University, Australia

Intravenous (IV) fluid administration in the perioperative setting must be justified on the basis of an existing or predicted fluid deficit. Like any drug, IV fluid can cause harmful side effects.

Fluid composition (Table 80.1)

Crystalloids

Isotonic crystalloids are solutions of sterile water containing ionised, water-soluble salts (electrolytes) to approximate the ion-water concentration of human plasma. The most commonly used crystalloid worldwide is 0.9% sodium chloride ('normal saline'). 0.9% saline is 'normal' because its tonicity is approximately equivalent to healthy extracellular compartment tonicity, meaning there should be no net movement of water into or out of cells with its administration.

Balanced salt solutions

Balanced salt solutions closely approximate normal physiological electrolyte concentrations and pH. Their electroneutrality is maintained with non-chloride anions (lactate, or gluconate and acetate), which are metabolised to bicarbonate following infusion; therefore the hyperchloraemic acidosis caused by 0.9% sodium chloride is avoided.

Colloids

Colloid fluids are composed of crystalloid solutions (usually saline) to which insoluble, high molecular weight (MW) substances are added. These substances are too large to permeate healthy vascular endothelium and hence exert oncotic pressure, with the theoretical advantage of retaining fluid volume in the intravascular space. Colloids are categorised below.

- Blood-derived proteins
  - Albumin (MW 69 kDa)

Perioperative Medicine for the Junior Clinician, First Edition. Edited by Joel Symons, Paul Myles, Rishi Mehra and Christine Ball.
© 2015 John Wiley & Sons, Ltd. Published 2015 by John Wiley & Sons, Ltd.
Companion website: www.wiley.com/go/perioperativemed

TABLE 80.1 Components and pH of different intravenous fluids

| | Plasma | Crystalloids | | | | Colloids | | |
| | | Saline 0.9% | Hartmann's | Plasma-Lyte | Albumex 4% | Voluven (6% HES 130/0.4) | Gelofusine |
	mmol/L	mmol/L	mmol/L	mmol/L	mmol/L	mmol/L	mmol/L
Sodium	136–145	154	129	140	140	154	154
Potassium	3.5–5.0		5.0	5.0			
Magnesium	0.8–1.0			1.5			
Calcium	2.2–2.6		2.5				
Chloride	98–106	154	109	98	128	154	120
Acetate				27			
Gluconate				23			
Lactate			29				
Osmolarity (mOsmol/L)	290–310	308	274	295			274
Colloid (g/L)	Predominantly albumin (35–45 g/L)	–	–	–	Albumin (40 g/L)	HES 130/0.4 (60 g/L)	Gelatin (40 g/L)
pH	7.4	5.5–6.2	5.5–6.2	7.4	5.5–6.2	5.5–6.2	7.4

HES, hydroxyethyl starch.

- Semi-synthetic
  - Hydroxyethyl starches (HES) of variable molecular weights (MW 70–670 kDa)
  - Gelatins (Gelofusine and Haemaccel)
  - Branched polysaccharides (dextrans – now rarely used)

Indications

Maintenance fluids

The perioperative neuroendocrine response to surgery results in retention of sodium and water, with a reduction in maintenance fluid requirements. Preoperative fluids for fasting patients are not routinely indicated. For most patients, operative fluid losses are replaced during surgery and oral intake is resumed promptly after surgery, so ongoing maintenance fluids are not required [1].

Where oral intake is delayed (e.g. gastrointestinal surgery), inadequate fluid replacement will result in reduced cardiac output and oxygen delivery. In this setting, IV fluids can help to maintain circulating volume state, and allow administration of electrolytes and nutritional substrates. Conversely, excessive fluid administration is also associated with adverse effects such as acidosis, oedema (peripheral and pulmonary) and increased patient mortality. Traditional estimates of fluid deficits and requirements are given in Table 80.2.

Bolus fluids

Rapid volume state expansion is generally regarded as first-line treatment in acute circulatory failure, and to reverse or prevent hypovolaemia from anaesthetic, surgical or illness factors. Patients with overt and subclinical shock, and who are assessed to be fluid responsive, should receive boluses of fluid. Volumes as high as 20–40 mL/kg have traditionally been prescribed.

Fluid is administered with the expectation that it will increase cardiac preload and cardiac output. However, only 50% of haemodynamically unstable, critically ill patients are volume responsive, indicating the need for accurate assessment of the patient's intravascular volume status and exclusion of other factors contributing to organ hypoperfusion (Figure 80.1). The loss of vascular tone that occurs with systemic inflammatory states or with epidural anaesthesia results in expansion of the intravascular space and thus a *relatively* low volume state; hence there is a physiological rationale for fluid administration in these conditions. However, fluid boluses should be discontinued once the patient is no longer fluid responsive,

TABLE 80.2 **Traditional estimates of fluid requirements**

Maintenance requirement	Clinical indicators of preoperative deficit (% circulating volume)	Intraoperative evaporative losses
1.5 mL/kg/hr (2–3 L/day)	• 10%: thirst, venous constriction • 20%: sweating, decreased urine output, mild tachycardia • 30%: heart rate > 120 beats per minute, moderate hypotension, pallor, cool peripheries, anuria • 40%: severe hypotension and tachycardia • 50%: loss of consciousness • > 50%: cardiac arrest	• 0.5–1.0 mL/kg/hr (dependent upon degree of visceral exposure)

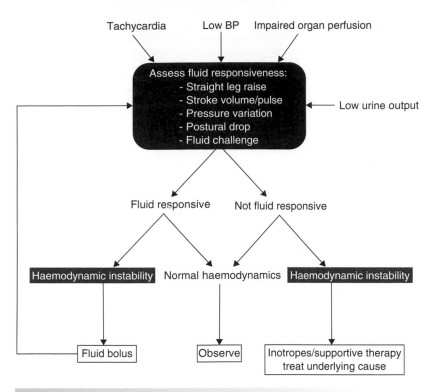

Tachycardia   Low BP   Impaired organ perfusion

Assess fluid responsiveness:
- Straight leg raise
- Stroke volume/pulse
- Pressure variation
- Postural drop
- Fluid challenge

Low urine output

Fluid responsive   Not fluid responsive

Haemodynamic instability   Normal haemodynamics   Haemodynamic instability

Fluid bolus   Observe   Inotropes/supportive therapy treat underlying cause

FIGURE 80.1 **Decision making in fluid resuscitation. BP, blood pressure.**

as numerous studies have found correlations between fluid overload and poor patient outcomes, including mortality.

Choice of fluid

Fluid selection should be based on physiological requirements; however, with a few exceptions (see below), there is little clinical evidence that any solution is more effective or safer than any other [2].

Conceptually, body fluids are divided between the intracellular compartment and the interstitial and intravascular components of the extracellular fluid compartment.

Crystalloids

Following administration, crystalloids quickly disperse between the interstitial and intravascular extracellular fluid compartments, resulting in interstitial oedema as well as increasing circulating volume.

Saline
The advantages of saline are that it is isotonic, readily available and of low cost. However, it can cause hyperchloraemic metabolic acidosis when administered in large volumes, and may impair renal function. The clinical consequences of these effects are unclear.

Balanced salt solutions

Balanced salt solutions are increasingly recommended as first-line fluids in surgical patients because their electrolyte composition approximates extracellular fluid. Although randomised evidence comparing saline with balanced salt solutions is pending, there is substantial observational evidence to support their use due to reductions in postoperative infections, reductions in renal impairment and the reduced need for blood transfusion [3].

Rare complications of excessive administration of balanced salt solutions include hyperlactaemia (particularly when lactate clearance is impaired, such as in liver failure), metabolic alkalosis and hypotonicity.

Colloids

Colloids are frequently prescribed due to their potential to remain in the intravascular space longer than crystalloids. However, in major surgery and critical illness, the capillary endothelial glycocalyx layer becomes more permeable and colloids may leak, with resultant loss of intravascular oncotic pressure [4].

Large randomised controlled trials have not confirmed any benefit of colloids over crystalloids for fluid resuscitation, and in specific populations some colloids have been shown to be harmful. Albumin is equivalent to saline with respect to patient outcomes, except in patients with severe traumatic brain injury where albumin increases mortality [5,6]. Hydroxyethyl starch solutions have been shown to cause kidney injury and increase mortality. Other semi-synthetic colloids such as gelatins or polygeline solutions have not been studied in high-quality, randomised controlled trials; their use is hard to justify in the absence of benefit seen with other colloids [7].

References

1. Chappell D, Jacob M, Hofmann-Kiefer K, Conzen P, Rehm M. A rational approach to perioperative fluid management. *Anesthesiology*, 2008;**109**(4):723–740. doi:10.1097/ALN.0b013e3181863117

2. Myburgh JA, Mythen MG. Resuscitation fluids. *New England Journal of Medicine*, 2013;**369**(13):1243–1251. doi:10.1056/NEJMra1208627

3. Shaw AD, Bagshaw SM, Goldstein SL, et al. Major complications, mortality, and resource utilization after open abdominal surgery: 0.9% saline compared to Plasma-Lyte. *Annals of Surgery*, 2012;**255**(5):821–829. doi:10.1097/SLA.0b013e31825074f5

4. Woodcock TE, Woodcock TM. Revised Starling equation and the glycocalyx model of transvascular fluid exchange: an improved paradigm for prescribing intravenous fluid therapy. *British Journal of Anaesthesia*, 2012;**108**(3):384–394. doi:10.1093/bja/aer515

5. Safe Study Investigators. Saline or albumin for fluid resuscitation in patients with traumatic brain injury. *New England Journal of Medicine*, 2007;**357**(9):874–884. doi:10.1056/NEJMoa067514

6. Finfer S, Bellomo R, Boyce N, et al. A comparison of albumin and saline for fluid resuscitation in the intensive care unit. *New England Journal of Medicine*, 2004;**350**(22):2247–2256. doi:10.1056/NEJMoa040232

7. Perel P, Roberts I, Ker K. Colloids versus crystalloids for fluid resuscitation in critically ill patients. *Cochrane Database of Systematic Reviews*, 2013;**2**:CD000567. doi:10.1002/14651858.CD000567.pub6

Ventilation strategies

John Botha

Monash University, Australia

Mechanical ventilation can be non-invasive through a facemask or invasive following tracheal intubation. It remains a treatment option when there are clinical signs or laboratory results indicating that a patient cannot protect their airway or maintain adequate gas exchange. Initiation of mechanical ventilation should be based on clinical judgement and indications include a respiratory rate >30/min, inability to maintain $SaO_2 > 90\%$ with $FiO_2 > 0.60$, a $PaCO_2 > 50$ mmHg or a pH < 7.25.

Physiology and physics of ventilation

Normal inspiration generates negative intrapleural pressure and in mechanical ventilation, the pressure gradient is a consequence of positive pressure provided by the ventilator.

The ventilated lungs can be thought of as a tube (large airways, tracheal tube, ventilator tubing) attached to an inflatable ball (alveoli). The pressure to move gas through the tube is determined by the resistance and the flow such that:

$$Pressure = flow \times resistance$$

The baseline pressure in the alveoli at the end of expiration is the PEEP. The inflation pressure is determined by the additional volume of gas pumped into the lung and the stiffness or compliance of the lung such that:

$$Alveolar\ pressure = volume / compliance + PEEP$$

Compliance is inversely proportional to the elastance of the lung.

Peak airway opening pressure (Pao) is measured at the airway opening and represents the total pressure required to deliver a volume of gas into the lung. This total pressure is determined by the inspiratory flow resistance (resistive pressure), the elastance of the lung and chest wall, and PEEP.

$$Airway\ pressure = flow \times resistance + volume / compliance + PEEP$$

Increased peak airway pressure requires measurement of the end-inspiratory pressure (plateau pressure) by an end-inspiratory hold manoeuvre to determine the relative contributions of resistive and elastic pressures (Figure 81.1). When airflow

Perioperative Medicine for the Junior Clinician, First Edition. Edited by Joel Symons, Paul Myles, Rishi Mehra and Christine Ball.
© 2015 John Wiley & Sons, Ltd. Published 2015 by John Wiley & Sons, Ltd.
Companion website: www.wiley.com/go/perioperativemed

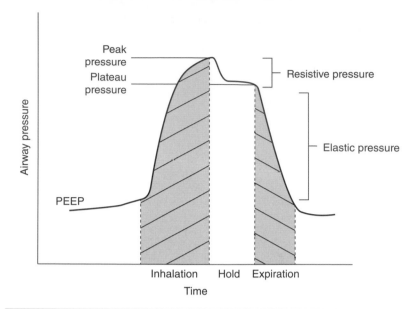

FIGURE 81.1 **Components of airway pressure during mechanical ventilation, illustrated by an inspiratory hold manoeuvre. PEEP, positive end-expiratory pressure.**

ceases, the airway pressure falls below its peak value. This end-inspiratory pressure reflects the elastic pressure once PEEP is subtracted and the difference between peak and plateau pressure is the resistive pressure.

Elevated resistive pressure implies that the tracheal tube is occluded or there is bronchoconstriction while an increase in elastic pressure suggests decreased lung compliance or limited chest wall or diaphragmatic movement.

Setting the ventilator

FiO_2 is initially set at 1.0 and is thereafter reduced to target the required oxygenation, and PEEP may be applied to reduce airspace closure at the end of expiration. Tidal volume and respiratory rate determine the minute ventilation. Large volumes may cause overinflation and small volumes atelectasis.

Mechanical ventilators may deliver a constant volume (volume cycled), a constant pressure (pressure cycled) or a combination of both with each breath. Because pressures and volumes are directly linked by the pressure–volume curve, any given volume will correspond to a specific pressure, and vice versa. Further ventilator settings may include respiratory rate, tidal volume, trigger sensitivity, flow rate, waveform and inspiratory/expiratory (I/E) ratio.

Manipulating oxygenation and ventilation

Oxygenation may be improved by increasing the PAO_2 or by improving the V/Q mismatch. Oxygenation is thus improved by increasing FiO_2, increasing PEEP, increasing inspiratory time and increasing tidal volume or inspiratory pressure. Carbon dioxide elimination is determined by alveolar ventilation.

$$\text{Alveolar ventilation} = \text{respiratory rate} \times (\text{tidal volume} - \text{dead space})$$

Carbon dioxide elimination is increased by increasing tidal volume, increasing respiratory rate and decreasing dead space.

Modes of mechanical ventilation [1]

Assist control (AC) modes

A breath may be delivered by the ventilator (control breath) or triggered by the patient (assisted breath). The characteristics of both breaths are identical and may be volume or pressure controlled. The tidal volume, duration of inspiration, inspiratory pause time and inspiratory flow can be set on the ventilator and are determined by the ventilator settings.

Synchronised intermittent mandatory ventilation (SIMV)

The ventilator delivers a set number of mandatory breaths which can be volume or pressure controlled. Any spontaneous breathing by the patient is possible and these spontaneous breaths may be pressure supported.

The differences between these two modes of ventilation are shown in Figure 81.2.

Pressure support mode (PS)

A level of inspiratory pressure is delivered every time the patient initiates a breath. There is no back-up mode so if a patient becomes apnoeic, no breaths are given. Tidal volumes may change if compliance and resistance change.

Pressure regulated volume control (PRVC)

The ventilator initially delivers a test breath and subsequently adjusts the pressure delivered so as to provide the set tidal volume. The ventilator varies the ventilator pressure to provide the preset volume.

Neurally adjusted ventilatory assist (NAVA)

When the ventilator is triggered by a pressure or flow change, there is delay between the initiation of effort by the respiratory muscles and the delivery of support. NAVA uses the neural stimulus to respiratory muscles to trigger the ventilator simultaneously with muscular effort measured using electrodes mounted on a nasogastric tube.

Airway pressure release ventilation (APRV) [2]

This mode delivers high levels of continuous positive airway pressure, often greater than 20 cmH_2O (P_{high}) alternating with time cycled releases at a lower pressure (P_{low}).

Proportional-assist ventilation (PAV+)

This is a mode of support in which the ventilator generates pressure proportional to the instantaneous flow (flow assist) and volume (volume assist) of a patient. The resistance and elastance of the respiratory system are constantly measured by the ventilator software and flow and volume are adjusted accordingly.

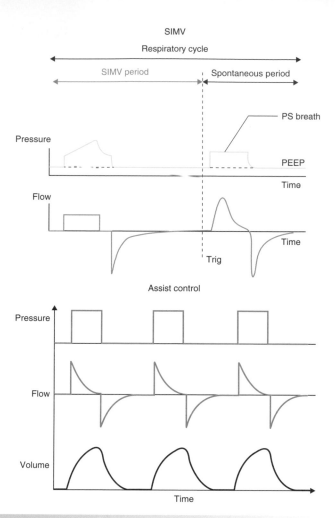

FIGURE 81.2 **Difference between synchronised intermittent mandatory ventilation (SIMV) (top) and assist control (bottom) mode of ventilation. PS, pressure support.**

High-frequency oscillatory ventilation (HFOV)

With this mode of ventilation, an oscillating piston pump and a bias gas (flow rate) of 20–40 L/min are used to generate a ventilator frequency typically between 180 and 900 bpm and a tidal volume typically 1–2 mL/kg.

Novel strategies to improve oxygenation
Recruitment

There are various recruitment methods that have been used in the past, including the static recruitment method, the dynamic recruitment method and the staircase recruitment method where incremental PEEP is applied to 'open' the lung.

Prone ventilation

Oxygen in prone patients is improved through alveolar recruitment, changes in lung position in the thorax allowing uniform lung distension and redirection of compressive force exerted by the heart on the lungs (preventing their expansion) toward the sternum, and a reduction in extravascular lung water [3].

References

1. Stewart NI, Jagelman TA, Webster NR. Emerging modes of ventilation in the intensive care unit. *British Journal of Anaesthesia*, 2011;**107**(1):74–82. doi:10.1093/bja/aer114

2. Stock MC, Downs JB, Frolicher DA. Airway pressure release ventilation. *Critical Care Medicine*, 1987;**15**(5):462–466. www.ncbi.nlm.nih.gov/pubmed/3552443

3. Tiruvoipati R, Botha J. Prone ventilation for severe hypoxic respiratory failure: lacking evidence but probably not efficacy. *British Journal of Intensive Care*, 2010;**20**(3):67–72.

81

82 Sepsis and the inflammatory response to surgery

Tomás Corcoran and Kajari Roy

Royal Perth Hospital, Australia

Pathophysiology

Neuroendocrine components of the surgical stress response include the following.

1. Sympathetic nervous system activation
   - Tachycardia, hypertension, glycolysis, increased cardiac output
2. Pituitary hormone secretion
   - ACTH: increased cortisol production, insulin resistance and glycolysis
   - Arginine vasopressin (AVP): promotes water retention in the distal nephron
   - Growth hormone (GH): glycolysis and insulin resistance
3. Adrenal gland activation
   - Catecholamine secretion
   - Cortisol secretion
   - Aldosterone: promotes renal sodium retention in the loop of Henle

Inflammatory components of the surgical stress response

Resolution of inflammation, when tissues have healed or an infection is eradicated, is an active process.

The acute phase response

This term is used to describe the changes involving organ systems distant from the site, or sites, of inflammation or infection. These manifestations result from inflammatory mediators and a series of proteins called acute phase reactants

Perioperative Medicine for the Junior Clinician, First Edition. Edited by Joel Symons, Paul Myles, Rishi Mehra and Christine Ball.
© 2015 John Wiley & Sons, Ltd. Published 2015 by John Wiley & Sons, Ltd.
Companion website: www.wiley.com/go/perioperativemed

(APRs). Most of these compounds increase with inflammation (positive APRs); a small number decrease (negative APRs). Procalcitonin is of particular interest as it may prove a useful marker to differentiate an inflammatory response due to infection from that caused by tissue injury (surgery, trauma, reperfusion). Albumin is the most notable negative APR. Hypoalbuminaemia is associated with severe inflammation and chronic disease, and predicts higher risk of poor outcome after surgery.

Counterinflammatory response to surgery (CARS) and illness

The counterinflammatory response to surgery is a systemic deactivation of the immune system that restores homeostasis from an inflammatory state. Sustained inflammation may provoke excessive CARS with the potential for severe infectious complications in the postoperative period, multiorgan failure and death [1].

Clinical features

Clinical features of the inflammatory response to surgery

The surgical stress response and clinical findings are usually proportionate to the extent of tissue injury (e.g. high in cardiac surgery with bypass, low in laparoscopic surgery). It should not persist beyond 24–48 hours [2].

The systemic inflammatory response syndrome (SIRS) is a non-specific, systemic clinical response to inflammation, commonly seen in postoperative surgical patients but also with diverse disorders such as pancreatitis, bowel ischaemia, multiple trauma and sepsis (Box 82.1). It is also the first stage of a continuum of disease that progresses in increasing severity from SIRS to septic shock, multiorgan dysfunction and potentially death.

Diagnosis of SIRS requires two or more of the following:

- body temperature $>38°C$ or $<36°C$
- heart rate >90/min (2 SD above the normal value for age)
- hyperventilation evidenced by a respiratory rate of >20 bpm or a $PaCO_2$ of <32 mmHg
- WCC of $>12,000$ cells/L or <4000/L.

Diagnostic criteria [3]

Sepsis is defined as SIRS *with* documented infection (such as positive blood cultures or consolidation on a CXR). A constellation of other clinical and laboratory findings is commonly seen (Box 82.2) [4].

Severe sepsis is associated with organ dysfunction, hypoperfusion abnormality (e.g. lactic acidosis, oliguria, acute alteration of mental status) or hypotension. It is critical to recognise it early as prompt, appropriate intervention can improve survival. Mortality is 10–40%.

Septic shock is sepsis with hypoperfusion and hypotension despite adequate fluid resuscitation. Patients who are receiving inotropic or vasopressor agents may not be hypotensive at the time that perfusion abnormalities are measured. Mortality is 30–60%.

BOX 82.1 Causes of SIRS

Infectious (sepsis = SIRS and infection)

Respiratory	Pneumonia Empyema
Abdominal	Cholecystitis Appendicitis Bacterial peritonitis Diverticulitis
Urinary	Pyelonephritis Urinary tract infection
Skin	Cellulitis Necrotising fasciitis Surgical wound infection
Cardiac	Infective endocarditis
Central nervous system	Meningitis Meningococcal septicaemia

Non-infectious

Trauma	Surgery Burns
Endocrine	Diabetic comas (ketoacidotic and hyperosmolar) Addisonian crisis Thyrotoxicosis Carcinoid syndrome
Cardiovascular	Myocardial infarction Myocarditis Pulmonary embolism
Drug reactions	Anaphylaxis Serotonin syndrome Hypersensitivity reactions
Miscellaneous	Acute pancreatitis Transfusion reactions Vasculitic crises (e.g. lupus)

Multiple organ dysfunction syndrome (MODS) has many manifestations. It is seen with and without sepsis (e.g. acute pancreatitis). There are two relatively distinct, although not mutually exclusive pathways by which MODS can develop.

- Primary MODS is an inflammatory response resulting from a direct insult to an organ (e.g. gastric aspiration in the lungs).
- Secondary MODS occurs when trauma or infection in one part of the body provokes a systemic inflammatory response and dysfunction of organs remote from the site of initial injury/inflammation.

BOX 82.2 Clinical and laboratory findings in sepsis

SIRS criteria plus infection plus *some* of the following

Cardiovascular and perfusion variables
  Hypotension (SBP <90 mmHg or MAP <70 mmHg)
  Elevated cardiac index (>3.5 L/min/m^2)
  Slow capillary refilling
  Increased lactate (>1 mmol/L)

Organ dysfunction variables
  Arterial hypoxaemia (PaO$_2$/FiO$_2$ <300)
  Acute oliguria (urine output <0.5 mL/kg/hr for at least 2 hr despite
  adequate fluid resuscitation)
  Creatinine increase >44.2 μmol/L
  Coagulation abnormalities (INR >1.5 or APTT >60 s)
  Thrombocytopenia (platelet count <100,000 μL)
  Hyperbilirubinaemia (plasma total bilirubin >70 μmol/L)
  Ileus (absent bowel sounds)

Inflammatory parameters
  Normal WBC count with greater than 10% immature forms
  Plasma C-reactive protein more than 2 SD above the normal value
  Plasma procalcitonin more than 2 SD above the normal value

APTT, activated partial thromboplastin time; INR, international normalised ratio; MAP, mean arterial pressure; SBP, systolic blood pressure; SD, standard deviation; WBC, white blood cell.

Distinction between the surgical inflammatory response, SIRS and sepsis [3]

There is extensive clinical overlap between the inflammatory response to surgery, SIRS and sepsis.

When a patient develops SIRS, the principal priority is to identify the cause and exclude infection; early identification and treatment of sepsis are critical to a successful outcome. SIRS and sepsis share many common clinical features and biochemical and inflammatory markers may not be helpful, especially in the early stages of sepsis. If the patient deteriorates rapidly, therapeutic measures often need to be introduced to support failing organ systems while the diagnostic process is under way.

Treatment [4]

The principal aims of treating sepsis are diagnosis, resuscitation, source control and treatment of complications. These are not mutually exclusive, but rather *should happen simultaneously.*

Diagnosis

Potentially infected, seriously ill patients should be screened routinely for severe sepsis to allow earlier implementation of therapy. This screening involves cultures of blood, sputum and urine and the imaging of possible sites of infection (CXR for pneumonia, echocardiograms for infective endocarditis, ultrasound and CT scan of abdomen for intra-abdominal collections).

Support/resuscitation

Initial management includes supplementary oxygen therapy and fluid administration (see below) to improve tissue perfusion. Escalation will require IV haemodynamic support (including pressors and inotropes), ventilatory support and transfer to an area of higher nursing and medical care.

Antimicrobial treatment

This involves initial broad-spectrum antimicrobial therapy and source control (such as surgery to remove infected foci). Effective antimicrobial administration within the first hour of documented hypotension is associated with increased survival to hospital discharge in adult patients with septic shock [5]. Specific treatments (e.g. renal replacement therapy for acute renal failure) will be determined by the organ failures that may develop.

Fluid therapy in SIRS and severe sepsis [6]

The choice of fluid used for initial resuscitation is contentious (refer to Chapter 74 Goal-directed therapy, Chapter 75 Fluids and electrolytes, and Chapter 80 Postoperative fluid therapy). Both crystalloid and colloid solutions have been recommended. Of the colloids, albumin is associated with a decrease in mortality when used for resuscitation but should be used with caution in patients with traumatic brain injury. Both HES and gelatins may cause renal injury. An initial fluid challenge of 20–30 mL/kg of crystalloids per kilogram of body weight is given, and continued as long as there is haemodynamic improvement.

References

1. Ward NS, Casserly B, Ayala A. The compensatory anti-inflammatory response syndrome (CARS) in critically ill patients. *Clinics in Chest Medicine*, 2008;**29**(4):617–625. doi:10.1016/j.ccm.2008.06.010

2. Menger MD, Vollmar B. Systemic inflammatory response syndrome (SIRS) and sepsis in surgical patients. *Intensive Care Medicine*, 1996;**22**(6):616–617. doi:10.1007/bf01708116

3. Levy MM, Fink MP, Marshall JC, et al. 2001 SCCM/ESICM/ACCP/ATS/SIS International Sepsis Definitions Conference. *Critical Care Medicine*, 2003;**31**(4):1250–1256. doi:10.1097/01.CCM.0000050454.01978.3B

4. Dellinger RP, Levy MM, Rhodes A, et al. Surviving sepsis campaign: international guidelines for management of severe sepsis and septic shock: 2012. *Critical Care Medicine*, 2013;**41**(2):580–637. doi:10.1097/CCM.0b013e31827e83af

5. Kissoon N, Carcillo JA, Espinosa V, et al. World Federation of Pediatric Intensive Care and Critical Care Societies: Global Sepsis Initiative. *Pediatric Critical Care Medicine*, 2011;**12**(5):494–503. doi:10.1097/PCC.0b013e318207096c

6. Raghunathan K, Shaw AD, Bagshaw SM. Fluids are drugs: type, dose and toxicity. *Current Opinion in Critical Care*, 2013;**19**(4):290–298. doi:10.1097/MCC.0b013e3283632d77

Nutritional support

Craig Walker

Monash Medical Centre, Australia

Malnourished patients are at increased risk of complications and mortality after surgery [1]. Nutrition for the surgical patient can be optimised by appropriate preoperative nutritional assessment, and ensuring adequate pre- and postoperative nutrition.

Preoperative assessment

Most patients presenting for elective surgery will have a normal nutritional status but if the patient's BMI is less than 20 kg/m², they have lost weight in the last three months or have had a reduced dietary intake in the last week then more detailed history and examination is required.

All patients who are critically ill or have been hospitalised for more than a week need a nutritional assessment [2], with attention to obese and oedematous patients, who may not appear to be malnourished but may have marked muscle wasting [3].

Patients at risk for severe malnutrition include those with the following.

- Weight loss >15% within six months (>5% in one month)
- BMI <18 kg/m²
- Reduced dietary intake (<25% of normal requirements in preceding week)
- Prolonged hospitalisation or nursing home
- Critical illness, malignancy, malabsorption
- Chronic organ failure (COPD, dialysis, HF)
- Recent major abdominal surgery

Preoperative nutrition

Patients who are severely malnourished should have their surgery delayed, if possible, to allow time for correction of their nutritional deficit [4]. Referral to an experienced dietitian or clinical nutrition team is essential. Preoperative nutritional support will be required for at least 10 days, preferably much longer. A few days are unlikely to achieve any benefit.

Perioperative Medicine for the Junior Clinician, First Edition. Edited by Joel Symons, Paul Myles, Rishi Mehra and Christine Ball.
© 2015 John Wiley & Sons, Ltd. Published 2015 by John Wiley & Sons, Ltd.
Companion website: www.wiley.com/go/perioperativemed

There is insufficient evidence to support delaying surgery solely for nutritional reasons if there is only mild or moderate malnutrition. However, if surgery is delayed for other reasons, it is important to maintain adequate nutritional support.

> One of the most common causes of malnutrition in hospitals is repeated fasting for procedures that are often delayed or postponed.

For most surgical procedures, prolonged fasting (>12 hr) is unnecessary and patients who have no specific risk of aspiration may be allowed solids up to six hours and clear fluids up to two hours prior to anaesthesia [5].

Modes of nutritional support

Delivery of nutrition can be in the form of oral supplementation (with dietary counselling if appropriate), tube feeding or parenteral nutrition. Tube and parenteral feeds can be delivered at home if prolonged nutritional support is required and appropriate back-up and expertise are in place.

Oral feeding

There are a wide variety of oral supplements available. Oral feeding has the advantage of allowing the patient a varied diet but requires the patient to have adequate swallowing. Prethickened feeds may be helpful in patients whose swallowing is impaired.

Enteral nutrition

Enteral nutrition (EN) can be given by a tube inserted directly into the gastrointestinal tract. While this overcomes any difficulty with swallowing or anorexia, the patient is still at risk of aspiration if they vomit or the tube is malpositioned.

Short-term EN is usually administered by the nasogastric route. Gastric tubes can be inserted percutaneously (either endoscopically or by surgery) if prolonged enteral feeding is expected. EN may be given as a bolus or as a continuous infusion, thereby reducing gastric distension and the risk of vomiting.

Hospitalised patients often develop some degree of gastric stasis. This may manifest as high residual gastric aspirates and can necessitate a pause or reduction in the rate of feeding. While this may be appropriate, it is important to restart feeds as soon as possible.

> Inappropriately prolonged pauses or reduction in feed administration are one of the major causes of malnutrition in the hospital setting.

While prokinetics such as metoclopramide or erythromycin may be helpful for gastric stasis, early placement of a postpyloric tube should be considered. These can be inserted radiologically, endoscopically or percutaneously if prolonged therapy is warranted.

Many surgeons performing major upper GI procedures, such as oesophagectomy or pancreatoduodenectomy, will insert a percutaneous jejunal feeding tube at the time of surgery. Jejunal feeds are usually given continuously.

Parenteral nutrition

Parenteral nutrition (PN) is when the patient is fed intravenously with solutions containing amino acids, glucose and lipid in various combinations, depending on the manufacturer. Usually vitamins and trace elements will be added to the solution or given IV by a separate route. When PN is the patient's sole source of nutrition, it is called total parenteral nutrition (TPN).

As it bypasses the gastrointestinal tract completely, PN is unaffected by gastric stasis, bowel obstruction, ileus or other conditions that prevent adequate EN. In addition, as it does not increase the risk of aspiration, it does not need to be stopped prior to procedures, thereby avoiding many of the pitfalls to delivering adequate nutrition to hospital patients.

However, there are considerable risks associated with PN (Box 83.1) and EN is preferred whenever possible. A combination of EN and PN may be required if the patient is not able to achieve adequate caloric intake by EN alone [4].

Postoperative management

In most patients, early feeding (<24 hr) after surgery is feasible, safe and probably beneficial [6]. If the patient is unable to tolerate oral feeding and is well nourished then an enteric tube is probably not indicated for the first five days. However, if the patient is malnourished or was tube fed prior to surgery, then EN can be commenced as soon as practicable.

Contraindications to early feeding include intestinal obstruction or ileus, intestinal ischaemia and severe sepsis/illness.

83

BOX 83.1 Risks and complications of parenteral nutrition

Central venous catheter related
  Insertion:
    Pneumothorax
    Haemothorax
    Arterial puncture
    Cardiac perforation
    Brachial plexus injury
  Venous thrombosis
  Air embolism
  Catheter site infection
  Septicaemia

Metabolic
  Hyperglycaemia
  Hypoglycaemia
  Electrolyte disturbances
  Fluid overload
  Hypertriglyceridaemia
  Hepatic dysfunction

Institution of EN may be complicated by gastrointestinal dysmotility due to intraoperative manipulation of the gut and opioid use for postoperative pain relief. Gastric distension may be overcome by insertion of a postpyloric feeding tube for jejunal feeds.

Given the complications, postoperative commencement of TPN should be avoided unless it is apparent that the patient will not be able to tolerate EN within 10 days after surgery. Earlier introduction of TPN may be warranted in the severely malnourished patient.

Patients who were on TPN prior to surgery can have their TPN reinstated within a few hours, but close attention needs to be paid to metabolic monitoring due to the increased stress of surgery.

References

1. Studley HO. Percentage of weight loss – a basic indicator of surgical risk in patients with chronic peptic ulcer. *JAMA*, 1936;**106**:458–460.

2. Weinsier RL, Hunker EM, Krumdieck CL, Butterworth CE Jr. Hospital malnutrition. A prospective evaluation of general medical patients during the course of hospitalization. *American Journal of Clinical Nutrition*, 1979;**32**(2):418–426. www.ncbi.nlm.nih.gov/pubmed/420132

3. Stenholm S, Harris TB, Rantanen T, Visser M, Kritchevsky SB, Ferrucci L. Sarcopenic obesity: definition, cause and consequences. *Current Opinion in Clinical Nutrition and Metabolic Care*, 2008;**11**(6):693–700. doi:10.1097/MCO.0b013e328312c37d

4. Weimann A, Braga M, Harsanyi L, et al. ESPEN guidelines on enteral nutrition: surgery including organ transplantation. *Clinical Nutrition*, 2006;**25**(2):224–244. doi: 10.1016/j.clnu.2006.01.015

5. Brady M, Kinn S, Stuart P. Preoperative fasting for adults to prevent perioperative complications. *Cochrane Database of Systematic Reviews*, 2003;**4**:CD004423. doi:10.1002/14651858.CD004423

6. Lewis SJ, Egger M, Sylvester PA, Thomas S. Early enteral feeding versus 'nil by mouth' after gastrointestinal surgery: systematic review and meta-analysis of controlled trials. *BMJ*, 2001;**323**(7316):773–776. doi:10.1136/bmj.323.7316.773

84 Postoperative surgical complications

Katherine Martin

The Alfred Hospital, Australia

This chapter will discuss common, important postoperative surgical complications.

Wound complications

Poor wound healing is more likely if there are patient risk factors (Table 84.1) or poor wound closure technique (Table 84.2). Skilled wound closure is pivotal to minimising wound complications [1,2]. Many patient factors are modifiable, if not reversible. A through history and physical examination allows for preoperative optimisation to limit wound complications.

Excessive scar formation results from a prolonged inflammatory state, e.g. infection. It may lead to keloid formation.

Wound dehiscence involves disruption through the full thickness of a sutured wound, classically within the first 10 days. It should be prevented by attention to surgical technique (see Table 84.1).

An incisional hernia is an abdominal wall defect, with or without a bulge, in an area of postoperative scar, detected clinically or radiologically. Most develop in the early postoperative period but may not become clinically apparent until much later. Hernias are prevented by good surgical technique and slow or non-absorbable suture material lasting for at least six weeks [1].

A wound infection or surgical site infection (SSI) commonly involves endogenous skin flora and may increase morbidity and mortality. It may be a superficial incisional (skin, subcutaneous tissue), deep incisional (e.g. fascia, muscle) or organ/space SSI (any area opened or manipulated during an operation, other than the incision).

Surgical site infections may result in hypertrophic scaring, keloid formation, delayed wound healing, wound dehiscence and incisional hernias. Necrotising infections reverse the wound healing process.

Preoperatively, SSIs can be minimised by optimisation of co-morbidities, screening for virulent and resistant micro-organisms and decolonising treatment or antimicrobials for

Perioperative Medicine for the Junior Clinician, First Edition. Edited by Joel Symons, Paul Myles, Rishi Mehra and Christine Ball.
© 2015 John Wiley & Sons, Ltd. Published 2015 by John Wiley & Sons, Ltd.
Companion website: www.wiley.com/go/perioperativemed

TABLE 84.1 Patient factors affecting wound healing

Modifiable	Non-modifiable
Cigarette smoking	Age >60 years
Obesity	Previous radiotherapy
Malnutrition and catabolism	Malignancy
Increased catecholamine levels associated with poor pain control	Previous surgery through same incision
Diabetes mellitus	Need for emergency surgery
Tissue oedema	Surgery for perforated viscus
Immunosuppression due to disease and/or drug therapy (e.g. glucocorticosteroids)	
Postoperative respiratory failure	
Postoperative ileus resulting in abdominal distension	
Colonisation with virulent or resistant micro-organisms	
Renal failure	
Liver failure with coagulopathy and/or jaundice	

TABLE 84.2 Technical aspects of wound closure that affect wound healing

Technique	Effect	Recommendation
Wound edge approximation	Allows wound healing to bridge the gap between opposite edges until adequate intrinsic strength develops	Wound edge approximation should be even, without visible gaps
Use of braided suture	Harbouring of bacteria within the suture material	Use of monofilament suture
Self-locking anchor knots	Lesser decrease in suture strength when compared to conventional knots	Use of self-locking knots to anchor suture
Suture line tension	Local tissue ischaemia and necrosis, leading to infection, tissue loss and subsequent loss of wound edge apposition	Minimisation of wound tension to allow for adequate wound edge approximation
Continuous or interrupted suture technique	Continuous suture shown to be stronger than interrupted technique	Continuous suture
Suture length to wound length ratio (SL:WL)	Tensile strength increases with higher SL:WL	SL:WL >4
Small stitches close together or larger stiches further apart	Larger stitches include muscle and peritoneum, resulting in tissue ischaemia, and are associated with increased incidence of dehiscence and hernia	Small stitches 5–8 mm from wound edge, in aponeurosis only, and 4–5 mm apart

Source: Israelsson and Millbourn [1]. Reproduced with permission from Elsevier Ltd.

active skin infection. Prophylactic antibiotics administered via strict guidelines ensure optimal tissue concentration at time of skin incision and, in certain circumstances, postoperatively (refer to Chapter 29 Antibiotic prophylaxis). Good surgical technique will minimise wound contamination and tissue ischaemia. Dressings should be occlusive yet absorptive and left intact for at least 24 hours. Soaked dressings should be changed under sterile conditions and strict hand hygiene practice maintained by all healthcare workers at all times. Nutrition, intravenous line management, catheter care, fluid balance and co-morbidities are all important factors.

Deep surgical site infection

Deep organ/space SSI involves the organs and tissue space manipulated intraoperatively and has similar risk factors to incisional SSI. Prostheses such as mesh and orthopaedic implants are contributing factors.

Symptoms and signs may become evident from the third postoperative day to months or years later. They include pain, purulent discharge from surgical drains, loss of appetite and failure to thrive, evidence of sepsis (fever, tachycardia, an increased WCC and C-reactive protein [CRP]) and septic shock.

Diagnosis is confirmed with the aspiration of pus, the identification of mico-organisms in aspirates or a fluid collection on imaging. Management is dependent on the location, extent, symptoms and signs, co-morbidities and original surgery. It includes antibiotic therapy, percutaneous aspiration and drainage under image guidance, and reoperation. The management of patient co-morbidities is important, particularly diabetes mellitus.

Anastomotic leak

Anastomotic leak occurs in approximately 7% of all colorectal anastomoses. It results in intra-abdominal and pelvic sepsis, poor long-term anorectal function, enterocutaneous fistulae, an increased incidence of permanent stoma and an increase in all-cause mortality. Local recurrence and cancer-free survival may be adversely affected [3].

Contributing factors include impaired blood flow at the anastomotic site, excessive tension, poor or improper suturing and stapler use, alteration of the normal intestinal flora and deep SSI. The incidence increases as the distance of the colorectal anastomoses from the anal verge decreases [3] and the stapled method for ileocolic anastomoses is associated with fewer leaks than the handsewn one [4].

Anastomotic leak usually becomes evident after the third postoperative day but symptoms may develop after discharge from hospital. They include increased abdominal pain, localised or generalised peritonitis, faecal or purulent discharge from intra-abdominal drains, loss of appetite, failure to thrive and evidence of sepsis. Diagnosis can be confirmed by endoscopy, imaging with intraluminal contrast, and reoperation.

Management is dependent on the clinical signs and complications, the location of the anastomosis and pre-existing co-morbidities.

Patients with peritonitis or septic shock require resuscitation and return to theatre for confirmation of diagnosis, peritoneal cavity washout and an end or defunctioning stoma. Patients with minimal symptoms may be managed with antibiotics and percutaneous drainage of any fluid collection that is found on imaging. Parenteral rather than enteric feeding may be required, particularly with higher gastrointestinal anastomotic leaks. Patient co-morbidities such as diabetes must be optimised.

Postoperative bleeding

Postoperative bleeding usually becomes evident within the first 24 hours. Delayed bleeding usually occurs three to seven days postoperatively, often associated with surgical site infection. Failure to secure vessels or identify areas of active bleeding, failure of sutures, knots and iatrogenic injury are technical causes. Patient factors include coagulopathy, antiplatelet and anticoagulant agents, clotting factor dilution, underlying bleeding disorder (often not previously identified) and friable tissue associated with ageing, malnutrition, chronic steroid use, previous surgery or an underlying inflammatory process, e.g. severe necrotising pancreatitis, deep SSI.

Rapid clinical diagnosis is essential to establish the following.

- Hypovolaemia: tachypnoea, tachycardia (supine or postural), decreased urine output and hypotension (supine or postural)
- Pallor, 'light-headedness', 'dizziness' or confusion (altered conscious state)
- Haematoma or swelling at the surgical site (especially post mastectomy, post thyroidectomy)
- Increased pain at or deep to the surgical incision
- Excessive blood loss from surgical drains

Relevant investigations include:

- FBE: note haemoglobin concentration may initially remain within normal limits
- ABG: base excess to assess tissue perfusion
- ultrasound, e.g. of the pericardium after cardiac surgery
- CT-angiography to identify active extravasation or increasing haematoma size.

Management priorities are as follows.

1. Airway, breathing and circulation. If these are compromised, seek urgent assistance and initiate resuscitation. Administer oxygen, nurse the patient supine and head down, insert two large-bore IV cannulae and commence a warmed crystalloid infusion. Apply pressure to any expanding wounds or external bleeding.
2. Assess immediate threat to airway, breathing or circulation, e.g. post-thyroidectomy haemorrhage. Opening of the surgical incision may be required before the patient returns to theatre. Reintubation may be difficult.
3. Inform the operating surgeon.
4. Subsequent management may include further investigations (e.g. CT-angiogram), return to theatre, administration of clotting factors, blood transfusion, ICU.

References

1. Israelsson LA, Millbourn D. Prevention of incisional hernias: how to close a midline incision. *Surgical Clinics of North America*, 2013;**93**(5):1027–1040. doi:10.1016/j.suc.2013.06.009
2. Becker JM, Stucchi AF. Wound healing. In: Essentials of Surgery. Philadelphia, PA: Elsevier, 2006, pp. 62–72.
3. Shogan BD, Carlisle EM, Alverdy JC, Umanskiy K. Do we really know why colorectal anastomoses leak? *Journal of Gastrointestinal Surgery*, 2013;**17**(9):1698–1707. doi:10.1007/S11605-013-2227-0
4. Choy PYG, Bissett IP, Docherty JG, Parry BR, Merrie A, Fitzgerald A. Stapled versus handsewn methods for ileocolic anastomoses. *Cochrane Database of Systematic Reviews*, 2011;**9**:CD004320. doi:10.1002/14651858.Cd004320.Pub3

85 Postoperative chest pain

Shane Nanayakkara[1] and Peter Bergin[2]

[1] The Alfred Hospital, Australia
[2] The Alfred Hospital and Monash University, Australia

Chest pain is a common complaint in the hospital environment. Although chest pain may be benign [1], in the postoperative setting it must be taken seriously and investigated. Due to the large variety and complexity of anatomical structures within the thoracic cavity, there are a multitude of aetiologies (Figure 85.1).

Investigation of postoperative chest pain must take into account several factors, including the type of operation performed, pre-existing patient co-morbidities and intraoperative complications (Table 85.1).

Myocardial ischaemia and infarction

Myocardial infarction (MI) in the non-operative setting is mainly precipitated by plaque rupture of a non-critical coronary stenosis, with a subsequent coronary thrombosis. Due to the stresses of an operation, however, several other factors can contribute to myocardial ischaemia. Importantly, most (>50%) myocardial injury is subclinical, without overt chest pain.

The Third Universal Definition of Myocardial Infarction [2] requires an elevated cardiac biomarker, with at least one of the following present.

- Symptoms of ischaemia
- New or presumed new ST-T wave changes
- New left bundle branch block
- Development of pathological Q waves
- Imaging evidence of new loss of viable myocardium or new regional wall motion abnormality
- Identification of an intracoronary thrombus by angiography or autopsy

Myocardial infarction is subcategorised into several different types (Box 85.1).

Previously it was thought that the majority of perioperative MIs were Type 2, but both cardiac and non-cardiac surgery can cause myocardial ischaemia in a number of ways, including:

- plaque rupture
- direct myocardial and coronary artery damage
- anaemia, particularly from significant blood loss
- coronary embolism

Perioperative Medicine for the Junior Clinician, First Edition. Edited by Joel Symons, Paul Myles, Rishi Mehra and Christine Ball.
© 2015 John Wiley & Sons, Ltd. Published 2015 by John Wiley & Sons, Ltd.
Companion website: www.wiley.com/go/perioperativemed

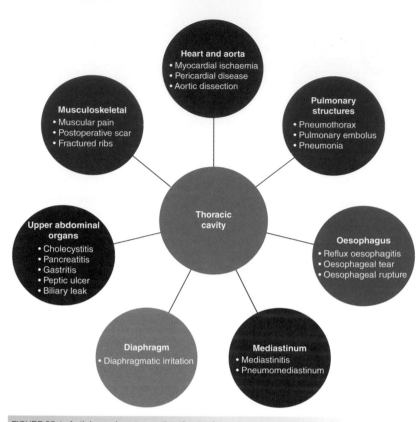

FIGURE 85.1 **Aetiology of postoperative chest pain.**

TABLE 85.1 **Causes of chest pain and their corresponding clinical symptoms**

Cause	Nature
Myocardial infarction	Central, crushing, radiating to left arm
Pericardial effusion	Worse with lying down, improved with sitting up
Pulmonary embolism	Sharp, pleuritic/worse with inspiration
Pneumothorax	Sudden onset, rapidly progressive, associated with dyspnoea
Aortic dissection	Tearing, interscapular, severe in nature
Musculoskeletal	Worse with palpation or movement

- toxic effects of circulating catecholamines
- hypotension
- arrhythmias
- respiratory failure and hypoxia.

Patients with known coronary artery disease should have had a preoperative cardiac risk assessment (refer to Chapter 11 The cardiac patient for non-cardiac surgery,

BOX 85.1 Categorisation of myocardial infarction

Type 1 Spontaneous myocardial infarction

Spontaneous myocardial infarction related to atherosclerotic plaque rupture, ulceration, fissuring, erosion or dissection with resulting intraluminal thrombus in one or more of the coronary arteries leading to decreased myocardial blood flow or distal platelet emboli with ensuing myocyte necrosis

Type 2 Myocardial infarction secondary to an ischaemic imbalance

In instances of myocardial injury with necrosis where a condition other than coronary artery disease contributes to an imbalance between myocardial oxygen supply and/or demand

Type 3 Myocardial infarction resulting in death when biomarker values are unavailable

Cardiac death with symptoms suggestive of myocardial ischaemia and presumed new ischaemic ECG changes or new LBBB, but death occurring before blood samples could be obtained, before cardiac biomarker could rise or in rare cases cardiac biomarkers were not collected

Type 4a Myocardial infarction related to percutaneous coronary intervention

Myocardial infarction associated with PCI is arbitrarily defined by elevation of cTn values >5 × 99th percentile URL in patients with normal baseline values, or a rise of cTn values >20% if the baseline values are elevated and are stable or falling. In addition, (i) symptoms suggestive of myocardial ischaemia or (ii) new ischaemic ECG changes or new LBBB, or (iii) angiographic loss of patency of a major coronary artery or a side branch or persistent slow- or no-flow or embolization, or (iv) imaging demonstration of new loss of viable myocardium or new regional wall motion abnormality are required

Type 4b Myocardial infarction related to stent thrombosis

Myocardial infarction associated with stent thrombosis is detected by coronary angiography or autopsy in the setting of myocardial ischaemia and with a rise and/or fall of cardiac biomarkers values with at least one value above the 99th percentile URL

Type 5 Myocardial infarction related to coronary artery bypass grafting (CABG)

Myocardial infarction associated with CABG is arbitrarily defined by elevation of cardiac biomarker values >10 × 99th percentile URL in patients with normal baseline cTn values (<99th percentile URL). In addition, (i) new pathological Q waves or new LBBB, or (ii) angiographic documented new graft or new native coronary occlusion, or (iii) imaging evidence of new loss of viable myocardium or new regional wall motion abnormality

Source: Thygesen et al. [2]. Reproduced with permission from Oxford University Press. ECG, electrocardiogram; LBBB, left bundle branch block; PCI, percutaneous coronary intervention; URL, upper reference limit.

Chapter 12 Cardiovascular risk assessment in cardiac surgery, Chapter 13 Preoperative cardiac testing and Chapter 16 Preoperative cardiopulmonary exercise testing). This should be reviewed when assessing the postoperative patient with chest pain. Preoperative troponin levels should be obtained where possible from any preoperative stored blood samples. Baseline ECGs should also be used for comparison.

Pericardial disease

Pericarditis and pericardial effusions can occur following many operations, either as a sympathetic response or due to direct entry of the pericardium. They are usually asymptomatic and picked up incidentally on echocardiography performed for another reason. However, occasionally they can be pathological.

Cardiac surgery is commonly associated with pericardial effusion. Features of tamponade such as hypotension, elevated jugular venous pressure (JVP) and muffled heart sounds must prompt early echocardiography and consideration of operative drainage. In many cases, however, these effusions resolve quickly and rarely are of significant consequence.

The postcardiac injury syndrome can occur with surprisingly little trauma, as a result of an immune phenomenon. It often occurs many weeks or even months after the initial injury.

Pulmonary embolism

The postoperative patient is at particularly high risk of PE (refer to Chapter 24 Thromboprophylaxis). Fewer than 50% of patients present with chest pain [3] and again a high degree of suspicion is required. Tests such as a D-dimer are not useful due to their low specificity in the postsurgical period, and early non-invasive imaging needs to be considered.

Pneumothorax

Pneumothorax is not uncommon after cardiothoracic surgery, with quoted rates of up to 1.4%. It is potentially fatal. Vigilance is the key, particularly if the patient has chest pain and desaturation. Clinical examination may reveal hyper-resonance over the region of the pneumothorax, but early radiographic assessment is critical.

Key steps in the evaluation and management of postoperative chest pain

Ensure oxygenation and haemodynamic stability; is there an immediate threat to life?

Call for help early.

Check blood pressure in both arms

Many causes of chest pain are associated with haemodynamic instability, and a blood pressure differential between arms is important if there is suspicion of aortic dissection.

Assess heart rate and rhythm

An early ECG is critical, and serial ECGs within a short time period may be useful if there is ongoing pain without obvious changes on the first ECG.

- *Myocardial ischaemia*: assess for ST elevation or depression, T wave inversion and pathological Q waves.
- *Pulmonary embolism*: although the most common feature is sinus tachycardia, features of right heart strain may be present, including S1Q3T3.
- *Arrhythmia*: tachyarrhythmias are often associated with chest pain, particularly if there is underlying coronary disease.
- *Pericarditis*: classically diffuse concave ST elevation is seen with PR depression.

Assess respiratory rate and work of breathing

Tachypnoea may suggest a respiratory cause.

Brief, focused examination

Chest
- Expansion may be unequal with pneumothorax or large effusion.
- Tracheal deviation is away from large pneumothoraces and towards collapse.
- Percussion is resonant over a pneumothorax and dull over an effusion.
- Auscultation reveals crackles with pneumonia, or diminished sounds over a pneumothorax.

Pulses
Radiofemoral or radio-radial delay; assess for differential blood pressure.

Cardiac
- Muffled heart sounds are present with a pericardial effusion.
- JVP may be elevated with acute myocardial infarction or with tamponade.
- RV heave is present with acute PE.
- An early diastolic murmur may be heard from aortic regurgitation as a result of an aortic dissection.
- A pansystolic murmur from mitral regurgitation secondary to myocardial infarction may be heard.

Abdomen
- Assess for peritonitic features.
- Epigastric tenderness may occur with peptic ulceration.

Establish initial investigations

Three tests are key early on.

1. Bloods
   - FBE to exclude anaemia
   - Biochemistry and liver function to assess organ dysfunction and electrolyte imbalance
   - Cardiac enzymes now and in six hours (depending on the assay used)
   - Cross-match if operative management suspected
2. ECG (ideally already taken)
3. CXR
   - Depending on the situation, a mobile study on the ward may be required
   - An erect CXR is most useful if aiming to exclude pneumothorax

ABG is not always required but consider supplemental investigations.

- Echocardiography
- CT pulmonary angiogram (CTPA) or CT aortogram

Review and reassess

Even if the diagnosis has not become clear early on, serial review and testing (serial cardiac enzymes and ECG) can be very useful in the short to medium term.

Postoperative troponin rise

One common difficult situation is that of a postoperative troponin rise in the absence of clinical symptoms, known as myocardial injury after non-cardiac surgery or MINS (refer to Chapter 88 Myocardial injury after non-cardiac surgery). It is important to exclude secondary causes of troponin rise, such as pulmonary embolus or renal dysfunction. Since there is a significant association between a raised postoperative troponin and mortality [4], these patients should be referred to a cardiologist and managed appropriately.

References

1. Klinkman MS, Stevens D, Gorenflo DW. Episodes of care for chest pain: a preliminary report from MIRNET. Michigan Research Network. *Journal of Family Practice,* 1994;**38**(4):345–352. www.ncbi.nlm.nih.gov/pubmed/8163958

2. Thygesen K, Alpert JS, Jaffe AS, et al. Third universal definition of myocardial infarction. *Circulation*, 2012;**126**(16):2020–2035. doi:10.1093/eurheartj/ehs184

3. McGee S. Pulmonary embolism. In: *Evidence Based Physical Diagnosis*, 3rd edn. Philadelphia, PA: Elsevier Saunders, 2007, pp. 283–287.

4. Botto F, Alonso-Coello P, Chan MT, et al. Myocardial injury after noncardiac surgery: a large, international, prospective cohort study establishing diagnostic criteria, characteristics, predictors, and 30-day outcomes. *Anesthesiology*, 2014;**120**(3):564–578. doi:10.1097/ALN.0000000000000113

86 Postoperative shortness of breath

KJ Farley[1] and Deirdre Murphy[2]

[1] The Alfred Hospital, Australia
[2] The Alfred Hospital and Monash University, Australia

Shortness of breath (dyspnoea/breathlessness) is defined as a subjective perception of difficulty breathing. Even without deranged vital signs (commonly decreased SpO_2 and tachypnoea), breathlessness disproportionate to the patient's level of exertion may indicate underlying pathology.

Breathlessness is common, and may indicate a life-threatening complication which is preventable and/or treatable [1]. Early detection and treatment of patients with respiratory deterioration, as well as escalation of management, may improve patient outcomes [2,3].

Assessment of the postoperative breathless patient

History

Relevant history includes the onset of breathlessness (time since surgery, gradual versus sudden) and the associated features/risk factors for specific aetiologies (Tables 86.1 and 86.2). Risk factors for postoperative breathlessness include the following.

- *Patient factors:* age, preoperative co-morbidities and medications (e.g. myocardial ischaemia, smoking, COPD, pulmonary fibrosis, pulmonary hypertension, immunosuppression)
- *Preoperative respiratory function and symptoms:* exercise tolerance, sputum volume and colour (refer to Chapter 15 Pulmonary risk assessment)
- *Surgical factors:* when and how long was the operation, mode of anaesthesia, analgesia administered and surgical site (high-risk surgery sites are chest and abdomen). It is also important to establish the volume of blood loss, fluid and blood products given, presence of a nasogastric tube, laparotomy versus laparoscopy, etc. [4,5].

Perioperative Medicine for the Junior Clinician, First Edition. Edited by Joel Symons, Paul Myles, Rishi Mehra and Christine Ball.
© 2015 John Wiley & Sons, Ltd. Published 2015 by John Wiley & Sons, Ltd.
Companion website: www.wiley.com/go/perioperativemed

TABLE 86.1 **An approach to common differential diagnoses for postoperative breathlessness**

Common causes of postoperative breathlessness	History/ examination clues	Key investigation clues	Initial treatment/s
Pneumonia	↑ sputum volume/ purulence Fever Sweats, chills, rigors Tachycardia, hypoxia, tachypnoea	↑ WCC ↑ CRP, procalcitonin CXR showing air bronchograms, consolidation Positive cultures (sputum, blood)	Start broad-spectrum antibiotics as soon as possible (refer to local antibiotic guidelines)
Lobar collapse (e.g. from sputum retention)	Uncontrolled pain → difficulty deep breathing/ coughing Focal ↓ air entry and dull percussion note	Lobar collapse on CXR	Analgesia Normal saline nebs Chest physiotherapy Consider bronchoscopy if no resolution with basic treatment
Pneumothorax	Neck/thoracic surgery Subclavian/internal jugular CVC Recent chest drain removal Pleuritic chest pain Hyper-resonant percussion note Ipsilateral ↓chest expansion and ↓ air entry Tracheal deviation to other side and haemodynamic compromise if tension pneumothorax	Erect CXR showing lung edge or deep sulcus sign Chest ultrasound showing absent pleural sliding (not specific) and lung point (specific)	Insert chest drain **Do NOT wait for CXR before treating a tension pneumothorax with immediate needle thoracostomy followed by a chest drain**
Exacerbations of COPD, asthma	History of respiratory diseases Wheeze	Clear CXR with hyperexpanded lung fields	Inhaled bronchodilators Steroids, e.g. oral prednisolone (IV hydrocortisone if cannot swallow or nil by mouth)
Myocardial ischaemia/ infarction	Central crushing chest pain (may radiate to back/ jaw/arm) Note: some patients may not have chest pain Sweating Nausea/vomiting Dizziness	ECG changes of STEMI or non-STEMI Raised CK/ troponin	Discuss with cardiologist Start aspirin if low risk bleeding (discuss with surgeon first) Revascularisation as soon as possible if STEMI (refer to Chapter 88)

TABLE 86.1 *(Continued)*

Common causes of postoperative breathlessness	History/examination clues	Key investigation clues	Initial treatment/s
Fluid overload/LVF	Orthopnoea PND Positive fluid balance Dependent pitting oedema (remember in the supine patient this will be the sacral region, not the ankles!) Features of underlying cause, e.g. myocardial ischaemia, arrhythmias	CXR (bilateral upper lobe venous diversion, Kerley B lines, interstitial or alveolar opacities, pleural effusions, may have underlying cardiomegaly) Features of underlying cause, e.g. myocardial ischaemia, arrhythmias ↑ BNP	Diurese Treat hypertension Treat underlying cause (arrhythmia, myocardial ischaemia, etc.) Consider CPAP
Pulmonary embolus	Pleuritic chest pain Haemoptysis or dry cough Calf pain	ECG changes Positive V/Q or CTPA DVT on lower limb ultrasound May have right heart dysfunction and dilation on echocardiography ↑ troponin (non-specific for establishing diagnosis; use for prognostication)	Continuous cardiac monitoring for massive/submassive PE Therapeutic anticoagulation (MUST discuss bleeding risk with surgeon first) Escalate if haemodynamic compromise? thrombolysis
Metabolic acidosis	Features of underlying cause, e.g. tissue ischaemia, hypotension, diabetes, diarrhoea Respiratory rate may be ↑/↓ Kussmaul breathing – deep sighing breaths Usually normal respiratory examination and SpO_2	↓ HCO_3^- ↓ $PaCO_2$ Normal or ↑ anion gap will help work out cause Evidence of underlying cause, e.g. ketones, renal failure, lactate, toxins	Treat underlying cause
Uncontrolled pain	Shallow respiratory pattern Inability to breathe deeply or cough	CXR showing poor inspiratory effort, atelectasis or lobar collapse	↑ analgesia

(Continued)

TABLE 86.1 (Continued)

Common causes of postoperative breathlessness	History/ examination clues	Key investigation clues	Initial treatment/s
Anxiety This should be a diagnosis of exclusion	History of anxiety May have features of hyperventilation (tingling fingers, tetany)	Respiratory alkalosis on ABG	Reassurance Anxiolytics (if safe) Consider liaising with psychiatrists if severe

ABG, arterial blood gas; CK, creatine kinase; COPD, chronic obstructive pulmonary disease; CPAP, continuous positive airway pressure; CRP, C-reactive protein; CTPA, CT pulmonary angiogram; CVC, central venous catheter; CXR, chest X-ray; DVT, deep vein thrombosis; ECG, electrocardiogram; IV, intravenous; LVF, left ventricular failure; PE, pulmonary embolus; PND, paroxysmal nocturnal dyspnoea; STEMI, ST elevation myocardial infarction; WCC, white cell count.

TABLE 86.2 An approach to rarer differential diagnoses for postoperative breathlessness

Rarer causes of postoperative breathlessness	History/examination clues	Key investigation clues	Initial treatment/s
Pleural effusion/ haemothorax	Neck/thoracic surgery Subclavian or internal jugular CVC placement Recent removal chest drain or drain output suddenly ↓ to zero Ipsilateral ↓ chest expansion and ↓ air entry Ipsilateral stony dull percussion note	Erect CXR showing pleural fluid (look for meniscus sign) Pleural fluid on chest ultrasound – can be quantified	Treat underlying cause, e.g. cardiac failure, coagulopathy, surgical bleeding May need pleural tap
Arrhythmias	Central chest pain Palpitations Dizziness, sweating, nausea Irregular/fast pulse	12-Lead ECG/rhythm strip Electrolyte disturbances (especially K^+, Mg^{2+}, PO_4^{3-})	Discuss with cardiologist May need continuous ECG monitoring Replace electrolytes Antiarrhythmic drug
Diaphragmatic dysfunction	Neck/thoracic/ abdominal surgery Poor cough strength/ shallow breathing despite apparent compliance	CXR showing raised hemidiaphragm Chest ultrasound showing failure of hemidiaphragm to contract	Chest physiotherapy Position sitting up for maximal mechanical advantage
Anaphylaxis	Urticaria Wheeze Hypotension, tachycardia Lip and tongue swelling	**This is a medical emergency – do not wait for investigations before initiating treatment (send serum tryptase)**	Advanced life support measures including intramuscular adrenaline (refer to Chapter 72)

TABLE 86.2 (Continued)

Rarer causes of postoperative breathlessness	History/examination clues	Key investigation clues	Initial treatment/s
Neuromuscular disease	History of neuromuscular disease, e.g. motor neurone disease, myasthenia gravis, multiple sclerosis		Liaise with neurologist
Large airway obstruction	Stridor Focal/unilateral wheeze		Call for help
Transfusion-related acute lung injury (TRALI)	Massive transfusion (especially plasma) Acute onset (within hours of blood product transfusion) of breathlessness, tachypnoea, hypoxia [6] (refer to Chapter 77)	Bilateral CXR opacities Normal left ventricular filling pressures No signs of other causes, e.g. infection, fluid overload May have transient leucopenia or thrombocytopenia	Supportive care
Acute respiratory distress syndrome (ARDS)	Extrapulmonary or pulmonary illnesses, e.g. sepsis, pancreatitis, pneumonia Acute onset (within 7 days) of respiratory symptoms and signs [7]	Bilateral CXR infiltrates and normal left ventricular filling pressures No signs of other causes	Supportive care Treat the underlying illness

CVC, central venous catheter; CXR, chest X-ray; ECG, electrocardiogram.

Examination of the patient with shortness of breath

Examination of the patient with shortness of breath is summarised in Figure 86.1.

Investigations

Useful blood tests which may be required include the following.

- *FBE:* polycythaemia from chronic hypoxia, severe anaemia, raised WCC with sepsis
- *U&E:* renal failure, electrolyte disturbances contributing to arrhythmias, low HCO_3^- in metabolic acidosis
- *Troponin:* myocardial ischaemia or injury (refer to Chapter 85 Postoperative chest pain and Chapter 88 Myocardial injury after non-cardiac surgery)
- *ABG:* helpful for oxygenation, ventilation and acid–base status. Remember that a normal oxygen saturation (SpO_2) does NOT exclude *ventilation* abnormalities; an ABG is needed to diagnose high or low arterial carbon dioxide ($PaCO_2$) levels
- *CRP, procalcitonin:* infection/inflammation
- *BNP:* left ventricular failure (refer to Chapter 35 Heart failure)
- *Coagulation profile, group and hold:* if bleeding is suspected or procedural intervention is anticipated

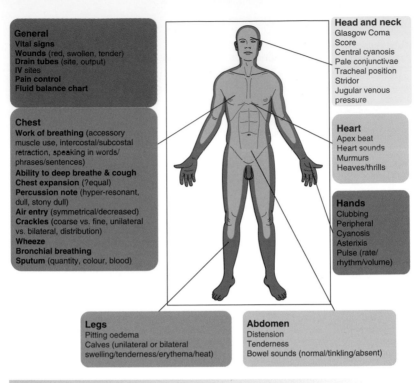

General
Vital signs
Wounds (red, swollen, tender)
Drain tubes (site, output)
IV sites
Pain control
Fluid balance chart

Head and neck
Glasgow Coma Score
Central cyanosis
Pale conjunctivae
Tracheal position
Stridor
Jugular venous pressure

Chest
Work of breathing (accessory muscle use, intercostal/subcostal retraction, speaking in words/phrases/sentences)
Ability to deep breathe & cough
Chest expansion (?equal)
Percussion note (hyper-resonant, dull, stony dull)
Air entry (symmetrical/decreased)
Crackles (coarse vs. fine, unilateral vs. bilateral, distribution)
Wheeze
Bronchial breathing
Sputum (quantity, colour, blood)

Heart
Apex beat
Heart sounds
Murmurs
Heaves/thrills

Hands
Clubbing
Peripheral Cyanosis
Asterixis
Pulse (rate/rhythm/volume)

Legs
Pitting oedema
Calves (unilateral or bilateral swelling/tenderness/erythema/heat)

Abdomen
Distension
Tenderness
Bowel sounds (normal/tinkling/absent)

FIGURE 86.1 **Focused examination of the patient with shortness of breath.**

Chest X-ray (CXR): look for pleural effusions, pneumothorax, consolidation, lobar collapse, cardiomegaly or heart failure.

ECG: look for myocardial infarction/ischaemia, LVH and arrhythmias (refer to Chapter 111 ECG interpretation).

Do not forget that isolated sinus tachycardia is the most common ECG abnormality in PE. There may be a right bundle branch block (RBBB) or right axis deviation. The 'classic' ECG findings of S1Q3T3 are rarely seen (Figure 86.2).

Other investigations

Review the patient's preoperative investigations for clues to the current diagnosis, e.g. spirometry (obstructive versus restrictive defect) chest radiology, echocardiography and prior ECGs for comparison.

Depending on history and examination findings, other useful investigations may include a septic screen (sputum, urine and blood cultures), lung pathology ultrasound (Video 86.1), echocardiography, D-Dimer, V/Q scan or CTPA.

Treatment

In addition to treating the specific underlying cause of breathlessness (see Tables 86.1 and 86.2), all breathless postoperative patients should have the following general treatments.

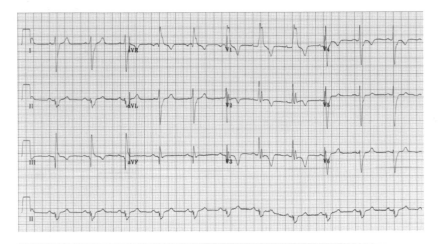

FIGURE 86.2 The ECG in pulmonary embolism. Although this ECG does not demonstrate a sinus tachycardia, there is a RBBB, right axis deviation, inverted T waves in V1–V4 and S1Q3T3 (a deep S wave in lead I, Q wave and inverted T wave in lead III).

www.wiley.com/go/perioperativemed

VIDEO 86.1 Lung pathology ultrasound. Ultrasound is an excellent point-of-care test that can be used to rapidly diagnose and confirm clinical examination of chest pathology.

- *Apply high-flow O₂*: the O_2 flow rate needs to match the patient's highest inspiratory flow rate to avoid the entrainment of room air (which will decrease the inspired O_2 concentration); this may be as high as 40 L/min or more in some patients. A non-rebreathing mask may be helpful.
- *Sit the patient up* if possible (the only patients who benefit from being supine are those with high spinal injuries).
- *Establish IV access* and send initial blood tests.
- *Call for help*/escalate management if needed, e.g. significantly deranged vital signs, rapid deterioration, meeting medical emergency team (MET) or Early Warning Score criteria, extreme pain.

- Ensure adequate analgesia.
- Encourage deep breathing and coughing exercises.

Conclusion

Breathlessness is a common problem in the postoperative patient, with many differential diagnoses. A systematic approach to the patient, with a thorough history and examination, as well as selected investigations, will assist in correctly establishing the cause/s of breathlessness. Prompt treatment is required in order to prevent further deterioration in this patient group. Ongoing, close monitoring is required.

References

1. Ferreyra G, Long Y, Ranieri VM. Respiratory complications after major surgery. *Current Opinion in Critical Care*, 2009;**15**(4):342–348. doi:10.1097/MCC.0b013e32832e0669

2. Jones DA, DeVita MA, Bellomo R. Rapid-response teams. *New England Journal of Medicine*, 2011;**365**(2):139–146. doi:10.1056/NEJMra0910926

3. Winters BD, Weaver SJ, Pfoh ER, Yang T, Pham JC, Dy SM. Rapid-response systems as a patient safety strategy: a systematic review. *Annals of Internal Medicine*, 2013;**158**(5):417.

4. Doyle RL. Assessing and modifying the risk of postoperative pulmonary complications. *Chest*, 1999;**115**(5 Suppl):77S–81S. doi:10.1378/chest.115.suppl_2.77s

5. Mitchell CK, Smoger SH, Pfeifer MP, et al. Multivariate analysis of factors associated with postoperative pulmonary complications following general elective surgery. *Archives of Surgery*, 1998;**133**(2):194–198. doi:10.1001/archsurg.133.2.194

6. Vlaar AP, Juffermans NP. Transfusion-related acute lung injury: a clinical review. *Lancet*, 2013;**382**(9896):984–994. doi:10.1016/S0140-6736(12)62197-7

7. Force ADT. Acute respiratory distress syndrome: the Berlin definition. *JAMA*, 2012;**307**(23):2526–2533. doi:10.1001/jama.2012.5669

Postoperative hypotension

Steven Fowler

The Alfred Hospital, Australia

Hypotension refers to a decrease in systemic blood pressure of more than 20% below preoperative baseline *or* MAP <60 mmHg *or* SBP <90 mmHg.

There is no single target BP appropriate for all patients – the value of BP in relation to the preoperative baseline and clinical scenario needs to be considered. The definition of hypotension varies widely between studies.

Epidemiology

Postoperative hypotension occurs commonly in association with drug treatment (e.g. general or neuraxial anaesthesia, antihypertensives, especially ACE inhibitors and ARBs), major fluid shifts (e.g. blood loss) and cardiovascular disease (e.g. poor LV function).

Pathophysiology

Mean pressure within the circulation is dependent on the pumping action of the heart (there are two pumps in series – LV and RV), the resistance of the arterial tree and filling (both volume and venous tone). The circulatory system is also pulsatile and elastic.

> Hypotension in the postoperative setting is a predictor of postoperative complications. It requires rapid and comprehensive assessment and management.

Compensatory tachycardia often occurs and may be associated with myocardial ischaemia. *Shock* is a syndrome of inadequate tissue perfusion and oxygen delivery leading to acidosis.

Perioperative Medicine for the Junior Clinician, First Edition. Edited by Joel Symons, Paul Myles, Rishi Mehra and Christine Ball.
© 2015 John Wiley & Sons, Ltd. Published 2015 by John Wiley & Sons, Ltd.
Companion website: www.wiley.com/go/perioperativemed

Aetiology

Hypotension (and shock) can be classified as hypovolaemic, distributive or cardiogenic. However, any clinical scenario may involve multiple contributing aetiologies (Table 87.1).

Consider discontinuing ACEIs and ARBs at least 10 hours before surgery, as these agents have been associated with intraoperative hypotension [1].

Assessment

* What is the heart rate and rhythm?
* Are pulses – peripheral and central – present?
* Is there a poor SpO_2 trace? Check capillary refill time.
* Check BP manually (beware automated BP malfunction).
* Measure JVP (intravascular volume status) and assess tissue turgor (dehydration).
* Check that invasive arterial BP reading equals the cuff reading and that transducer height is at the level of the heart.
* Check temperature, respiratory rate and cognition.
* Consider inserting a urinary catheter and assess urine output.
* Quickly scan for an obvious cause – bleeding/drains, fluid balance, drugs administered.
* Routine investigations include full blood count, coagulation screen, U&E, ionised calcium and group and antibody screen.
* Consider 12-lead resting ECG, troponin, CXR and screening TTE.

TABLE 87.1 **Aetiology of hypotension**

Reduced preload ('hypovolaemic')	Reduced afterload/ systemic vascular resistance ('distributive')	Reduced contractility ('cardiogenic')
Blood loss	Sepsis	Myocardial ischaemia/ infarction
Dehydration/replacement deficit	Systemic inflammatory response syndrome (SIRS)	Valvular disease
Gastrointestinal tract losses, burns, other insensible losses	Residual anaesthetic effect	Arrhythmias
Polyuria	Drugs (e.g. antihypertensives)	Other ventricular failure (e.g. cardiomyopathy)
Patient positioning	Anaphylaxis	Negatively inotropic drugs
Heart transplant	Acute adrenocorticoid insufficiency	Neurohumoral component of shock states
Pericardial tamponade	Carcinoid	
Tension pneumothorax	Neurogenic (e.g. 'spinal shock')	
Embolism		

Management

The management of hypotension includes both resuscitation and stabilisation (Figure 87.1), and frequently drug therapy (Table 87.2).

Blood pressure can be supported with drug therapy but it is important to first treat the cause (see Aetiology above). Treatment should begin with a less potent agent that is more easily titrated and with fewer side effects. More potent vasopressor agents such as adrenaline and noradrenaline can be given if necessary via central venous access. Note that blood pressure is often used as a surrogate measure of organ blood flow but is different from cardiac output.

Complications

Hypotension is an important factor in the development of postoperative complications. One important study found that periods of clinically significant hypotension (SBP < 90 mmHg requiring treatment) were strongly correlated with postoperative death resulting from myocardial ischaemia, cerebral ischaemia, renal failure and rebound hypertension or heart failure [2]. Perioperative hypotension may

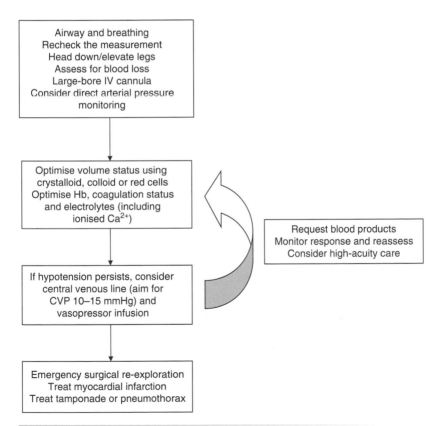

FIGURE 87.1 **Algorithm for resuscitation and stabilisation of the hypotensive patient. CVP, central venous pressure; Hb, haemoglobin; IV, intravenous.**

TABLE 87.2 **Drug therapy for the hypotensive patient**

Drug	Dose	Side effects	Comments
Phenylephrine *Pure alpha-1 agonist*	100–200 mcg IV bolus +/– 0.5–5 mg/hr IVI	Bradycardia	Mild effect Widely available
Metaraminol *alpha > beta agonist*	0.5 mg IV bolus +/– 1–5 mg/hr IVI	Bradycardia: ↓ cerebral blood flow; hyperglycaemia	Intermediate potency beta effect is helpful
Ephedrine *Non-selective alpha- and beta-agonist*	3–6 mg IV bolus up to 30 mg	Tachycardia, myocardial ischaemia, arrhythmias	Prolonged effect Helpful in bradycardia Tachyphylaxis Effect resembles adrenaline but 250× less potent
Noradrenaline *alpha-1 > beta-1 agonist*	2–20 mcg/min IVI	Bradycardia Arrhythmias GI tract ischaemia	Use central venous access
Adrenaline *Non-selective alpha- and beta-agonist*	5–50 mcg IV bolus +/– 2–20 mcg/min IVI	Tachycardia, myocardial ischaemia, arrhythmias, hyperglycaemia	Potent agent Bronchodilator Difficult to titrate (profound hypertension) Use central venous access
Milrinone *PDI inodilator*	50 mcg/kg IV bolus + 5–50 mcg/ min IVI	Hypotension, arrhythmias, myocardial ischaemia	↑ CO and ↓ SVR without ↑ myocardial O₂ demand May worsen supraventricular tachyarrhythmias Caution in renal impairment
Isoprenaline *Pure beta-agonist*	1–10 mcg/min IVI	Tachycardia, myocardial ischaemia, hyperglycaemia	Bronchodilator Indicated for bradyarrhythmias
Dobutamine *beta-1 > beta-2-agonist*	2.5–10 mcg/min IVI	Myocardial ischaemia Arrhythmias	Improves systolic heart failure
Vasopressin Smooth muscle vasoconstrictor *(V1a receptor)*	2–4 units/hr IVI	Myocardial ischaemia, water intoxication	Reduces vasoplegia in refractory shock Specialist usage only

CO, carbon monoxide; GI, gastrointestinal; IV, intravenous; IVI, intravenous infusion; SVR, systemic vascular resistance.

also cause *ischaemia-reperfusion injury* which may manifest as dysfunction of any vital organ. Among the most sensitive organs to be affected in this way are the kidneys and the heart [3].

References

1. Comfere T, Sprung J, Kumar MM, et al. Angiotensin system inhibitors in a general surgical population. *Anesthesia and Analgesia*, 2005;**100**(3):636–644. doi:10.1213/01. ANE.0000146521.68059.A1

2. Devereaux PJ, Yang H, Yusuf S, et al. Effects of extended-release metoprolol succinate in patients undergoing non-cardiac surgery (POISE trial): a randomised controlled trial. *Lancet*, 2008;**371**(9627):1839–1847. doi:10.1016/S0140-6736(08)60601-7

3. Walsh M, Devereaux PJ, Garg AX, et al. Relationship between intraoperative mean arterial pressure and clinical outcomes after noncardiac surgery: toward an empirical definition of hypotension. *Anesthesiology*, 2013;**119**(3):507–515. doi:10.1097/Aln.0b013e3182a10e26

Myocardial injury after non-cardiac surgery

Fernando Botto[1] and PJ Devereaux[2]

[1] Estudios Clinicos Latino America (ECLA), Argentina
[2] McMaster University, Canada

Myocardial injury after non-cardiac surgery (MINS) is defined as myocardial cell injury caused by ischaemia (that may or may not result in necrosis), has prognostic relevance (i.e. independently impacts 30-day mortality), and occurs during or within 30 days after non-cardiac surgery [1]. MINS does not include perioperative myocardial injury that is due to pulmonary embolism, sepsis, cardioversion, chronic troponin elevation or another known non-ischaemic aetiology.

The Vascular events In non-cardiac Surgery patIents cOhort evaluatioN (VISION) Study [2] was a large international prospective cohort study evaluating complications after non-cardiac surgery. VISION established the diagnostic criterion for MINS as a troponin T (TnT) measurement ≥0.03 ng/mL judged as resulting from myocardial ischaemia (i.e. no evidence of a non-ischaemic aetiology causing the troponin elevation).

The definition of MINS is broader than the definition of myocardial infarction (MI) in that it includes not only MI but also the other prognostically relevant perioperative myocardial injuries due to ischaemia. A majority of patients suffering MINS will not fulfil the criteria of the universal definition of MI [3].

An example of MINS

A 79-year-old woman with a history of hypertension, diabetes mellitus and hypercholesterolaemia underwent elective hip replacement surgery. She participated in a prospective study that measures perioperative cardiac biomarkers. On the second day after surgery, the patient had an elevated TnT measurement of 0.05 ng/mL. She did not experience any ischaemic symptoms (i.e. chest pain or shortness of breath) and her ECG showed no ischaemic changes. A medical consultant wrote tropinitis in her chart as the explanation for her TnT elevation. The following day the patient was discharged home on analgesic medication plus her usual losartan and oral hypoglycaemic drug.

Two days later the patient developed progressive shortness of breath and on presentation to the hospital was found to have acute pulmonary oedema. An ECG showed inverted T waves in leads V1 to V6, and her TnT measurement was 1.7 ng/mL. The patient suffered a cardiac arrest two days later and died.

Perioperative Medicine for the Junior Clinician, First Edition. Edited by Joel Symons, Paul Myles, Rishi Mehra and Christine Ball.
© 2015 John Wiley & Sons, Ltd. Published 2015 by John Wiley & Sons, Ltd.
Companion website: www.wiley.com/go/perioperativemed

Epidemiology

Worldwide, more than 100 million adults >45 years of age undergo a major non-cardiac surgery annually [4,5]. Approximately 2 million patients die within 30 days of surgery based on the largest international perioperative prospective cohort study [2].

The VISION Study included patients >45 years of age who underwent major non-cardiac surgery that required at least an overnight hospital admission. VISION demonstrated an 8% incidence of MINS, and 10% of patients suffering MINS died within 30 days. These data suggest that worldwide, 8 million patients suffer MINS annually, and 800,000 die as a result of MINS [1].

Clinical findings

The VISION Study showed that the vast majority of MINS complications occur within the first three days after surgery (87% within two days and 96% within three days), when patients are receiving analgesic medications that can mask ischaemic symptoms. Only 16% of MINS patients experience ischaemic symptoms (e.g. chest pain, dyspnoea), and only 35% have documented ischaemic ECG abnormalities (e.g. ST elevation or depression, T wave inversion). The lack of symptoms and identified ischaemic ECG changes can inappropriately lull physicians into a false sense of security that the event is not prognostically relevant. Regarding the universal definition of MI, only 42% of MINS patients fulfilled its requirements [1].

Pathophysiology

Existing evidence shows that during the perioperative period of non-cardiac surgery, two mechanisms may produce ischaemic events:

- myocardial oxygen supply–demand mismatch that can occur as a consequence of surgical stress (i.e. surgical trauma, anaesthesia/analgesia, pain, bleeding, hypothermia, fasting, intubation/extubation) in patients with chronic significant coronary artery disease
- a sudden coronary blood flow reduction caused by a coronary artery thrombus that can occur due to the inflammatory and hypercoagulable environment.

Independent preoperative predictors of MINS

Factors that increase the risk of MINS [1].
1. Age ≥75 years old
2. Male gender
3. Current atrial fibrillation
4. eGFR <60 mL/minute/1.73 m²
5. History of:
   ○ diabetes
   ○ hypertension
   ○ congestive heart failure
   ○ coronary artery disease
   ○ peripheral vascular disease
   ○ stroke
6. Urgent/emergency surgery

Clinical outcomes in patients suffering MINS

Refer to Table 88.1.

Scoring system to predict the risk of 30-day mortality in patients suffering MINS

There are three independent predictors of 30-day mortality in patients suffering MINS [1].

• Age ≥75 years old	1 point
• Anterior ischaemic ECG findings	1 point
• ST elevation or new LBBB	2 points

Table 88.2 shows 30-day mortality rates in patients suffering MINS based on the scoring system.

Management

Observational data from the international POISE trial [6] suggest that patients suffering MINS benefit from aspirin and statin therapy and that these drugs reduce the 30-day risk of mortality [7]. The ongoing MANAGE trial is randomising patients to receive a new oral anticoagulant versus placebo on top of aspirin in patients suffering MINS. Further research is required to test other cardiovascular interventions to improve the outcome of patient suffering MINS.

TABLE 88.1 Clinical outcomes at 30 days after non-cardiac surgery in patients suffering MINS

	Patients who did not suffer MINS	Patients who suffered MINS
Mortality	1.1%	9.8%
Stroke	0.4%	1.9%
Non-fatal cardiac arrest	0.06%	0.8%
Congestive heart failure	1.0%	9.4%
Combined major events	2.4%	18.8%

TABLE 88.2 Thirty-day mortality rates in patients suffering MINS

MINS score	Expected 30-day mortality
0	5%
1	10%
2	19%
3	33%
4	50%

References

1. Botto F, Alonso-Coello P, Chan MT, et al. Myocardial injury after noncardiac surgery: a large, international, prospective cohort study establishing diagnostic criteria, characteristics, predictors, and 30-day outcomes. *Anesthesiology*, 2014;**120**(3):564–578. doi:10.1097/ALN.0000000000000113

2. Devereaux PJ, Chan MTV, Alonso-Coello P, et al. Association between postoperative troponin levels and 30-day mortality among patients undergoing noncardiac surgery. *JAMA*, 2012; **307**(21):2295–2304.

3. Thygesen K, Alpert JS, Jaffe AS, et al. Third universal definition of myocardial infarction. *European Heart Journal*, 2012;**33**(20):2551–2567. doi:10.1093/eurheartj/ehs184

4. Weiser TG, Regenbogen SE, Thompson KD, et al. An estimation of the global volume of surgery: a modelling strategy based on available data. *Lancet*, 2008;**372**(9633):139–144. doi: 10.1016/S0140-6736(08)60878-8

5. Devereaux PJ. Major vascular complications in patients undergoing noncardiac surgery: the magnitude of the problem, risk prediction, surveillance, and prevention. In: Yusuf S, Cairns JA, Camm AJ et al., editors. *Evidence based Cardiology*, 3rd edn. London: BMJ Books, 2009.

6. Devereaux PJ, Yang H, Yusuf S, et al. Effects of extended-release metoprolol succinate in patients undergoing non-cardiac surgery (POISE trial): a randomised controlled trial. *Lancet*, 2008;**371**(9627):1839–1847. doi:10.1016/S0140-6736(08)60601-7

7. Devereaux PJ, Xavier D, Pogue J, et al. Characteristics and short-term prognosis of perioperative myocardial infarction in patients undergoing noncardiac surgery: a cohort study. *Annals of Internal Medicine*, 2011;**154**(8):523–528. doi:10.7326/0003-4819-154-8-2011 04190-00003

89

Aspiration

Alan Kakos

The Alfred Hospital, Australia

Pulmonary aspiration can be defined as the inhalation of gastric contents into the respiratory tract. It is potentially fatal, and can occur in anyone with a full stomach and an altered conscious state. It is of particular concern with anaesthesia, and should receive due consideration when planning anaesthesia and airway management.

In the British Fourth National Audit Project of the Royal College and Difficult Airway Society (NAP4), a prospective registry of major airway complications over 12 months in every NHS hospital in Britain, aspiration was the primary event in 17% of adverse event reports, and the most common cause of anaesthesia deaths (50%) and brain damage (53%) [1].

Pathophysiology

The aspiration of gastric contents induces a chemical burn, which triggers an inflammatory response in the airways. The hypothesis that the volume of gastric contents and their pH are the two main determinants of injury severity is being challenged, and the key determinant is now thought to be the presence of food particulate in the aspirate [2].

Aspiration can induce a variety of clinical complications, from bronchial obstruction due to the presence of solid material in the airway, to bronchoconstriction, chemical pneumonitis, infectious pneumonia, acute lung injury and acute respiratory distress syndrome (ARDS) [3].

Risk factors

In most reported cases of perioperative aspiration, one or more risk factors are present. These can be considered in the groups shown in Box 89.1.

Prevention

At present, no clear guidelines exist for the care of a patient with one or more risk factors for aspiration. Assessment and management must occur on an individual basis.

Perioperative Medicine for the Junior Clinician, First Edition. Edited by Joel Symons, Paul Myles, Rishi Mehra and Christine Ball.
© 2015 John Wiley & Sons, Ltd. Published 2015 by John Wiley & Sons, Ltd.
Companion website: www.wiley.com/go/perioperativemed

BOX 89.1 Risk factors for aspiration

Type of surgery	Emergency surgery
	Trauma
	Intra-abdominal surgery
	Surgery in lithotomy position
Patient factors	Unfasted
	Altered conscious state
	Obesity
	Pregnancy (post first trimester)
	Age >60 years
	Gastro-oesophageal reflux disease and
	oesophageal disorders, e.g. achalasia
	Hiatus hernia
	Prior laparoscopic band/gastric bypass surgery
	Gastroparesis
	• Opioids
	• Sepsis
	• Extensive burns
	• Pain
	• Diabetes
	• Intestinal obstruction
	• Post trauma/immediately post surgery
Anaesthetic factors	Inadequate anaesthesia
	Coughing and straining
	Inadequate airway protection

Fasting guidelines

Preoperative fasting guidelines have been modernised over the last 15 years and fasting periods considerably shortened [4] (Box 89.2). Reduced fasting times for surgery have beneficial effects on postoperative glucose and protein metabolism, while conferring no increased risk of aspiration in low-risk patients. Enhanced recovery programmes in abdominal surgery, which include a reduced fasting period, have demonstrated an attenuation of surgical stress and improved functional recovery of surgical patients [5].

In the emergency surgical patient, the time from last oral intake to time of trauma or commencement of pain/pathology where gastric emptying becomes impaired should be considered. Persistent nausea and vomiting and the absence of hunger despite prolonged fasting should also alert the clinician to a potentially 'full stomach' and increased risk of aspiration.

Pharmacotherapy

Antacids, H2 receptor antagonists, proton pump inhibitors and prokinetic drugs have all been postulated to have a role in the reduction of aspiration risk. There is no clear evidence that any of these drugs improves outcomes in low-risk adults. Given that each of these drugs has potential side effects and a cost burden if used on a large scale, their use is not recommended as routine aspiration prophylaxis. In patients at risk of aspirating, such as those with known gastroparesis, these drugs may confer a benefit, though this has not been proven in good-quality, large randomised trials. As such, their use must be determined on an individual basis.

Rapid sequence induction

Rapid sequence induction (RSI) is an induction technique for general anaesthesia which minimises the time from loss of awake, protective airway reflexes to intubation and airway protection with a tracheal tube. Drug and dose selection, patient positioning, the use of positive pressure ventilation before tracheal intubation and the role of cricoid pressure are all aspects of the procedure subject to ongoing debate. Most debate surrounds cricoid pressure, the application of 30 N of backwards force to the cricoid cartilage against the cervical vertebrae to occlude the upper oesophagus and prevent regurgitation. Critics argue that it is frequently performed incorrectly, that it can impair laryngeal visualisation and that fatal regurgitation has occurred despite its application. Proponents contend that it is a low-risk intervention, which may protect against aspiration and should continue to be integral to RSI.

Anaesthetic technique

Appropriate anaesthetic technique is vital in decreasing aspiration risk. To facilitate surgical procedures, avoiding general anaesthesia by using a regional technique may be indicated. For general anaesthetics, selection of tracheal intubation (and RSI) over an LMA or Proseal® Mask airway is advised in cases where risk is present. Awake intubation techniques may be considered in particularly high-risk cases. Since increased intra-abdominal pressure in the supine patient with a full stomach can still cause micro-aspiration despite the placement of a tracheal tube, the avoidance of coughing and straining, and ensuring appropriate tracheal tube position and cuff inflation, is mandatory.

Outside the operating theatre, 'conscious sedation' in the unfasted patient is potentially dangerous. Sedation, without definitive airway protection, of unfasted patients in the emergency department for minor procedures such as the relocation of dislocated joints is one such example. Similarly, allowing a patient with an altered conscious state and unclear fasting status to remain with an 'unprotected airway' also presents an aspiration risk. Unfasted patients with an acute head injury, patients who have ingested sedating drugs or those with a decreased GCS for any other reason should be considered for intubation and definitive airway protection.

Management

If aspiration is suspected in an unprotected airway, immediate suctioning of gastric contents followed by securing of the airway with a tracheal tube should occur to prevent further aspiration. Bronchoscopy should be performed and any particulate matter lavaged. Bronchospasm should be treated with bronchodilators as required.

Routine commencement of antibiotics is not indicated in the acute phase, though targeted antibiotic therapy should be initiated after positive culture of bronchoalveolar lavage fluid or if significant particulate aspiration has occurred [6]. Corticosteroids are thought to be of little benefit.

A baseline CXR should be arranged in recovery, though initial CXR will be normal in 25% aspiration cases. If the patient is extubated and remains asymptomatic two hours after the event, they can be transferred for ward care. Patients with SpO_2 <94% on supplemental oxygen, tachypnoea or tachycardia should be referred to the ICU. If an acute lung injury develops, intensive care management including protective ventilatory strategies is essential.

Significant morbidity and occasional mortality can ensue from aspiration. A small number of patients may die rapidly from airway obstruction. Those requiring ICU admission usually either recover within 72 hours or deteriorate to develop one or more of pneumonitis, pneumonia, ARDS and potentially fatal multiorgan failure. Since the management of perioperative aspiration is largely supportive and the consequences potentially severe, it is essential to consider the risk and to formulate a safe perioperative plan.

References

1. Cook TM, MacDougall-Davis SR. Complications and failure of airway management. *British Journal of Anaesthesia*, 2012;**109**(Suppl 1):i68–i85. doi:10.1093/bja/aes393

2. Beck-Schimmer B, Bonvini JM. Bronchoaspiration: incidence, consequences and management. *European Journal of Anaesthesiology,* 2011;**28**(2):78–84. doi:10.1097/EJA.0b013e32834205a8

3. Marik PE. Aspiration pneumonitis and aspiration pneumonia. *New England Journal of Medicine*, 2001;**344**(9):665–671. doi:10.1056/NEJM200103013440908

4. Soreide E, Ljungqvist O. Modern preoperative fasting guidelines: a summary of the present recommendations and remaining questions. *Best Practice and Research in Clinical Anaesthesiology*, 2006;**20**(3):483–491. doi:10.1016/j.bpa.2006.03.002

5. Nygren J. The metabolic effects of fasting and surgery. *Best Practice and Research in Clinical Anaesthesiology*, 2006;**20**(3):429–438. doi:10.1016/j.bpa.2006.02.004

6. Janda M, Scheeren TW, Noldge-Schomburg GF. Management of pulmonary aspiration. *Best Practice and Research in Clinical Anaesthesiology*, 2006;**20**(3):409–427. doi:10.1016/j.bpa.2006.02.006

90 Postoperative delirium and postoperative cognitive dysfunction

Brendan Silbert and Lisbeth Evered

St Vincent's Hospital, Australia
The University of Melbourne, Australia

Perioperative neuropsychiatric syndromes can be classified as:
- emergence delirium
- postoperative delirium
- postoperative cognitive dysfunction (POCD).

Since anaesthesia and surgery invariably accompany each other, it is difficult to attribute neuropsychiatric consequences to either component.

Emergence delirium

Emergence delirium, or agitation, occurs immediately after general anaesthesia, resolves within minutes to hours and is akin to a substance-induced delirium. The incidence is about 3% in adults but is more common in children and younger adults. It is associated with emerging consciousness, tracheal tubes, pain, full bladder or urinary catheter, factors which are easily identified and managed. In children it is associated with preoperative anxiety and responds to behavioural preparation and preoperative sedation [1]. Although dramatic and disruptive, it is generally short-lived and managed with appropriate analgesia or sedation. Most episodes resolve before the patient leaves the recovery room.

Postoperative delirium

Postoperative delirium is of greater duration and is associated with postoperative morbidity and mortality [2]. It often goes unnoticed but its identification is important as it is a significant risk factor for both institutionalisation and dementia. Patients are

Perioperative Medicine for the Junior Clinician, First Edition. Edited by Joel Symons, Paul Myles, Rishi Mehra and Christine Ball.
© 2015 John Wiley & Sons, Ltd. Published 2015 by John Wiley & Sons, Ltd.
Companion website: www.wiley.com/go/perioperativemed

often initially lucid before the delirium sets in over the following days, often manifesting at night (decreased sensory input). It has an acute onset and a variable course, and mostly affects the elderly. The incidence is high and is related to the type and urgency of surgery (repair of fractured neck of femur >50%, very common after abdominal, cardiac and peripheral vascular surgery) [2]. Preoperative risk factors include prior cognitive impairment, physical function, alcohol abuse, polypharmacy, bladder catheterisation, psychoactive drugs and dehydration.

There are three types of postoperative delirium.

- Hyperactive (~25%), characterised by agitation (most easily recognised)
- Hypoactive (~50%), characterised by lethargy (higher mortality, most often missed)
- Mixed (~25%)

The diagnosis is often made using the Confusion Assessment Method (CAM), a four-question screening tool (94% sensitivity, 89% specificity administered by trained individuals). A variation (CAM-ICU) is often used for sedated or intubated patients [3].

Diagnosis requires the presence of Feature 1 *plus* Feature 2 and either Feature 3 or Feature 4.

- Feature 1. Acute onset and fluctuating course of change in mental status
- Feature 2. Inattention evidenced by being easily distracted
- Feature 3. Disorganised thinking (rambling, unclear, illogical)
- Feature 4. Altered level of consciousness (either hyperalert or lethargic)

Treatment of postoperative delirium includes prevention of sleep deprivation (maintenance of circadian cues), prevention of sensory deprivation (glasses, hearing aids), pain management, preventing dehydration or other physiological perturbations [2]. Orientation with clocks and calendars may help. Pharmacological interventions, if indicated, target agitation and the underlying condition; anxiolytics and sedatives such as haloperidol [1] and dexmeditomidine are recommended [4].

Studies of general versus regional anaesthesia have not demonstrated a difference in rates of delirium [5]. While physicians are unable to find a unifying theory for the basis of delirium, identification and management remain purely empirical.

Clinical studies distinguish postoperative delirium from POCD and to date there is limited evidence suggesting an association between the two.

Postoperative cognitive dysfunction

The term POCD is used to describe an objectively measurable decline in cognition at some time point following anaesthesia and surgery. The presence of a substantial decline in performance, relative to the change seen in non-surgical individuals (controls), implies that POCD is present (Figure 90.1) [6].

Postoperative cognitive dysfunction can only be reliably detected by administering a cognitive test battery to patients before and after surgery, so that any change in performance can be measured. Such cognitive batteries are not used routinely, so subtle decline in cognition in patients usually goes undetected. Detecting POCD is important because it increases length of hospital stay, increases mortality and decreases quality of life, but currently assessment for POCD remains purely a research tool.

Postoperative cognitive dysfunction is associated with increasing age and inversely with education (or intelligence) and at three months is 16–21% in patients over 65 years.

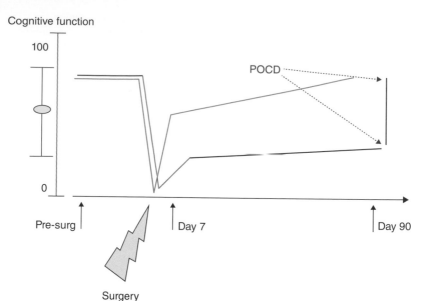

Cognitive function

100

0

Pre-surg | Day 7 | Day 90

Surgery

FIGURE 90.1 **Representation of postoperative cognitive dysfunction [6].** Assuming a starting point for an individual subject of nearly 100% cognition before surgery, subsequent assessment and analysis of cognition may show a decline at day 7 postoperatively which may improve over the following 90 days (*red line*); if the cognitive tests at 90 days show that there is a significant decline in cognition (*black line*), the patient is said to suffer from postoperative cognitive dysfunction.

Postoperative cognitive dysfunction was originally believed to be a consequence of cardiac surgery, specifically the heart-lung machine. It was subsequently shown that off-pump surgery did not decrease the incidence, and POCD risk is similar after non-cardiac surgery and investigations under sedation, such as coronary angiography [7].

The cause may be anaesthesia, surgery, patient vulnerability/susceptibility, or some combination of all three. Current theories suggest that acute inflammation in vulnerable patients is most likely, although there is a constant shift in causation theories in response to accumulating data [6].

Tests of cognition

The test battery administered to detect POCD usually comprises a number (eight to ten most frequently) of pen and paper cognitive tests, which each probe specific neuropsychological domains (Table 90.1). Generally a change in an individual is compared against a non-surgical control group so that the impact of the surgery and anaesthesia can be interpreted independently of known (practice) or unknown (time) effects.

Dysfunction

An arbitrary definition has been proposed to define when an individual has deteriorated enough to be classified as having POCD. This is generally considered to be a significant decline (≥ 1.96 SD) below the control group on two or more tests, or on a composite score of all the tests. This is a very conservative requirement

TABLE 90.1 Cognitive tests and neuropsychological domains commonly employed to detect POCD

Test	Domain
Verbal learning	Memory
Digit symbol substitution	Attention/executive function
Trail making A	Attention
Trail making B	Attention/executive function
Controlled oral word association	Executive function
Semantic fluency test	Verbal fluency
Grooved peg board	Manual dexterity

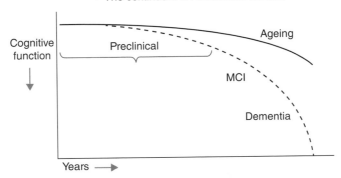

FIGURE 90.2 **Hypothetical model of the clinical trajectory of Alzheimer's disease. The stage of preclinical AD (biomarker or imaging postive) precedes mild cognitive impairment (MCI) many years before the onset of dementia [8].**

compared to the definition of mild cognitive impairment (MCI) used as a measure of subtle decline in cognition in population studies (a decline compared to population norms >1.5 SD on one test).

Alzheimer's disease

This neurodegenerative disease has a high prevalence in the elderly and the disease process commences many years before cognitive symptoms become apparent. Biomarkers (CSF proteins) and neuroimaging may detect Alzheimer's disease years (or decades) before the first subtle memory loss appears. Since the prodromal state of MCI is known to precede frank dementia by many years, anaesthesia is being administered to many elderly patients who are asymptomatic but will inevitably suffer cognitive decline in the future. Whether anaesthesia and surgery hasten this decline remains uncertain (Figure 90.2) [8].

References

1. Deiner S, Silverstein JH. Postoperative delirium and cognitive dysfunction. *British Journal of Anaesthesia*, 2009;**103**(Suppl 1):i41–46. doi:10.1093/bja/aep291

2. Rudolph JL, Marcantonio ER. Review articles: postoperative delirium: acute change with long-term implications. *Anesthesia and Analgesia*, 2011;**112**(5):1202–1211. doi:10.1213/ANE.0b013e3182147f6d

3. Inouye SK, van Dyck CH, Alessi CA, Balkin S, Siegal AP, Horwitz RI. Clarifying confusion: the confusion assessment method. A new method for detection of delirium. *Annals of Internal Medicine*, 1990;**113**(12):941–948. doi:10.7326/0003-4819-113-12-941

4. Zhang H, Lu Y, Liu M, et al. Strategies for prevention of postoperative delirium: a systematic review and meta-analysis of randomized trials. *Critical Care*, 2013;**17**(2):R47. doi:10.1186/cc12566

5. Bryson GL, Wyand A. Evidence-based clinical update: general anesthesia and the risk of delirium and postoperative cognitive dysfunction. *Canadian Journal of Anaesthesia*, 2006;**53**(7):669–677. doi:10.1007/BF03021625

6. Silbert B, Evered L, Scott DA. Cognitive decline in the elderly: is anaesthesia implicated? *Best Practice and Research in Clinical Anaesthesiology*, 2011;**25**(3):379–393.

7. Evered L, Scott DA, Silbert B, Maruff P. Postoperative cognitive dysfunction is independent of type of surgery and anesthetic. *Anesthesia and Analgesia*, 2011;**112**(5):1179–1185. doi:10.1016/j.bpa.2011.05.001

8. Sperling RA, Aisen PS, Beckett LA, et al. Toward defining the preclinical stages of Alzheimer's disease: recommendations from the National Institute on Aging-Alzheimer's Association workgroups on diagnostic guidelines for Alzheimer's disease. *Alzheimer's and Dementia*, 2011;**7**(3):280–292. doi:10.1016/j.jalz.2011.03.003

91 Postoperative hyperthermia

Glenn Downey

The Alfred Hospital and Monash University, Australia

Normal thermoregulation

Normal human core temperature of 36.3–37.1°C (measured orally) is kept within a narrow range by a highly efficient thermoregulatory system (Figure 91.1). There is circadian variation of 0.6°C, plus variation with the menstrual cycle and exercise.

Mechanisms of hyperthermia

There are two mechanisms for hyperthermia. The first is an imbalance between heat production and heat loss. Such patients complain of being hot and sweating, and have a warm periphery. The second is an elevation of the core temperature 'set-point' of the hypothalamus by pyrogenic cytokines (Figure 91.2) released through inflammatory and infective disease states. It is this second process that is correctly referred to as fever or pyrexia; these patients complain of chills, display a cold periphery and shiver.

Postoperative hyperthermia

The 'normal' inflammatory response to major surgery raises patient temperatures in the early postoperative period by about 1.5°C, more than 50% of patients recording temperatures above 38°C and 25% above 38.5°C [1]. This mechanism appears to be a resetting of the core temperature by pyrogenic cytokines, particularly IL-6, released in response to tissue damage and stresses of surgery. The degree of fever is proportional to the extent and duration of surgery.

Inflammation is the most common cause of hyperthermia on the first two postoperative days. Unless there are clinical signs strongly suggesting an alternative cause of the hyperthermia, no further investigations or treatment, other than symptomatic relief with antipyretics, are indicated.

Contrary to previously held dogma, there is little evidence to support the notion that atelectasis causes postoperative hyperthermia.

There are many other causes of hyperthermia in the postoperative period (Table 91.1). The most important are as follows.

Perioperative Medicine for the Junior Clinician, First Edition. Edited by Joel Symons, Paul Myles, Rishi Mehra and Christine Ball.
© 2015 John Wiley & Sons, Ltd. Published 2015 by John Wiley & Sons, Ltd.
Companion website: www.wiley.com/go/perioperativemed

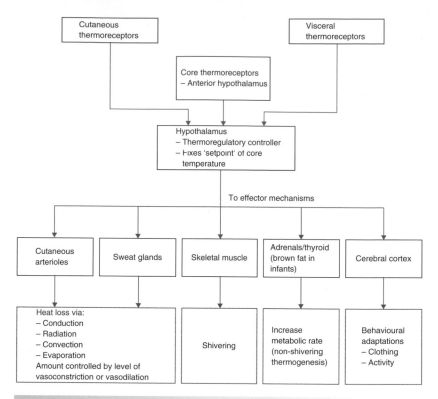

FIGURE 91.1 **Thermoregulatory system.**

- Bacteraemia
  - ○ Bacteria or toxins released into circulation directly from surgical manipulations
  - ○ Common after surgeries with infected/colonised fields, e.g. bowel surgery
- Postoperative sepsis
  - ○ Most common of the treatable causes
  - ○ Of all postoperative infections, the four most likely are:
    - (a) surgical site infection (SSI)
    - (b) urinary tract infection (UTI)
    - (c) pneumonia
    - (d) septicaemia
- Excessive intraoperative heating (passive hyperthermia)
  - ○ More common in infants and children
  - ○ More likely if no temperature monitoring employed with effective heating modalities, e.g. forced air warmer
- Pre-existing infection
  - ○ For example, intercurrent viral upper respiratory tract infection
  - ○ Evidenced by preoperative temperature and symptomatology
- Drug induced
  - ○ There are at least seven drug toxicity syndromes that can cause hyperthermia [2]. Those most relevant to the postoperative period are described in Table 91.2
  - ○ Serotonin syndrome is the most common
  - ○ Malignant hyperthermia (MH) is the most important to diagnose (see below)

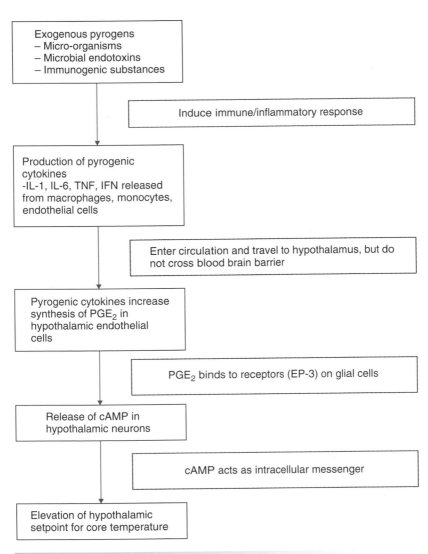

91

FIGURE 91.2 **Cytokines and proposed pathway of fever production.** cAMP, cyclic adenosine monophosphate; IFN, interferon; IL, interleukin; PGE, prostaglandin E; TNF, tumour necrosis factor.

- Venous line-related infection
  - Peripheral and central venous catheters
- DVT/PE
- Blood product administration
- Allergic reactions
  - To drugs, contrast media, skin preparations, latex or wound dressings
- Drug withdrawal
  - Opioids, benzodiazepines, alcohol
  - Temperature usually only mildly raised

TABLE 91.1 Postoperative inflammatory response/sepsis characteristics

Source	Onset	Temp (°C)	Features
Inflammatory response	POD1–2	37.5–39	Lack of other obvious cause
Bacteraemia	POD1	>38.5	Short-lived, high spiking temperatures
SSI (2–5% of all surgeries)	POD3–5	37.5–38.5	Increasing pain at wound site +/– wound discharge Can later develop into more serious deep wound infection/abscess if untreated. Confirmed by examination and imaging
UTI (5% even when urinary catheter *in situ* for less than 48 hours)	POD3–5	37.5–38.5	Suspected with IDC and cloudy urine High fever (>38.5) and rigors only if develop into pyelonephritis or prostatitis Confirmed by urinalysis and culture
Pneumonia	POD3–5	>38	More common after abdominal/major surgery Predisposed by pre-existing airway disease Symptoms and signs of collapse/consolidation, +/– hypoxaemia Confirmed by CXR, sputum microscopy and culture
Septicaemia	POD5–30	>38.5	Usually develops later Patient generally unwell Can be associated with CVS collapse Confirmed by blood cultures

CVS, cardiovascular system; CXR, chest X-ray; IDC, indwelling catheter; POD, postoperative day; SSI, surgical site infection; UTI, urinary tract infection.

- Intracranial haemorrhage and neurotrauma
  - Fever is very common after neurosurgery and neurotrauma, and is probably related to cytokines being released directly from cerebral tissue
- Endocrine disorders
  - Rare
  - Hyperthyroidism and 'thyroid storm'
  - Phaeochromocytoma

Management

This will depend upon the underlying cause and severity of the hyperthermia. Principles of treatment include the following.

- Stop any active warming measures.
- Increase heat loss.
  - Remove blankets and clothing.
  - Reduce ambient temperature and humidity.
  - Fans.
  - Cold compresses to scalp, neck, groin, axillae.
- Treat underlying cause.
  - Cease causative agents.
  - Antibiotics if indicated.
- Antipyretics: paracetamol/acetaminophen, NSAIDs, or aspirin if fever (not effective for other causes of hyperthermia).

TABLE 91.2 Drug-induced hyperthermic syndromes

Syndrome	Common agents	Onset	Characteristics
Central anticholinergic syndrome	Atropine Scopolamine Antihistamines Psychotropics Benzodiazepines Volatile anaesthetics Nitrous oxide Propofol Ketamine Opioids	Usually becomes evident on emergence from anaesthesia	CNS depression is most common (85%) postoperative presentation with delayed emergence from anaesthesia, stupor and coma Can get excitatory phenomena with agitation, confusion, hallucinations. Hyperthermia in 25%, and usually mild Diagnosis confirmed by reversal with physostigmine [4]
Neuroleptic malignant syndrome (antidopaminergic fever)	Phenothiazines Butyrophenones (haloperidol, droperidol) Atypical antipsychotics (olanzapine, quetiapine) Metoclopramide Withdrawal of anti-Parkinson's medications (L-dopa)	Usually days after exposure, but can occur at any time during treatment	Symptoms and signs evolve over 1–3 days Encephalopathy with delirium, stupor and coma Progressive generalised rigidity, which responds to non-depolarising muscle relaxants Autonomic dysfunction Temp >38°C Elevated creatinine phosphokinase
Serotonin syndrome	Interaction between any of: SSRI MAOI TCA Tramadol Metoclopramide Linezolid (antibiotic)	Usually minutes to hours after exposure	CNS effects: agitation, akathisia, pressured speech, delirium, seizures, coma Autonomic hyperactivity: diarrhoea, mydriasis, hypertension, tachycardia, sweating Neuromuscular: clonus, hyper-reflexia, rigidity predominantly in lower limbs
Malignant hyperthermia (MH)	Volatile anaesthetic agents (sevoflurane, isoflurane, desflurane) Succinylcholine	See MH section	See MH section

CNS, central nervous system; MAOI, monoamine oxidase inhibitor; SSRI, selective serotonin reuptake inhibitor; TCA, tricyclic antidepressant.

- Monitor temperature and vital signs appropriately.
- Ensure adequate hydration.
- Treat any associated complications.

Malignant hyperthermia

Malignant hyperthermia is a pharmacogenetic disorder of calcium handling in the sarcoplasmic reticulum of skeletal muscle. On exposure to triggering agents, which include all volatile anaesthetic agents and the depolarising muscle relaxant succinylcholine, sustained release of calcium leads to continuous muscle activity, producing a hypermetabolic state. It has also rarely been reported in response to exercise and stress. If left untreated, death will ensue in over 70% of cases, but since the advent of dantrolene the mortality of MH episodes has fallen to 5–15%.

Malignant hyperthermia is an autosomally dominant inherited condition, with incomplete penetrance and highly variable expressivity. Its incidence varies worldwide, but its prevalence is about 1 in 100,000 anaesthetics in the USA. In approximately 70% of cases an abnormality in the ryanodine (RYR1) receptor, responsible for calcium homeostasis in skeletal muscle, can be identified. It has also been linked to mutations in the dihydropyridine receptor (DHPR).

There is an association with several other genetically determined myopathic conditions, the most common being central core disease [3]. Patients with these conditions should be considered as being MH susceptible.

Presentation

> **Malignant hyperthermia is a medical emergency** and early diagnosis is imperative (Table 91.3). Any suspicion of MH should be treated immediately.

Malignant hyperthermia typically becomes apparent shortly after the induction of anaesthesia. Occasionally it can present in the postoperative period or recrudesce after seemingly successful initial treatment. While it is called malignant hyperthermia, elevated temperature is not an early sign and is not required to make the diagnosis.

TABLE 91.3 **Presentation of malignant hyperthermia [5]**

Early	Late
Masseter spasm with succinylcholine; more prevalent in children	Hyperkalaemia
Tachypnoea and hypercarbia	Hyperthermia
Tachycardia	Rhabdomyolysis with markedly raised creatine phosphokinase (CPK) levels
Hypoxaemia	Markedly raised myoglobin levels and myoglobinuria
Generalised muscle rigidity	
Mixed metabolic and respiratory acidosis	Malignant ventricular dysrhythmias
Profuse sweating	Cardiac arrest
Mottled skin	Disseminated intravascular coagulation
Ventricular ectopic beats and ventricular bigeminy	
Cardiovascular instability	

www.wiley.com/go/perioperativemed

VIDEO 91.1 **Malignant hyperthermia management.**

Marked hyperventilation, or hypercarbia, and generalised muscle rigidity are the two hallmarks of early MH.

Management (Video 91.1)

In the postoperative setting, call the anaesthetic department *immediately* to co-ordinate treatment and resuscitation. Activate the department malignant hyperthermia protocol and call for the 'malignant hyperthermia box' which will contain all the equipment, medications and instructions necessary. Enlist extra assistance immediately as the management of MH requires several people. Refer to www.anaesthesia.mh.org.au/mh-resource-kit/w1/i1002692/ for more information on the management of MH.

Cessation of triggering agents is imperative, and supportive measures, such as hyperventilation with 100% oxygen and treatment of dysrhythmias and hyperkalaemia, are vitally important.

Dantrolene is the only known medication that will switch off the hypermetabolic process within skeletal muscle cells. Commence administration of dantrolene as quickly as possible, and arrange for extra supplies from nearby hospitals as each hospital usually only stocks enough to initiate treatment.

References

1. Frank SM, Kluger MJ, Kunkel SL. Elevated thermostatic setpoint in postoperative patients. *Anesthesiology*, 2000;**93**(6):1426–1431. doi:10.1097/00000542-200012000-00014

2. McAllen KJ, Schwartz DR. Adverse drug reactions resulting in hyperthermia in the intensive care unit. *Critical Care Medicine*, 2010;**38**(6 Suppl):S244–252. doi:10.1097/CCM.0b013e3181dda0d4

3. Klingler W, Rueffert H, Lehmann-Horn F, et al. Core myopathies and risk of malignant hyperthermia. *Anesthesia and Analgesia* 2009; **109**(4): 1167–1173. doi: 10.1213/ANE. 0b013e3181b5ae2d

4. Brown DV, Heller F, Barkin R. Anticholinergic syndrome after anesthesia: a case report and review. *American Journal of Therapeutics*, 2004;**11**(2):144–153. doi:10.1097/00045391-200403000-00010

5. Glahn KPE, Ellis FR, Halsall PJ, et al. Recognizing and managing a malignant hyperthermia crisis: guidelines from the European Malignant Hyperthermia Group. *British Journal of Anaesthesia*, 2010;**105**(4):417–420. doi:10.1093/Bja/Aeq243

92 Perioperative hypothermia

John Monagle[1] and Shashikanth Manikappa[2]

[1] Monash Health and Monash University, Australia
[2] Dandenong Hospital, Australia

Maintenance of normal body temperature during surgery is important for optimal patient recovery and prevention of complications.

Body temperature

Core body temperature is maintained in a narrow range and reflects highly perfused tissues, primarily the thoracic and abdominal organs, and the central nervous system. Reliable semi-invasive sites for measurement of core body temperature are the nasopharynx, the lower end of the oesophagus and the tympanic membrane.

Body temperature is considered normal at 36.3–37.1°C (measured orally) and this will vary with the 24-hour circadian rhythm (lowest just before awakening), as well as with activity and hormonal cycles. An individual's normal range varies by about 0.6°C before the autonomic responses of shivering or sweating intervene. Temperature is maintained primarily by behavioural responses and to a lesser degree by autonomic responses. Behavioural changes are driven by changes sensed in body surface receptors. Autonomic reactions result from changes detected by core body sensors. Anaesthesia renders behavioural responses ineffective.

The thermoneutral zone (the environmental temperature at which heat is neither lost nor gained) is approximately 27°C for a naked resting adult (28–32°C), and lower for lightly clothed individuals (about 21°C). This assumes a still environment, to minimise heat loss. Operating rooms frequently have high-flow dry air conditioning set to about 21°C, making them hostile sites in which to maintain body temperature.

Risk factors for hypothermia

Individual temperature compensating factors include amount of body fat, the ability of the individual to protect themselves from the cold, the body's capacity to compensate for heat loss and the surface/mass ratio [1]. Children and elderly people have less ability to compensate for heat loss.

Perioperative Medicine for the Junior Clinician, First Edition. Edited by Joel Symons, Paul Myles, Rishi Mehra and Christine Ball.
© 2015 John Wiley & Sons, Ltd. Published 2015 by John Wiley & Sons, Ltd.
Companion website: www.wiley.com/go/perioperativemed

Hypothermia in the perioperative patient

Patients are often hypothermic on arrival in the operating room, in particular trauma patients. Inadvertent hypothermia occurs in 50–90% of patients undergoing surgery [2]. Core body temperature decreases most in the first hour of general anaesthesia, then decreases more slowly for another three to five hours [2]. Altered vasomotor tone is the primary trigger for enhanced heat loss; the degree of change is less with major regional anaesthesia.

Consequences of hypothermia

Intraoperative body temperatures down to 33°C are well tolerated, often with no obvious physiological effects [3] other than impairment of the coagulation system. Physiological effects will usually be evident at temperatures below 33°C.

Metabolic rate slows approximately 6% for each 1°C decrease in core body temperature [4]. Obvious signs of hypothermia are outlined in Table 92.1.

Below 32°C cardiac conduction is impaired. Atrial fibrillation occurs in about half of patients with a core temperature less than 30°C, and serious arrhythmias occur more commonly below 28°C. Contractility is severely depressed at core temperatures less than 28°C [5]. Resuscitation is difficult below 32°C, as the ventricle is non-compliant, making CPR ineffective.

There are no significant mechanical respiratory system changes until below 30°C. Carbon dioxide and oxygen are more soluble in plasma at lower temperatures, resulting in lower PCO_2 and PO_2 levels, with an increased pH [3]. Patient temperature at the time of sampling for blood gas analysis should be noted on the request slip so that appropriate corrections can be made to guide patient management.

Hypothermia decreases the activity of clotting factors and impairs platelet function [5]. *Beware*: clotting tests remain normal, as they are usually conducted at 37°C regardless of patient temperature [6].

Mild hypothermia may provide neuroprotection from local or global insults, down to about 34°C. This is due to a combination of lowered cerebral metabolic rate and lowered cerebral blood flow. Below 34°C, any benefits may be offset by adverse cardiovascular effects [3].

TABLE 92.1 **Stages of hypothermia. Signs may vary in onset. Temperature thresholds are arbitrary**

Core temperature (°C)	Stage of hypothermia	Possible signs
32–35	Mild	Shivering, acrocyanosis, pallor, slurred speech, increasing clumsiness
28–32	Moderate	Confusion, compensatory signs disappear
25–28	Severe	Muscle rigidity, flushing, oedema, stupor
<25	Profound	Coma, clinical appearance of death

Source: Corneli [4]. Reproduced with permission from Wolters Kluwer Health.

Glomerular filtration rate falls steadily with declining temperature (to 50% at 30°C). Urine output decreases steadily but more slowly, due to impaired reabsorption in proximal tubules associated with the lowered metabolism of hypothermia [3].

Hypothermia reduces mobilisation of acetylcholine at the neuromuscular junction and will enhance the action of neuromuscular blockers. At core temperatures of less than 28°C, ability to spontaneously return body temperature to normal is lost.

Complications related to hypothermia

Postoperative shivering is the most obvious consequence of intraoperative hypothermia. Intraoperative shivering can occur in patients receiving spinal or epidural anaesthesia. Shivering increases metabolic rate. In the face of impaired cardiorespiratory function postoperatively, many surgical patients cannot meet the oxygen demands of such activity and may present as hypoxic in the recovery room [3].

Renal drug excretion can decrease by up to 10% for each 0.6°C temperature drop; hepatic clearance is also reduced in hypothermia [3]. This may exaggerate the sedative effects of anaesthetic agents and opioids, and prolong the action of neuromuscular blockers.

Hypothermia mediates vasoconstriction and decreases blood flow to surgical sites, increasing the risk of surgical site infections. A temperature drop of approximately 2°C is associated with a three-fold increase in the incidence of infection after colorectal surgery [6]. Avoiding hypothermia with forced air warming can reduce surgical site infection rates by up to two-thirds.

Prevention of hypothermia (Video 92.1)

92

The operating suite holding area should be temperature controlled, and preoperative patients kept covered. Preventive strategies in the operating room need to commence as early as possible – most heat loss occurs in the first hour. Prewarming may

www.wiley.com/go/perioperativemed

VIDEO 92.1 **This video discusses the importance of preventing hypothermia in the perioperative period.**

provide a buffer against the operating room environmental factors inherent with the commencement of an operation (anaesthetic induction, removal of patient coverings, surgical positioning and surgical site preparation).

Type and duration of surgery should dictate the active warming strategies required, especially in vulnerable groups. While heat loss prevention methods such as blankets or other insulation slow heat loss, active warming methods are superior in maintaining body temperature (Figure 92.1). Forced air warming (Figure 92.2) is a good primary strategy [2] but can be more effective at maintaining normal core body temperature when combined with fluid warming (Figure 92.3).

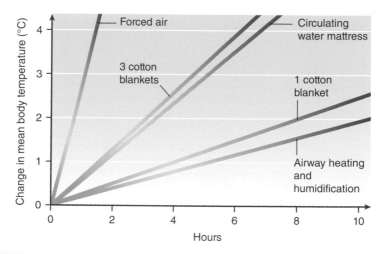

FIGURE 92.1 **Forced air warming (especially when combined with fluid warming) is superior to other methods in maintaining normal core body temperature.**

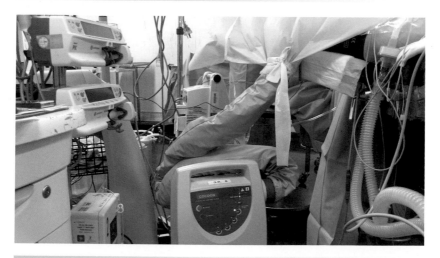

FIGURE 92.2 **Forced air warmer.** Forced air warming devices consist of a heating element which forces warmed air into an air blanket that sits on the surface of the body. This device can assist in conserving body heat.

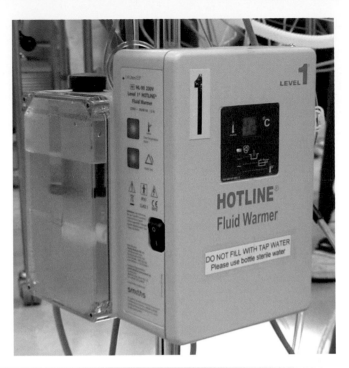

FIGURE 92.3 A fluid warmer is used to warm intravenous fluids to 37–42°C. It connects to the intravenous line attached to the patient.

References

1. Turk EE. Hypothermia. *Forensic Science, Medicine and Pathology*, 2010;**6**(2):106–115. doi:10.1007/s12024-010-9142-4

2. Moola S, Lockwood C. Effectiveness of strategies for the management and/or prevention of hypothermia within the adult perioperative environment. *International Journal of Evidence-Based Healthcare*, 2011;**9**(4):337–345. doi:10.1111/j.1744-1609.2011.00227.x

3. Morley-Forster PK. Unintentional hypothermia in the operating room. *Canadian Anaesthetists' Society Journal*, 1986;**33**(4):515–528. doi:10.1007/bf03010982

4. Corneli HM. Accidental hypothermia. *Pediatric Emergency Care*, 2012;**28**(5):475–480; quiz 481–482. doi:10.1097/PEC.0b013e3182539098

5. Thorsen K, Ringdal KG, Strand K, Soreide E, Hagemo J, Soreide K. Clinical and cellular effects of hypothermia, acidosis and coagulopathy in major injury. *British Journal of Surgery*, 2011;**98**(7):894–907. doi:10.1002/bjs.7497

6. Sessler DI. Complications and treatment of mild hypothermia. *Anesthesiology*, 2001;**95**(2):531–543. doi:10.1097/00000542-200108000-00040

Part VII
Pain management

93 Acute pain

Alex Konstantatos

The Alfred Hospital and Monash University, Australia

Pain is defined as 'an unpleasant sensory and emotional experience associated with actual or potential tissue damage, or described in terms of such damage' [1]. Pain is not just a physical phenomenon, and may not necessarily arise from visible injury. It has psychological components and both influences and is influenced by behaviour.

Acute pain typically lasts less than three months, has a clear cause, arising from a surgical procedure, injury or medical condition, responds well to therapy and heals predictably. Damage to the neurological system and significant psychological overlay are infrequent accompaniments. Importantly, acute pain can progress to chronic pain in situations where the cause is significant or where acute pain is inadequately managed.

Classification of pain

Pain can be broadly classified as nociceptive or neuropathic. Nociceptive pain occurs in a normally functioning nervous system and may arise from superficial structures (e.g. skin, muscle) or deeper structures such as viscera. Acute postoperative pain is nociceptive pain and may be somatic (e.g. orthopaedic surgery) or combined somatic and visceral pain, for example after colorectal surgery involving a large surgical incision. Nociceptive visceral pain may be dull or colicky and poorly localised, while nociceptive somatic pain is often sharp and well localised.

Neuropathic pain exists together with evidence of a lesion or inflammation affecting the nervous system. Neuropathic pain is intermittent, electric shock-like, and may radiate along the anatomical course of the affected nerve. Differentiation of nociceptive and neuropathic pain is challenging but has important implications (refer to Chapter 94 Neuropathic pain).

Pain of purely psychological origin can occur but more commonly psychological factors can intensify acute pain.

Pain history

A specific pain history is vitally important, both on initial contact with patients and when reviewing treatment. It is important to establish a patient profile, past history, anatomical site, presence of radiation, intensity, specific characteristics (dull, sharp, colicky, throbbing, shooting), factors that influence intensity, and associated symptoms such as nausea or vomiting.

Functional effects must also be considered such as breathing freely, drinking, eating, physical activity, sleep, ability to return to work, and psychological state.

Perioperative Medicine for the Junior Clinician, First Edition. Edited by Joel Symons, Paul Myles, Rishi Mehra and Christine Ball.
© 2015 John Wiley & Sons, Ltd. Published 2015 by John Wiley & Sons, Ltd.
Companion website: www.wiley.com/go/perioperativemed

Review of pain treatment is also important to assess efficacy and side effects, and progress of the underlying condition. Pain may increase because of inadequate treatment, unexpected deterioration or unanticipated patient factors.

Uncomplicated acute pain should respond to appropriate therapy and improve in accordance with expectations.

Aspects of examination

A physical examination can elucidate the context, aetiology and progression of pain. General observation including vital signs is important before focusing on the site of the pain. 'Look, feel, move' and if necessary continue with an examination of a related system (e.g. neurological/vascular system of a limb, abdominal examination). This may uncover a surgical complication such as concealed haemorrhage, infection or ischaemia.

Special measures of pain

Evaluating pain intensity is important. It can be subjective: *'How effective is your medication in relieving your pain?'* 1 = excellent, 2 = good, 3 = satisfactory, 4 = poor, 5 = very poor, or a pain scale can be used, e.g. the 10 cm Visual Analogue Scale, numeric rating scale [2] or the Functional Activity Score (FAS) where FAS A represents no limitation, FAS B represents mild limitation and FAS C represents severe limitation of function relative to the patient's baseline [3].

While most postoperative evaluations focus on optimisation and timing of analgesia therapies (Table 93.1), special attention should be given to consideration of treatment-related side effects (Table 93.2).

TABLE 93.1 **Typical postoperative evaluations**

Patient presentation	History and examination	Analgesia therapy
Middle-aged patient; day 2 post laparotomy. PCA morphine plus IV NSAID	Wound pain improving 3/10, more with coughing. Normal vital signs, minimal tenderness over wound only	Wean to oral opioid (24 h dose 20% <PCA dose over preceding 24 hr) and oral NSAID
Middle-aged patient; day 1 post laparotomy. PCA morphine plus IV NSAID	Severe pain 7/10 preventing coughing/deep breathing. Tachycardic, hyperalgesia over wound. Using PCA appropriately. No signs peritonitis or wound haematoma/infection	Inadequate analgesia. Continue PCA, add non-opioid analgesia. Explain use of PCA pre-emptively before coughing, physiotherapy or mobilisation
Elderly patient with epidural analgesia 4 days after abdominal aortic aneurysm surgery	Wound pain 2/10. Slight increase with deep breathing and coughing, minimal tenderness over wound only. Epidural site and neurological exam normal	Cease epidural block, remove catheter at appropriate time from last anticoagulant dose. Commence oral multimodal analgesia
Elderly patient with epidural analgesia 2 days after abdominal aortic aneurysm surgery	Wound pain 7/10, increased with deep breathing/coughing. Tenderness over wound, epidural site clean, demonstrable block to touch but doesn't cover wound dermatomes completely. Lower limb neurological exam normal	Epidural bolus and increased background infusion rate. Consider adding non-opioid analgesics

IV, intravenous; NSAID, non-steroidal anti-inflammatory drug; PCA, patient-controlled analgesia.

TABLE 93.2 Postoperative pain evaluation reviewing effects of treatment

Patient presentation	Management	Analgesia therapy
Elderly patient 24 h post laparotomy. Opioid infusion. Abdominal wound pain, previously 1–2/10. Increasing sedation, now semi-responsive. RR 10/min	Opioid-induced respiratory depression. Cease opioid infusion immediately; refer to HDU for ongoing monitoring of sedation	Once patient improves use opioid-sparing analgesic regimen
Elderly patient 48 h after abdominal surgery with epidural analgesia. No pain (0/10) but continued numbness affecting lower abdomen and both lower limbs	Non-tender abdomen with reduced motor function and reflexes affecting both lower limbs. Cease epidural infusion immediately and review in 1 h. **If unresolved, requires emergency MRI looking for epidural haematoma or abscess. Emergency neurosurgical decompression**	May need systemic analgesia therapy
Young patient 3 days post shoulder surgery involving single interscalene local anaesthetic block. Good analgesia first 24 hr (1/10). Ongoing numbness affecting upper limb	Neurological examination shows persistence of patchy upper limb block. Continue observations to exclude neural complication of block. Likely diagnosis is abnormally long persistence of block with full resolution. Will require neurologist referral if persists	Commence oral analgesia
Elderly patient 4 days after hip surgery receiving multimodal oral analgesia with opioid and NSAID. Good analgesia (2/10) but onset of epigastric pain	Stable vital signs, epigastric tenderness. May need gastroscopy to investigate gastritis/peptic ulceration	Cease NSAID, replace with other analgesic, e.g. paracetamol. Commence proton pump inhibitor

HDU, high-dependency unit; RR, respiratory rate; MRI, magnetic resonance imaging; NSAID, non-steroidal anti-inflammatory drug.

When to investigate and refer

Investigations to assess acute pain and related consequences should be considered in certain situations, e.g. chest X-ray for suspected peritonitis or an urgent MRI scan of the spinal cord for suspected epidural haematoma. Complicated acute pain, such as in those with chronic pain or drug dependency, requires referral to a specialist pain service.

Treatment

A key principle of pain treatment is to match the intensity, pattern and type of pain. Strong pain will require analgesics such as opioids or local anaesthetic block (such as an epidural or regional anaesthetic block). Continuous pain will require therapeutic levels of analgesia to be maintained, e.g. infusion of local anaesthetic with an epidural catheter (Figure 93.1; Video 93.1) or opioid, with strict oral dosing of short-acting or sustained-release formulations. Intermittent pain will respond to as required (p.r.n.) analgesic administration, e.g. PCA opioid (Figure 93.2; Video 93.2), or local anaesthetic or oral breakthrough analgesia. Nociceptive pain will respond well to combined opioid

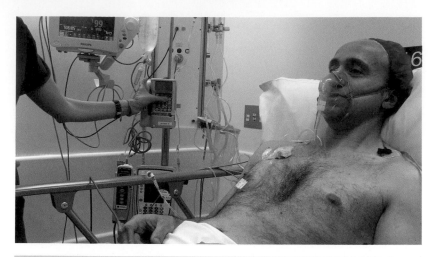

FIGURE 93.1 Epidural analgesia is a continuous infusion of local anaesthesia administered by a programmed delivery system into the epidural space. It is important to perform serial assessments of quality of analgesia as well as looking for motor block or other complications of the technique.

www.wiley.com/go/perioperativemed

VIDEO 93.1 **Epidural analgesia.**

and non-opioid analgesics (NSAIDs, paracetamol), while neuropathic pain is more likely to respond to drugs with membrane-stabilising properties.

Combining multiple analgesia therapies (multimodal analgesia) can improve quality of pain relief through action at multiple sites in pain pathways and reduce the side effects of individual agents related to high doses.

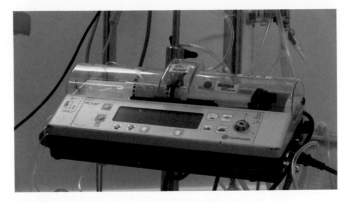

FIGURE 93.2 **Patient-controlled analgesia (PCA) devices can provide an excellent method of controlling pain in the postoperative period.**

www.wiley.com/go/perioperativemed

VIDEO 93.2 **Patient-controlled analgesia.**

Managing opioid therapy

While there are many different opioids, all have similar effects; they differ mainly in their speed of onset and duration of action. When prescribing opioids, the aim should be to rapidly achieve and maintain therapeutic levels. In most situations, rapid onset can be achieved with careful IV or rapid-onset oral dosing. Longer acting oral opioids are used for maintenance, with PCA a reasonable alternative for those unable to take oral medications. PCA allows a reasonable calculation of the correct opioid dose requirement for a particular patient but should be replaced as soon as possible with oral opioid therapy.

Opioid therapy should be part of a multimodal analgesia plan including non-opioid analgesics or local anaesthetic techniques (Table 93.3). The opioid component of

TABLE 93.3 Commonly used analgesics

Analgesic	Indications and mode of action	Common or important side effects
Opioid	Severe nociceptive pain. Reduction of neural transmission (potassium conductance)	Nausea/vomiting, sedation, respiratory depression
Local anaesthetic block	Inhibition of nerve transmission (sodium conductance)	Lowered threshold for CNS excitation, fitting, cardiac arrest
NSAIDs and COX-2 inhibitors	Mild-to-moderate, nociceptive pain. Inhibition of prostaglandin synthesis	Peptic ulceration, renal impairment, bronchospasm, platelet dysfunction
Paracetamol (acetaminophen)	Mild nociceptive pain. Inhibition of prostaglandin synthesis	Liver toxicity in overdose
Tramadol	Mild-to-moderate, nociceptive or ?neuropathic pain. Reduction of neural transmission (potassium conductance), descending inhibition via noradrenaline and serotonin potentiation	Nausea/vomiting, rash, diarrhoea, dizziness, reduced threshold to fitting
Ketamine	Moderate-to-severe nociceptive or neuropathic pain. NMDA inhibition at dorsal horn	Hallucinations, vivid dreams, elevated BP and HR
Pregabalin and gabapentin	Moderate neuropathic or ?nociceptive pain. Reduction of neural transmission (calcium conductance)	Drowsiness, fatigue, blurred vision, dry mouth, weight gain
Clonidine	Moderate nociceptive and neuropathic pain. Reduced presynaptic noradrenaline release, decreased sympathetic tone	Hypotension, bradycardia, drowsiness

BP, blood pressure; HR, heart rate; CNS, central nervous system; COX, cyclo-oxygenase; NMDA, N-methyl-D-aspartate; NSAID, non-steroidal anti-inflammatory drug.

any analgesic plan should be reviewed daily with a view to minimising opioids and limiting unfavourable effects. Prolonged opioid requirement may be indicative of emerging opioid dependence, neuropathic pain, psychogenic pain or surgical complication (refer to Chapter 28 Opioids and opioid addiction). These patients need specialist assessment. Patients discharged home on opioid therapy must have a weaning plan implemented or otherwise, in consultation with a specialist pain service, a pain management plan.

References

1. Merskey H, Bogduk N. Pain terms. A current list with definitions and notes of usage. In: *Classification of Chronic Pain*, 2nd edn. Seattle, WA: IASP Press, 1994.
2. Macintyre PE, Scott D, Schug S, Visser E, Walker S. *Acute Pain Management: Scientific Evidence*. Melbourne, Australia: ANZCA and FPM, 2010.
3. Scott D, McDonald W. *Acute Pain Management Measurement Toolkit*. Melbourne, Australia: Rural and Regional Health and Aged Care Services Division, Victorian Government Department of Human Services, 2007.

94 Neuropathic pain

Tim Hucker

Monash University, Australia

It is important that all medical staff are aware of the problems of neuropathic pain: when to anticipate it, how to diagnose it and the fundamental principles of treatment.

Pain states are predominantly nociceptive (normal) pain, neuropathic or a mixed picture. Neuropathic pain is defined as: 'Pain caused by a lesion or disease of the somatosensory nervous system' [1] and further divided into peripheral or central depending on the aetiology.

Neuropathic pain is a highly prevalent problem (e.g. affecting 8% of Europeans) [1] that is frequently poorly understood and inadequately managed. It consists of a spectrum of highly heterogeneous disorders ranging from poststroke pain, which can affect half the body, to trigeminal neuralgia which usually only affects one branch of the trigeminal nerve.

It is important to recognise neuropathic pain and commence management promptly because it is frequently severe and highly distressing for patients. Common analgesics such as NSAIDs are ineffective. Uncontrolled pain affects many domains of living, from quality of life to mood and employment. Early recognition and institution of correct treatment prevent the transition from acute to chronic, preventing chronic pain that is disabling, life-limiting and becomes immune to treatment. Neuropathic pain can be a symptom of other disease, e.g. a new presentation of multiple sclerosis.

Clinical features

Correct management of neuropathic pain requires a low index of suspicion for diagnosis; clinical features must then be elicited through the normal processes of history and examination. Once diagnosed, the aetiology must be established.

History

Broadly, symptoms and signs can be divided into positive or negative features.

Positive

- *Paraesthesia* (tingling)
- *Dysaesthesia*. An unpleasant or abnormal sensation, e.g. formication – the feeling of ants moving on the affected body part

Perioperative Medicine for the Junior Clinician, First Edition. Edited by Joel Symons, Paul Myles, Rishi Mehra and Christine Ball.
© 2015 John Wiley & Sons, Ltd. Published 2015 by John Wiley & Sons, Ltd.
Companion website: www.wiley.com/go/perioperativemed

- *Spontaneous pain*, e.g. the characteristic spontaneous 'lancinations' of trigeminal neuralgia
- *Character of the pain*: frequently described as burning or electric shock-like.

Negative

- *Principally numbness*: pain occurring paradoxically in an area that is numb is a classic feature.

Examination

Neurological examination is indicated in any patient with neuropathic features. This should be a detailed examination looking for signs of motor and sensory dysfunction and relating it to potential causes. For instance, neuropathic leg pain (Video 94.1) could be:

- in a stocking distribution from diabetic neuropathy
- in the distribution of a peripheral nerve such as the common peroneal nerve
- from a large nerve such as the sciatic nerve, commonly injured in traumatic pelvic fracture
- dermatomal, such as nerve root entrapment
- unilateral poststroke pain.

So, mapping out the area of sensory and/or motor dysfunction will assist in determining aetiology as well as diagnosis. In particular, determining the areas of altered sensation is vital to establish allodynia, hypo- or hyperaesthesia, hypo- or hyperalgesia: classic signs of neuropathic pain.

- *Allodynia*: pain response to a non-painful stimulus (passing cotton wool over the affected area will be painful).

www.wiley.com/go/perioperativemed

VIDEO 94.1 **A detailed neuropathic pain examination is required to differentiate the causes of neuropathic pain.**

- *Hypo- /hyperaesthesia*: reduced or increased sensitivity to stimulation (feeling of numbness or sensitivity to cotton wool).
- *Hypo- /hyperalgesia*: reduced or increased pain response to a stimulus that normally provokes pain (altered pain response to pinprick).

The simplest way of diagnosing is with a validated screening tool such as the DN4 (Douleur Neuropathique en 4) questionnaire. Refer to http://www.cheo.on.ca/uploads/1199%20DN4NeuropathicDiagnosticQuestionnaireFinal.pdf [2]. This can also be useful in assessing efficacy of treatment.

Common neuropathic pain conditions

Neuropathic pain is extremely common in community and hospital settings. Diagnosing some of the classic neuropathic conditions is important for management and to exclude other concerning differential diagnoses. In addition, many of the individual neuropathic pain conditions have specific treatments.

Trigeminal neuralgia is a condition that often presents with classic neuropathic symptoms. It is more common in older patients, particularly females, who report brief, excruciating and often highly distressing 'lancinations', usually in the distribution of the maxillary or mandibular branches of the trigeminal nerve unilaterally. Investigation with cerebral MRI is mandatory to investigate the vascular abnormality that frequently causes it and exclude tumour or multiple sclerosis. Carbamazepine is the mainstay of treatment [2].

Diabetic polyneuropathy is extremely common, affecting 16–49% of diabetics [2]. Patients usually report tingling, burning and 'electric shock' type pain more often in the feet and then the hands. Allodynia or hyperalgesia occurs in the paradoxically numb areas. Duloxetine is approved for the treatment of painful diabetic neuropathy.

Postherpetic neuralgia is a common neuropathic condition of pain in a unilateral dermatome beyond three months after the onset of a herpes zoster infection. The site is usually truncal and thoracic with similar positive clinical signs often evident. The mainstay of treatment is amitriptyline.

Management of neuropathic pain

Recognising that pain is difficult to measure, is subjective and has a significant psychological component [3] is the first step in its management. The domains of management are pharmacological, physical (e.g. spinal cord stimulation) and psychological (e.g. cognitive behavioural therapy). Pharmacological management should be initiated quickly.

The two main classes of drugs used are the gabapentinoids (gabapentin or pregabalin) and the tricyclic antidepressants in most neuropathic pain (except for the abovementioned conditions). Unfortunately, both groups of drugs are often limited by their interactions and side effects so a careful drug history is needed and therapy should be started at low dose, with a slow and steady dose increase.

NICE guidelines suggest offering a choice of amitriptyline, duloxetine, gabapentin or pregabalin and if not efficacious or well tolerated, offer one of the other three [4]. It is not uncommon to need a combination from each group when efficacy is limited by side effects.

94

Opioids are not indicated in the treatment of neuropathic pain without additional pain specialist/neurologist review. A recent Cochrane summary states 'We cannot say whether opioids are better than placebo for neuropathic pain over the long term' [5]. When factoring in the long list of opioid side effects and all the problems of addiction, there is rarely a case for their use (refer to Chapter 93 Acute pain and Chapter 95 The chronic pain patient).

References

1. Attal NF, N. Pharmacological management of neuropathic pain. Clinical updates. www.iasp-pain.org.

2. Votrubec M, Thong I. Neuropathic pain – a management update. *Australian Family Physician*, 2013;**42**(3):92–97.

3. Baron R, Binder A, Wasner G. Neuropathic pain: diagnosis, pathophysiological mechanisms, and treatment. *Lancet Neurology*, 2010;**9**(8):807–819. doi:10.1016/S1474-4422(10)70143-5

4. National Institute for Health and Clinical Excellence (NICE). Neuropathic pain – pharmacological management. NICE Clinical Guideline 173. www.nice.org.uk/guidance/cg173

5. McNicol ED, Midbari A, Eisenberg E. Opioids for neuropathic pain. *Cochrane Database of Systematic Reviews*, 2013;**8**:CD006146. doi:10.1002/14651858

95 The chronic pain patient

Carolyn Arnold

The Alfred Hospital and Monash University, Australia

Chronic pain is defined as continuous, long-term pain of more than 12 weeks' duration or pain persisting beyond the expected healing time. In Australia, Europe and the United States, 19–31% of adults suffer chronic pain, with a greater incidence in the over-65s age group. Patients already suffering chronic pain risk uncontrolled acute pain, unintended medication withdrawal syndromes and additional chronic pain when undergoing surgery.

Common causes include:

- musculoskeletal pain, e.g. osteoarthritis, low back pain
- persistent postsurgical pain (PPSP): up to 40% of patients attending chronic pain clinics
- neuropathic pain (rare but severe), e.g. postherpetic neuralgia, diabetic neuropathy (refer to Chapter 94 Neuropathic pain).

Effective management of chronic pain patients perioperatively can result in improved pain control, facilitate earlier functional recovery and shorten hospital stay. Chronic pain reduces quality of life, inhibits participation in family, social and working life, increases health service utilisation and places economic burdens on individuals and communities.

Preoperative management

Assess the patient's current pain status.

- History of pain and injury
- Expectations/fears about surgery
- Mood: preoperative anxiety, depressed mood and catastrophising are associated with higher postoperative pain levels
- Current medications and those not tolerated in the past
- Whether they have an appropriate expectation of outcome

Educate the patient, explain, listen, give clear expectations and aim to reduce anxiety.

Plan pre-, intra- and postoperative pain management in consultation with the patient (refer to Chapter 93 Acute pain).

Consent for regional anaesthesia if planned.

Perioperative Medicine for the Junior Clinician, First Edition. Edited by Joel Symons, Paul Myles, Rishi Mehra and Christine Ball.
© 2015 John Wiley & Sons, Ltd. Published 2015 by John Wiley & Sons, Ltd.
Companion website: www.wiley.com/go/perioperativemed

Plan analgesic management, e.g. preventive analgesics and regional analgesia. Importantly, continue regular analgesics even if the patient is fasting (or replace with parenteral equivalents).

Intraoperative management

Administer local anaesthesia, regional anaesthesia and analgesics as appropriate.

Postoperative management

Multimodal analgesia (parenteral and oral) should be used. Continue the patient's normal pain medications as baseline, including opioids, antidepressants and anticonvulsants. Monitor, review and adjust management frequently. Switch to oral analgesia as early as possible, and plan weaning analgesics for acute pain over 24–72 hours.

Special cases

* Management of the opioid-tolerant patient undergoing surgery (refer to Chapter 28 Opioids and opioid addiction)
* Persistent postsurgical pain

Persistent postsurgical pain

Surgery and injury are major risk factors for chronic pain. The incidence of PPSP varies from 10% to 80% and is increased with nerve injury (Table 95.1) [1].

Severe acute postoperative pain is the most significant risk factor for PPSP.

> Pain persisting two months after surgery warrants re-evaluation and multidisciplinary care by pain experts.
>
> Failure of acute pain to resolve is not an indication to continue opioid therapy.

Persistent postsurgical pain is usually multifactorial [2] (Figure 95.1). Modifiable risk factors include severe postoperative pain, surgical techniques (improving and using nerve-sparing approaches where possible) and adopting strategies to reduce and

TABLE 95.1 **Incidence of persistent postsurgical pain after common procedures [2,3]**

Surgery	Incidence %
Thoracotomy	50
Amputation	30–85
Mastectomy	30
Hip arthroplasty	12
Inguinal hernia repair	10

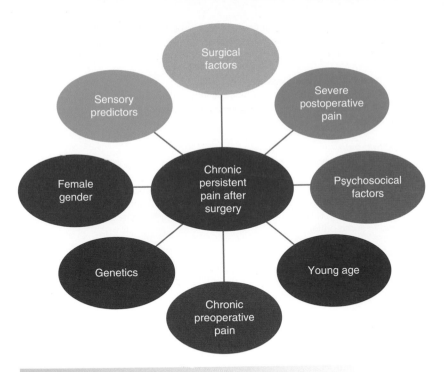

FIGURE 95.1 **Risk factors for PPSP.**

manage mood and anxiety by explaining and planning postoperative pain management to the patient, considering anxiolytic medications and follow-up.

Screening for high-risk cases ensures the most effective analgesic techniques are planned and tailored to the individual patient [3,4].

Avoid futile surgery. Consider alternatives including rehabilitation and non-surgical management options.

> Although nerve injury increases the risk of neuropathic pain postoperatively, it is not a given, and other factors are involved in addition to nerve injury. If surgical technique cannot be modified, greater care is required to address the other factors (see Figure 95.1).

In the future, application of pharmacogenomics principles will guide specific treatments, surgical techniques will improve and better analgesics will be available (refer to Chapter 9 Perioperative genomics).

Some general evidence-based guidance on techniques to reduce the development of chronic pain after surgery comes from Cochrane reviews [4,5] but suggest the available evidence is weak and more research is needed. Epidural anaesthesia may reduce the risk of development of chronic pain after thoracotomy in approximately one patient out of four. Paravertebral block may reduce chronic pain after breast surgey in one in five women. Ketamine use produces a modest but significant reduction in the incidence of chronic pain after surgery but this is not seen with pregabalin and gabapentin.

Specific types of persistent postsurgical pain

Persistent postsurgical pain can be nociceptive and/or neuropathic. Pain conditions arising as a result of surgical nerve injuries are a significant cause of PPSP, and neuropathic pain is a challenge to manage.

Neuropathic pain

Neuropathic pain needs to be recognised and treated promptly in the perioperative period (refer to Chapter 94 Neuropathic pain). Some surgery is inevitably associated with nerve injury and therefore a greater risk of persistent neuropathic pain, e.g. amputation, mastectomy and thoracotomy. 'Unintentional' nerve injuries can occur with any surgery, e.g. inguinal herniorrhaphy. Surgical decompression may be warranted in some patients.

Complex regional pain syndrome type 1

Complex regional pain syndrome type 1 (CRPS1), previously called reflex sympathetic dystrophy, is characterised by unexpectedly severe and prolonged pain following a minor or moderate trauma (such as fracture, soft tissue injuries or surgery) and usually affects a limb peripherally.

There is marked hypersensitivity to touch (allodynia – sensory dysfunction) swelling, redness, sweating (autonomic disturbances), inability to bear weight (if the leg is affected) or use the upper limb normally. There is occasionally tremor or dystonia (motor dysfunction). The area affected is greater than expected from the underlying condition (Figure 95.2).

Diagnosis of CRPS1 is clinical, with exclusion of other causes of pain presenting similarly, e.g. DVT, infections or missed musculoskeletal or nerve injuries. There are no specific objective tests for CRPS.

Features of CRPS1 following distal radial fractures (Colles' fractures) can occur in 32% of patients three weeks after cast removal, but more than 80% resolve by 18 months [6].

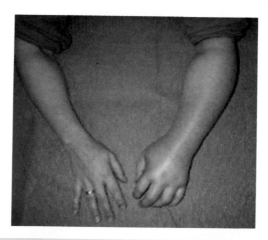

FIGURE 95.2 **CRPS1 in the left arm.**

Complex regional pain syndrome type 2

Complex regional pain syndrome type 2 (CRPS 2) includes all of the above symptoms and signs, and an identifiable nerve injury (previously called causalgia). The picture of the nerve injury will require careful evaluation as the allodynia and sensitivity may extend beyond the margins of the peripheral nerve sensory innervation. Management is similar, with additional care to restore muscle tendon length and joint range of movement where weakness exists, and nerve repair if indicated (plastics and neurosurgery evaluation, and nerve conduction studies may assist).

A small number of sufferers of CRPS go on to severe disability and chronic pain.

> Recognise CRPS early and refer to pain management services. Plan for early intervention: analgesia to control pain, oedema and hypersensitivity accompanied by early rehabilitation of function.

References

1. Crombie IK, Davies HTO, Macrae WA. Cut and thrust: antecedent surgery and trauma among patients attending a chronic pain clinic. *Pain*, 1998;**76**(1-2):167–171. doi:10.1016/S0304-3959(98)00038-4

2. Perkins FM, Kehlet H. Chronic pain as an outcome of surgery. A review of predictive factors. *Anesthesiology*, 2000;**93**(4):1123–1133. doi:10.1097/00000542-200010000-00038

3. Kehlet H, Jensen TS, Woolf CJ. Persistent postsurgical pain: risk factors and prevention. *Lancet*, 2006;**367**(9522):1618–1625. doi:10.1016/S0140-6736(06)68700-X

4. Andreae MH, Andreae DA. Local anaesthetics and regional anaesthesia for preventing chronic pain after surgery. *Cochrane Database of Systematic Reviews*, 2012;**10**:CD007105. doi:10.1002/14651858.CD007105.pub2

5. Chaparro LE, Smith SA, Moore RA, Wiffen PJ, Gilron I. Pharmacotherapy for the prevention of chronic pain after surgery in adults. *Cochrane Database of Systematic Reviews*, 2013;**7**:CD008307. doi:10.1002/14651858.Cd008307.Pub2

6. Jellad A, Salah S, Ben Salah Frih Z. Complex regional pain syndrome type I: incidence and risk factors in patients with fracture of the distal radius. *Archives of Physical Medicine and Rehabilitation*, 2014;**95**(3):487–492. doi:10.1016/j.apmr.2013.09.012

Index

Note: Page numbers in *italics* refer to Figures; those in **bold** to Tables.

Perioperative Medicine for the Junior Clinician, First Edition. Edited by Joel Symons, Paul Myles, Rishi Mehra and Christine Ball.
© 2015 John Wiley & Sons, Ltd. Published 2015 by John Wiley & Sons, Ltd.
Companion website: www.wiley.com/go/perioperativemed